Heart Diseases & Disorders
Sourcebook, 2nd Edition

Household Safety Sourcebook

Immune System Disorders Sourcebook

Infant & Toddler Health Sourcebook

Injury & Trauma Sourcebook

Kidney & Urinary Tract Diseases &
Disorders Sourcebook

Learning Disabilities Sourcebook,
2nd Edition

Leukemia Sourcebook

Liver Disorders Sourcebook

Lung Disorders Sourcebook

Medical Tests Sourcebook, 2nd Edition

Men's Health Concerns Sourcebook,
2nd Edition

Mental Health Disorders Sourcebook,
2nd Edition

Mental Retardation Sourcebook

Movement Disorders Sourcebook

Obesity Sourcebook

Osteoporosis Sourcebook

Pain Sourcebook, 2nd Edition

Pediatric Cancer Sourcebook

Physical & Mental Issues in Aging
Sourcebook

Podiatry Sourcebook

Pregnancy & Birth Sourcebook,
2nd Edition

Prostate Cancer

Public Health Sourcebook

Reconstructive & Cosmetic Surgery
Sourcebook

Rehabilitation Sourcebook

Respiratory Diseases & Disorders
Sourcebook

Sexually Transmitted Diseases
Sourcebook, 2nd Edition

Skin Disorders Sourcebook

Sleep Disorders Sourcebook

Sports In [...]

Stress-Re [...]

Stroke Sourcebook

Substance Abuse Sourcebook

Surgery Sourcebook

Transplantation Sourcebook

Traveler's Health Sourcebook

Vegetarian Sourcebook

Women's Health Concerns Sourcebook,
2nd Edition

Workplace Health & Safety Sourcebook

Worldwide Health Sourcebook

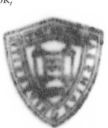

## Teen Health Series

Cancer Information for Teens

Diet Information for Teens

Drug Information for Teens

Mental Health Information
for Teens

Sexual Health Information
for Teens

Skin Health Information
for Teens

Sports Injuries Information
for Teens

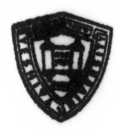

# Men's Health Concerns SOURCEBOOK

*Second Edition*

Health Reference Series

*Second Edition*

# Men's Health Concerns SOURCEBOOK

*Basic Consumer Health Information about the Medical and Mental Concerns of Men, Including Theories about the Shorter Male Lifespan, the Leading Causes of Death and Disability, Physical Concerns of Special Significance to Men, Reproductive and Sexual Concerns, Sexually Transmitted Diseases, Men's Mental and Emotional Health, and Lifestyle Choices That Affect Wellness, Such as Nutrition, Fitness, and Substance Use*

*Along with a Glossary of Related Terms and a Directory of Organizational Resources in Men's Health*

*Edited by*
**Robert Aquinas McNally**

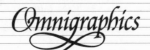

*Omnigraphics*

615 Griswold Street • Detroit, MI 48226

Bibliographic Note

Because this page cannot legibly accommodate all the copyright notices, the Bibliographic Note portion of the Preface constitutes an extension of the copyright notice.

Edited by Robert Aquinas McNally

*Health Reference Series*

Karen Bellenir, *Managing Editor*
David A. Cooke, MD, *Medical Consultant*
Elizabeth Barbour, *Permissions Associate*
Dawn Matthews, *Verification Assistant*
Laura Pleva Nielsen, *Index Editor*
EdIndex, Services for Publishers, *Indexers*

* * *

Omnigraphics, Inc.

Matthew P. Barbour, *Senior Vice President*
Kay Gill, *Vice President—Directories*
Kevin Hayes, *Operations Manager*
Leif Gruenberg, *Development Manager*
David P. Bianco, *Marketing Consultant*

* * *

Peter E. Ruffner, *Publisher*

Frederick G. Ruffner, Jr., *Chairman*

Copyright © 2004 Omnigraphics, Inc.

ISBN 0-7808-0671-9

Library of Congress Cataloging-in-Publication Data

Men's health concerns sourcebook : basic consumer health information about the medical and mental concerns of men ... / [edited by] Robert Aquinas McNally.-- 2nd ed.
    p. cm. -- (Health reference series)
    Previous ed. edited by Allan R Cook.
    Includes bibliographical references and index.
    ISBN 0-7808-0671-9
    1. Men--Health and hygiene--Popular works. I. McNally, Robert Aquinas. II. Health reference series (Unnumbered)

RA776.5M457 2004
613'.04234--dc22

                                                                    2004041520

# Table of Contents

*Part II: Other Physical Concerns of Special Significance for Men*

## Part III: Reproductive and Sexual Concerns

## Part IV: Mental and Emotional Health

## Part V: Wellness and Appearance

# Preface

## About This Book

Men are different from women, a distinction that is particularly apparent in the area of health. The differences between the genders are often startling, and they point to areas where greater awareness of men's unique health concerns can increase quality of life and prevent premature death:

- On average men die six years earlier than women.

- Men are far more likely than women to die from automobile accidents, industrial mishaps, or alcohol abuse.

- Men are four times more likely than women to kill themselves. In addition, white males over the age of 85 have the highest suicide rate of any group.

- While men suffer from a variety of diseases unique to their anatomy—such as prostate and testicular cancer—they are also subject to a number of maladies commonly considered "women's diseases"— such as osteoporosis, eating disorders, and even breast cancer.

*Men's Health Concerns Sourcebook, Second Edition* offers basic, reliable information about the diseases that most afflict men and the health concerns that are likely to affect their lives. In addition, the book offers ways of meeting men's key health challenges and lowering their risk of death and disability. The book deals with the leading causes of mortality in men; discusses key issues in reproductive and sexual health, including sexual dysfunction, sexually transmitted diseases, and family planning; addresses mental and emotional health; and provides information about nutrition, exercise, and appearance. The final portion of the book provides sources of additional help and information.

## How to Use This Book

This book is divided into parts and chapters. Parts focus on broad areas of interest. Chapters are devoted to single topics within a part.

*Part I: Leading Causes of Death and Disability in Men* looks first at the differences in disease patterns in men and women, then investigates the 12 leading killers of males: heart disease, cancer, stroke, accidents, chronic obstructive pulmonary disease, diabetes, pneumonia and influenza, suicide, chronic kidney disease, cirrhosis and chronic liver disease, assault and homicide, and HIV/AIDS.

*Part II: Other Physical Concerns of Special Significance for Men* looks at a variety of diseases that are unique to men, affect them disproportionately, or are common causes of male concern. Information is provided on hypertension, athlete's foot, Duchenne-Becker muscular dystrophy, Klinefelter syndrome, hemophilia, sleep apnea, and "women's diseases" that also affect men.

*Part III: Reproductive and Sexual Concerns* begins with a look at the male reproductive system, sexual orientation, and circumcision, then covers a variety of conditions affecting the genitals, including sexually transmitted diseases. The last chapter in this section offers extensive information on contraception and family planning.

*Part IV: Mental and Emotional Issues* focuses on health issues to which men often pay too little attention. This section's chapters look at stress, post-traumatic stress syndrome, depression, domestic violence, and male rape.

*Part V: Wellness and Appearance* provides information about preventive health and life-style choices. These chapters cover nutrition, tobacco, alcohol, recreational drugs, exercise, and hair loss.

*Part VI: Additional Help and Information* offers a glossary of terms related to men's health and a directory of organizational resources that can provide further information and help in specific areas.

## Bibliographic Note

This volume contains documents and excerpts from publications issued by the following U.S. government agencies: Centers for Disease Control and Prevention (CDC); Department of Justice; Food and Drug Administration (FDA); National Cancer Institute (NCI); National Heart, Lung, and Blood Institute (NHLBI); National Institute of Allergy and Infectious Disease; National Institute of Arthritis and Musculoskeletal and Skin Diseases (NIAMS); National Institute of Child Health and Development; National Institute of Diabetes and Digestive and Kidney Disorders (NIDDK); National Institute on Aging; National Institute on Alcohol Abuse and Alcoholism; National Institute on Drug Abuse; and the National Institute on Mental Health (NIMH).

In addition, this volume contains copyrighted documents from the following organizations and individuals: Academy of General Dentistry; American Academy of Family Physicians; American College of Emergency Physicians; American Dietetic Association; American Hair Loss Council; American Heart Association; American Lung Association; American Psychological Association; American Urological Association; Cancer Care, Inc.; Harvard Office of News and Public Affairs; Magee Rehabilitation; Medical College of Wisconsin; Multicultural Health Communication Service (New South Wales, Australia); Muscular Dystrophy Association Australia; National Center for the Victims of Crime; National Hemophilia Foundation; National Mental Health Association; National Safety Council; National Sleep Foundation; Nemours Foundation; New York City Department of Health and Mental Hygiene; San Francisco AIDS Foundation; Sexuality Information and Education Council of the United States (SIECUS); and WebMD Corporation.

Full citation information is provided on the first page of each chapter. Every effort has been made to secure all necessary rights to reprint the copyrighted material. If any omissions have been made, please contact Omnigraphics to make corrections for future editions.

## Acknowledgements

Thanks go to the many organizations, agencies, and individuals who have contributed materials for this *Sourcebook* and to medical consultant Dr. David Cooke, verification assistant Dawn Matthews, and document engineer Bruce Bellenir. Special thanks go to managing editor Karen Bellenir and permissions specialist Liz Barbour for their help and support.

# Note from the Editor

This book is part of Omnigraphics' *Health Reference Series*. The *Series* provides basic information about a broad range of medical concerns. It is not intended to serve as a tool for diagnosing illness, in prescribing treatments, or as a substitute for the physician/patient relationship. All persons concerned about medical symptoms or the possibility of disease are encouraged to seek professional care from an appropriate health care provider.

## Our Advisory Board

The *Health Reference Series* is reviewed by an Advisory Board comprised of librarians from public, academic, and medical libraries. We would like to thank the following board members for providing guidance to the development of this *Series*:

Dr. Lynda Baker,
Associate Professor of Library and Information Science,
Wayne State University, Detroit, MI

Nancy Bulgarelli,
William Beaumont Hospital Library, Royal Oak, MI

Karen Imarisio,
Bloomfield Township Public Library, Bloomfield Township, MI

Karen Morgan,
Mardigian Library, University of Michigan-Dearborn,
Dearborn, MI

Rosemary Orlando,
St. Clair Shores Public Library, St. Clair Shores, MI

## Medical Consultant

Medical consultation services are provided to the *Health Reference Series* editors by David A. Cooke, M.D. Dr. Cooke is a graduate of Brandeis University, and he received his M.D. degree from the University of Michigan. He completed residency training at the University of Wisconsin Hospital and Clinics. He is board-certified in Internal Medicine. Dr. Cooke currently works as part of the University of Michigan Health System and practices in Brighton, MI. In his free time, he enjoys writing, science fiction, and spending time with his family.

# Health Reference Series *Update Policy*

The inaugural book in the *Health Reference Series* was the first edition of *Cancer Sourcebook* published in 1989. Since then, the *Series* has been enthusiastically received by librarians and in the medical community. In order to maintain the standard of providing high-quality health information for the layperson the editorial staff at Omnigraphics felt it was necessary to implement a policy of updating volumes when warranted.

Medical researchers have been making tremendous strides, and it is the purpose of the *Health Reference Series* to stay current with the most recent advances. Each decision to update a volume will be made on an individual basis. Some of the considerations will include how much new information is available and the feedback we receive from people who use the books. If there is a topic you would like to see added to the update list, or an area of medical concern you feel has not been adequately addressed, please write to:

Editor
*Health Reference Series*
Omnigraphics, Inc.
615 Griswold Street
Detroit, MI 48226
E-mail: editorial@omnigraphics.com

# Part One

# Leading Causes of
# Death and Disability in Men

# Chapter 1

# Gender Patterns of Health and Disease

## Chapter Contents

## Section 1.1

## *The Shorter Male Lifespan*

"The Next Endangered Species—Men?" by Daniel DeNoon, reviewed by Michael Smith, MD, WebMD Medical News, © 2001 WebMD Corporation. All rights reserved.

The health gap between men and women widens every year. Men die sooner. Each of the 15 leading causes of death is more likely to kill them. Men have growing rates of psychological problems. Men are more likely to die as crime victims. Men shun doctors when they are sick and avoid checkups when they are well.

Are men going extinct? That's the provocative question posed by the 2001 First World Congress on Men's Health, an annual meeting of men's health experts.

"Will men be needed at all?" wonders conference chairman Siegfried Meryn, M.D., in the November 3 issue of the *British Medical Journal*. "With the advent of sperm banks, in vitro fertilization, sex-sorting techniques, sperm-independent fertilization of eggs with somatic cells, human cloning, and same-sex marriage, it is reasonable to wonder about the future role of men in society."

The problem doesn't seem to be in men's genes. When figures first started being kept in 1920, women only outlived men by one year. Ever since, women's life expectancy has increased faster than that of men.

"The question is not why women live longer than men. It's why did the increase in male life expectancy fail to keep pace with improvements in women's life expectancy," Emory University researcher Jean Bonhomme, M.D., M.P.H., tells WebMD. Bonhomme is a board member of the nonprofit Men's Health Network and president of the National Black Men's Health Network.

The answer, Bonhomme suggests, is that men don't get the same kinds of regular, preventive health care as women. They don't get it partly because they don't seek it.

"Since childhood, the sexes are taught to deal with physical pain differently," Bonhomme says. "A boy who scrapes his knee is told to stop crying and be a man. But when that boy is 50 years old and having chest pain, he will say, 'It's just indigestion,' because he's been taught to minimize his pain.... A lot of men who don't feel good don't pay it any mind. When it comes to disease, early treatment is critical. Men miss out on this opportunity."

A lot of this has to do with how men define themselves in Western culture.

"Part of what we consider manliness has a lot to do with being free and in charge of one's own destiny—and there's a certain stoicism," historian and American culture expert John F. Kasson, Ph.D., tells WebMD. "Men are taught not to complain, to grin and bear it. That has implications for how men see health care."

And yes, men's famous unwillingness to grapple with their emotions plays a role.

"Often for both physical issues and emotional issues, men have trouble dealing with their emotions," says Kasson, professor at the University of North Carolina, Chapel Hill. "I don't go along with all the men-are-from-Mars-women-are-from-Venus stuff, but it is true, by and large, that men find it difficult to get in touch with their own emotions and confide in others. There is this problem with admitting the need for help and seeking help—it isn't seen as manly."

Bonhomme says men are more likely than women to have jobs requiring dangerous and/or strenuous exertion. When this is the case, denying pain becomes a necessary part of earning a living—and it carries over into the rest of a man's life. This helps explain why black men tend to have poorer health and shorter life expectancy than white men.

"Not only do men have more dangerous jobs than women, but African American men have more dangerous jobs than white men," Bonhomme notes. "To do some work, you have to detach from your pain. African American men are overrepresented in manual labor that necessitates indifference to pain. And for African American men, there is also an element of distrust in the health care system."

What can be done? Fear campaigns will backfire, Bonhomme predicts. It is not honorable for men to be afraid. Instead, the health care system has to become more relevant to men.

"Men want to be better men," Bonhomme says. "We have to reverse the paradigm. Men see going to a doctor now to be admitting some kind of weakness or personal failure. Instead, they should see it as an ally of masculinity, something that can help you manage their independence, their vigor, and their functionality. And we need to stop shaming men and boys to always have to deny their pain."

## Section 1.2

# Why Are Men Less Healthy Than Women?

© 1998 NSW Multicultural Health Communications Service, New South Wales, Australia. Reprinted with permission. Reviewed by David A. Cooke, M.D., July 12, 2003.

**Summary:** The reasons why men are less healthy than woman.

Although men are usually physically stronger than women, they're not always healthier—and are more likely to die sooner. A new report on men's health from the NSW Department of Health highlights some alarming differences between men and women:

• On average, men die six years earlier than women.

• After the first year of life, the death rate for boys is 35 percent higher than girls.

• Fifty percent of men in Australia are overweight, compared to one-third of women.

• Men are more likely to have heart disease and cancer.

• Around twice as many men die of skin cancer as women.

• In people under 65, cigarette smoking causes around 40 percent of deaths in men, compared to 20 percent of deaths in women.

• Men are more likely to die or be seriously injured as a result of road accidents, falls, drownings, accidents at work, or violence. They are more likely to die of alcohol abuse.

• Men are three times more likely to commit suicide than women.

What are the reasons for these dramatic differences? One is that men typically take more risks than women. They're more likely to work in hazardous occupations, for instance—which helps explain why 93 percent of deaths at work happen to men. Sometimes taking risks can be a good thing, of course—where would we be without people willing to do risky jobs like firefighting? But too often, men take unnecessary risks—on the roads, for example—which cause harm to themselves and others.

Another reason is that men generally don't care for their health as much as women do. They're more likely to smoke or to drink too much alcohol, and eat a poorer diet—compared to women, men eat less fruit and more fat, for instance. They're also more likely to ignore health problems rather than see a doctor.

How do we improve men's health? A good place to start is in families. Women have traditionally looked after the health of their partners and sons and encouraged them to take care of themselves—and probably always will. But now it's time for men to take action themselves, not only for their own sake, but for the sake of their children. Fathers who set a good example with a healthy lifestyle, and safe behavior in areas like driving, drinking, and sport are more likely to raise healthier sons.

Some men think caring for health isn't "masculine." But the truth is that men who eat healthy food, exercise regularly, and get prompt treatment for health problems have a better chance of staying strong and active than men who don't.

# Section 1.3

# *Why Women Live Longer Than Men*

By William J. Cromie, in *Harvard University Gazette*,
October 1, 1998, © 1998 President and Fellows of Harvard College.
Reviewed and revised by David A. Cooke, M.D., on July 8, 2003.

Studying people who live 100 years and more leads Harvard researchers to conclude that menopause is a major determinant of the lifespans of both women and men.

Women's lifespan depends on the balance of two forces, according to Thomas Perls, a geriatrician at Harvard Medical School. One is the evolutionary drive to pass on her genes; the other is the need to stay healthy enough to rear as many children as possible. "Menopause draws the line between the two," Perls says. It protects older women from the risks of bearing children late in life, and lets them live long enough to take care of their children and grandchildren.

As for men, Perls believes "their purpose is simply to carry genes that ensure longevity and pass them on to their daughters. Thus, female longevity becomes the force that determines the natural lifespan of both men and women."

"Most animals do not undergo menopause," adds Ruth Fretts, an obstetrician-gynecologist at Harvard-affiliated Beth Israel Deaconess Medical Center in Boston. "It seems that menopause evolved in part as a response to the amount of time that the young remain dependent on adults to ensure their survival."

Pilot whales, for example, suckle their young until age 14, and they, along with humans, are two of the few species that menstruate.

Human females eventually become so frail that bearing children involves a high risk of death. Earlier in evolution, that was as young as 35 to 40 years old. "Anyone who developed a genetic alteration that caused infertility, i.e., menopause, obtained a survival advantage over females who continued to be fertile and died bearing children," Perls says.

## *The Gender Gap*

This reasoning, however, does not explain why women live so much longer than men. "In all developed countries and most undeveloped

8

ones, women outlive men, sometimes by a margin of 10 years," Perls and Fretts note. "In the U.S., average life expectancy at birth is about 79 years for women and about 72 years for men."

The gender gap is most pronounced in those who live 100 years or more. Among centenarians worldwide, women outnumber males nine to one. Perls and Fretts are studying all centenarians from eight cities and towns around Boston, 100 people in all. Eighty-five are women.

The mortality gap varies during other stages of life. Between ages 15 and 24 years, men are four to five times more likely to die than women. This time frame coincides with the onset of puberty and an increase in reckless and violent behavior in males. Researchers refer to it as a "testosterone storm." Most deaths in this male group come from motor vehicle accidents, followed by homicide, suicide, cancer, and drownings.

After age 24, the difference between male and female mortality narrows until late middle age. In the 55- to 64-year-old range, more men than women die, due mainly to heart disease, suicide, car accidents, and illnesses related to smoking and alcohol use. Heart disease kills five of every 1,000 men in this age group.

"It seems likely that women have been outliving men for centuries and perhaps longer," say Perls and Fretts. Even with the sizable risk conferred by childbirth, women have outsurvived men at least since the 1500s, although, in the United States between 1900 and the 1930s, the death risk for women of childbearing age was as high as that for men. Since then, improved health care, particularly in childbirth, has put women ahead of men again in the survival struggle, as well as raising life expectancy for both sexes.

A longer life doesn't necessarily mean a healthier life, however. While men succumb to fatal illnesses like heart disease, stroke, and cancer, women live on with nonfatal conditions such as arthritis, osteoporosis, and diabetes. "While men die from their diseases, women live with them," Perls comments.

It has been speculated that one contributor to the gender difference in lifespan is the influence of sex hormones. The male hormone testosterone not only increases aggressive and competitive behavior in young men, it increases levels of harmful cholesterol (low-density lipoprotein), raising a male's chances of getting heart disease or stroke.

On the other hand, the female hormone estrogen lowers harmful cholesterol and raises "good" cholesterol (high-density lipoprotein). However, studies of postmenopausal women have shown an increased rate of heart attacks and strokes in those given estrogen and progesterone. While it is clear that premenopausal women have lower rates

9

of cardiovascular disease than men of similar age, it is unknown whether this relates to sex hormones or some other factor.

Perls and Fretts believe that longer life means survival of the fittest, and women, evolutionarily speaking, are more fit than men. The longer a woman lives and the more slowly she ages, the more offspring she can produce and rear to adulthood. Therefore, evolution would naturally select the genes of such women over those who die young.

Long-lived men would also have an evolutionary advantage over their shorter-lived brethren. However, says Perls, "studies of chimps, gorillas, and other species closely related to humans suggest that a male's reproductive capacity is actually limited more by access to females than by lifespan. And because men have not been involved in child care as much as females, survival of a man's offspring, and thus his genes, depended not so much on how long he lived, but on how long the mother of his children lived."

In their studies of centenarians, Perls and Fretts found that a surprising number of women who lived to be 100 or more gave birth in their forties. These 100-year-old women were four times as likely to have given birth in their forties as women born in the same year who died at age 73. A study of centenarians in Europe by the Max Planck Institute of Demography in Germany found the same relationship between longevity and fecundity.

This does not mean that having a child in middle age makes a woman live longer. Rather, Perls says, "the factors that allow certain older women to bear children—a slow rate of aging and decreased susceptibility to disease—also improve a woman's chances of living a long time. Extending that idea, we argue that the driving force of human lifespan is maximizing the time during which woman can bear children. The age at which menopause eliminates the threat of female survival by ending further reproduction may therefore be the determinant of subsequent lifespan."

## Closing the Gap

If this is true, then the genes of female centenarians hold the secrets of a longer, healthier life. And these are no ordinary genes. Whether the average person drinks, smokes, exercises, or eats her vegetables adds or subtracts five to ten years to or from her life. But to live an additional 30 years requires the kind of genes that slow down aging and reduce susceptibility to conditions such as Alzheimer's disease, stroke, heart disease, and cancer.

Clues about what those genes are and how they work could come from studying those who survive 100 years or more, Perls believes. The New England Centenarian Study he runs is the only scientific investigation of the oldest oldsters being done in the United States. He has now expanded it to include all centenarians in the city of Boston, about 100 more people.

"We think that centenarians are a tremendous resource for the discovery of genes responsible for aging and the ways in which aging occurs," says Perls. "Finding these genes could lead to testing people and determining who might be disposed to accelerated aging via diseases such as Alzheimer's, cancer, heart disease, and stroke. Such individuals might eventually be treated to extend the prospect of their living longer."

The oldest person for which reliable records exist was a woman who recently died in France at the age of 123. "Reaching such an age is like winning the lottery," Perls comments. "The odds are about one in 6 billion. From a practical point of view, we can consider 100 years as the average maximum of human life. We're not there yet, of course. At present, average life expectancy for those born after 1960 is about 85 years."

Although women can expect to live longer than men, the gap is closing. Death rates have begun to converge in the past 20 years. Some researchers attribute the convergence to women taking on the behaviors and stresses formerly considered the domain of males—smoking, drinking, and working outside the home.

For example, Perls and Fretts point out that deaths from lung cancer have almost tripled in women in the past 20 years. One study concluded that, on average, middle-aged female smokers live no longer than male smokers.

"Smoking," Perls and Fretts conclude, "seems to be the 'great equalizer.'"

*—by William J. Cromie*

# Chapter 2

# Heart Disease

## Chapter Contents

# Section 2.1

## *Coronary Heart Disease*

Excerpted from "Facts about Coronary Heart Disease," National Heart, Lung, and Blood Institute, National Institutes of Health (NIH), NIH Pub. No. 02-2265, originally printed 1990, revised July 1993 and March 2003.

Coronary heart disease (CHD) is the most common form of heart disease, the leading cause of death for Americans. About 12.6 million Americans suffer from CHD, which often results in a heart attack. About 1.1 million Americans suffer a heart attack each year; about 515,000 of these heart attacks are fatal.

Fortunately, CHD can be prevented or controlled. This chapter gives an overview of CHD and its prevention, diagnosis, and treatment. It describes the steps that Americans can take to protect their heart health.

### What Is CHD?

The heart is a muscle that works 24 hours a day. To perform well, it needs a constant supply of oxygen and nutrients, which is delivered by the blood through the coronary arteries.

That blood flow can be reduced by a process called atherosclerosis, in which plaques or fatty substances build up inside the walls of blood vessels. The plaques attract blood components, which stick to the inside surface of the vessel walls. Atherosclerosis can affect any blood vessels and causes them to narrow and harden. It develops over many years and can begin early, even in childhood.

In CHD, atherosclerosis affects the coronary arteries. The fatty buildup, or plaque, can break open and lead to the formation of a blood clot. The clot covers the site of the rupture, also reducing blood flow. Eventually, the clot becomes firm. The process of fatty buildup, plaque rupture, and clot formation recurs, progressively narrowing the arteries. Ever less blood reaches the heart muscle.

When too little blood reaches a part of the body, the condition is called ischemia. When this occurs with the heart, it's called cardiac ischemia. If the blood supply is nearly or completely, and abruptly, cut

14

off, a heart attack results, and cells in the heart muscle that do not receive enough oxygen begin to die. The more time that passes without treatment to restore blood flow, the greater the damage to the heart. Because heart cells cannot be replaced, the cell loss is permanent.

## Who Gets CHD?

Certain behaviors and conditions increase the risk that someone will develop CHD. They also can increase the chance that CHD, if already present, will worsen. They are called "risk factors" and, while some cannot be modified, most can.

- *Risk factors that cannot be modified are:* age (45 or older for men; 55 or older for women) and a family history of early CHD (a father or brother diagnosed before age 55, or a mother or sister diagnosed with heart disease before age 65)

- *Factors that can be modified are:* cigarette smoking, high blood cholesterol, high blood pressure, overweight, obesity, physical inactivity, and diabetes

Risk factors do not add their effects in a simple way. Rather, they multiply each other's effects. Generally, each risk factor alone doubles a person's chance of developing CHD. Someone who has high blood cholesterol and high blood pressure and smokes cigarettes is eight times more likely to develop CHD than someone who has no risk factors. So, *it is important to prevent or control risk factors that can be modified.* See the "Life-style" section below for how to do this.

## What Are the Symptoms of CHD?

Symptoms of CHD vary. Some persons feel no discomfort, while others have chest pain or shortness of breath. Sometimes, the first symptom of CHD is a heart attack or cardiac arrest (a sudden, abrupt loss of heart function).

Chest pain also can vary in its occurrence. It happens when the blood flow to the heart is critically reduced and does not match the demands placed on the heart. Called angina, the pain can be mild and intermittent, or more pronounced and steady. It can be severe enough to make normal every-day activities difficult. The same inadequate blood supply also may cause no symptoms, a condition called silent ischemia.

Often, particularly in men, angina is felt behind the breastbone and may radiate up the left arm or neck. It may also be felt in the shoulder, elbows, jaw, or back. Angina is usually brought on by exercise, lasts two to five minutes, does not change with breathing, and is eased by rest.

A person who has any symptoms should talk with his or her doctor. Without treatment, the symptoms may return, worsen, become unstable, or progress to a heart attack.

## What Are the Tests for CHD?

There is no single, simple test for CHD. Which diagnostic tests are done depends on a number of factors, especially the severity of the symptoms and the likelihood that their cause is CHD. After taking a careful medical history and doing a physical examination, the doctor may use some of the following tests to rule out other causes for the symptoms, and to confirm the presence and check the severity of CHD.

### Electrocardiogram (ECG or EKG)

This is a graphic record of the electrical activity of the heart as it contracts and relaxes. The ECG can detect abnormal heartbeats, some areas of damage, inadequate blood flow, and heart enlargement.

### Stress Test

The stress test is used to check for problems that show up only when the heart is working hard. There are different types of stress test. One is called the exercise test (also called a treadmill test or bicycle exercise ECG); another uses a drug instead of exercise to increase blood flow. The latter is used for persons, such as those with arthritis, who cannot exercise. In both cases, the blood pressure and heartbeat response are continuously monitored and periodically recorded. An ECG rate and blood pressure are taken before, during, and after the test. For an exercise stress test, breathing and oxygen consumption also may be measured.

Still another type of stress test uses a nuclear scan (see next test) to assess heart muscle contraction or blood flow in the heart.

Stress tests are useful but not 100 percent reliable. False positives (showing a problem where none exists) and false negatives (showing no problem when something is wrong) can occur. For instance, gender and race can affect the measurements of exercise stress tests.

### Nuclear Scan

This also is called a thallium stress test. It is sometimes used to show areas of the heart that lack blood flow and are damaged, as well as problems with the heart's pumping action. A small amount of a radioactive material called thallium is injected into a vein, usually in the arm. A scanning camera positioned over the heart records whether the nuclear material is taken up by the heart muscle (healthy areas) or not (damaged areas). The camera also can evaluate how well the heart muscle pumps blood. This test can be done during both rest and exercise, enhancing the usefulness of its results.

### *Coronary Angiography (or Arteriography)*

This test is used to detect blockages and narrowed areas inside coronary arteries. A fine tube (catheter) is threaded through an artery of an arm or leg into position in the heart vessel. A dye that shows up on x-ray is then injected into the blood vessel, and the vessels and heart are filmed as the heart pumps. The picture is called an angiogram or arteriogram.

### *Ventriculogram*

This is a picture of the heart's main pumping chamber, the left ventricle. It is taken by following a procedure similar to the one described for an angiogram. For a ventriculogram, the catheter is positioned in the left ventricle.

### *Intracoronary Ultrasound*

This uses a catheter that can measure blood flow. It gives a picture of the coronary arteries that shows the thickness and character of the artery wall. This lets the doctor assess blood flow and blockages.

## *How Is CHD Treated?*

There are three main types of treatment for CHD: life-style, medication, and, for advanced atherosclerosis, special procedures. The first two types of treatment also can help prevent the development of CHD.

### *Life-Style*

Six key steps can help prevent or control CHD: stop smoking cigarettes, lower high blood pressure, reduce high blood cholesterol, lose extra weight, become physically active, and manage diabetes.

**Cigarette Smoking**. There is no safe way to smoke. Although low-tar and low-nicotine cigarettes may somewhat reduce the risk for lung cancer, they do not lessen the risk for CHD. In fact, smoking accelerates atherosclerosis. It also increases the risk for stroke.

The risk for CHD increases along with the number of cigarettes smoked daily. Quitting sharply lowers the risk, even in the first year and no matter what a person's age. Quitting also reduces the risk for a second heart attack in those who have already had one.

The U.S. Food and Drug Administration has approved five medications that can help persons stop smoking and lessen the urge to smoke. These are: bupropion SR (available only by prescription), which has no nicotine and reduces the craving for cigarettes; nicotine supplements, which include gum (available over the counter); a nicotine patch (available both over the counter and by prescription); a nicotine inhaler (available only by prescription); and a nicotine nasal spray (available only by prescription).

For more about how to stop smoking, check the Virtual Office of the U.S. Surgeon General at www.surgeongeneral.gov/tobacco.

**High Blood Pressure**. Also known as hypertension, high blood pressure usually has no symptoms. Once developed, it typically lasts a lifetime. If uncontrolled, it can lead to heart and kidney diseases and stroke.

Blood pressure is given as two numbers—the systolic pressure over the diastolic pressure—and both are important. A measurement of 140/90 mmHg (millimeters of mercury) or above is called high blood pressure but if either number is high, that too is hypertension. A healthy blood pressure is around 120/80.

Life-style steps often can prevent or control high blood pressure: lose excess weight, become physically active, follow a healthy eating plan, including foods lower in salt and sodium, and limit alcohol intake.

**High Blood Cholesterol**. Cholesterol is a soft, waxy substance involved in normal cell function. Normally, the body makes all the cholesterol it needs. Excess saturated fat and cholesterol in the diet cause the fatty buildup in blood vessels, which contributes to atherosclerosis.

Cholesterol travels through the blood in packages called lipoproteins. There are two main types of lipoprotein that affect the risk for CHD: low-density lipoprotein (LDL), also called the "bad" cholesterol, which causes deposits in blood vessels; and high-density lipoprotein (HDL), also called the "good" cholesterol, which helps remove cholesterol from the blood. It's important to have a low level of LDL and a high level of HDL.

**Overweight and Obesity.** About 65 percent of American adults are overweight or obese. Being overweight or obese increases the risk not only for heart disease, but also for other conditions, including stroke, gallbladder disease, arthritis, and breast, colon, and other cancers.

Overweight and obesity are determined by two key measures— body mass index, or BMI, and waist circumference. BMI relates height to weight. A normal BMI is 18.5–24.9; an overweight BMI is 25–29.9; and an obese BMI is 30 and over. For waist circumference, heart disease risk increases if it is greater than 35 inches for women or greater than 40 inches for men.

Those who are overweight or obese should aim for a healthy weight in order to reduce CHD risk. Even a small weight loss of just 10 percent of current weight will help to lower CHD risk and that of the other conditions too. Those who cannot lose should at least try not to gain more weight.

There are no quick fixes to lose weight. To be successful, weight loss must be viewed as a change of life-style and not as a temporary effort to drop pounds quickly. Otherwise, the weight will probably be regained. Do not try to lose more than 1/2 to 2 pounds a week.

To lose weight, follow a heart-healthy eating plan. Eat a variety of nutritious foods in moderate amounts. Choose foods that are lower in calories and fat. It's also important to become physically active. This helps use calories and aids weight loss. It also helps keep the weight off for life.

**Physical Activity**. Physical activity is one of the best ways to help prevent and control CHD. It can lower LDL and raise HDL. It also lowers blood pressure for those who are overweight.

To become physically active, do 30 minutes of a moderate activity on most, and preferably all, days. Examples of moderate activities are brisk walking and dancing. If 30 minutes is too much time, break it up into periods of at least 10 minutes each. Those who have been inactive should start slowly. Begin at a lower level of physical activity and slowly increase the time and intensity of the effort.

Those with CHD or who have a high risk for it should check with their doctor before starting a physical activity program. Others who should consult a doctor first include those with chronic health problems, men over age 40, and women over age 50. The doctor can give advice on how rigorous the exercise should be.

Those who have had a heart attack benefit greatly from physical activity. Many hospitals have a cardiac rehabilitation program. The doctor can offer advice about a suitable program.

**Diabetes.** Diabetes mellitus affects more than 17 million Americans. It damages blood vessels, including the coronary arteries of the heart. Up to 75 percent of those with diabetes develop heart and blood vessel diseases. Diabetes also can lead to stroke, kidney failure, and other problems.

Because of the link with heart disease, it's important for those with diabetes to prevent or control heart disease and its risk factors. Fortunately, new research shows that the same steps that reduce the risk of CHD also lower the chance of developing type 2 diabetes. And, for those who already have diabetes, those steps, along with taking any prescribed medication, also can delay or prevent the development of complications of diabetes, such as eye or kidney disease and nerve damage.

## *Medications*

Sometimes, in addition to making life-style changes, medications may be needed to prevent or control CHD. For instance, medications may be used to control a risk factor such as high blood pressure or high blood cholesterol and so help prevent the development of CHD. Or medication may be used to relieve the chest pain of CHD.

If prescribed, medications must be taken as directed. Drugs can have side effects. If side effects occur, they should be reported to the doctor. Often, a change in the dose or type of a medication, or the use of a combination of drugs, can stop the side effect.

Drugs used to treat CHD and its risk factors include:

- *Aspirin* helps to lower the risk of a heart attack for those who have already had one. It also helps to keep arteries open in those who have had a previous heart bypass or other artery-opening procedure such as coronary angioplasty (see next section). Because of its risks, aspirin is not approved by the Food and Drug Administration for the prevention of heart attacks in healthy persons. It may be harmful for some persons, especially those with no risk of heart disease. Patients must be assessed carefully to make sure the benefits of taking aspirin outweigh the risks. Each person should talk to his or her doctor about whether or not to take aspirin. Aspirin also is given to patients who arrive at a hospital emergency department with a suspected heart attack.

- *Digitalis* helps the heart contract better and is used when the heart's pumping function has been weakened; it also slows some fast heart rhythms.

- *ACE (angiotensin converting enzyme) inhibitor* stops production of a chemical produced by the body that makes blood vessels narrow. It is used for high blood pressure and damaged heart muscle. It also can prevent kidney damage in some patients with diabetes.

- *Beta blocker* slows the heart and makes it beat with less force, lowering blood pressure and making the heart work less hard. It is used for high blood pressure, chest pain, and to prevent a repeat heart attack.

- *Nitrate* (including nitroglycerin) relaxes blood vessels and stops chest pain/angina.

- *Calcium channel blocker* relaxes blood vessels, and is used for high blood pressure and chest pain/angina.

- *Diuretic* decreases fluid in the body and is used for high blood pressure. Diuretics are sometimes referred to as "water pills."

- *Blood cholesterol–lowering agents* decrease LDL levels in the blood. Some can increase HDL.

- *Thrombolytic agents*, also called "clot-busting drugs," are given during a heart attack to dissolve a blood clot in a coronary artery in order to restore blood flow. They must be given immediately after heart attack symptoms begin. To be most effective, they need to be given within one hour of the start of heart attack symptoms.

### Special Procedures

Advanced atherosclerosis may require a special procedure to open an artery and improve blood flow. This is usually done to ease severe chest pain or to clear major or multiple blockages in blood vessels. Two commonly used procedures are coronary angioplasty and coronary artery bypass graft operation:

**Coronary Angioplasty, or Balloon Angioplasty**. In this procedure, a fine tube, or catheter, is threaded through an artery into the narrowed heart vessel. The catheter has a tiny balloon at its tip. The balloon is repeatedly inflated and deflated to open and stretch the artery, improving blood flow. The balloon is then deflated, and the catheter is removed.

Doctors often insert a stent during the angioplasty. A wire mesh tube, the stent is used to keep an artery open after an angioplasty. The stent stays in the artery permanently.

Angioplasty is not surgery. It is done while the patient is awake and may last one to two hours.

In about one third of those who have an angioplasty, the blood vessel becomes narrowed or blocked again within six months. Vessels that reclose may be opened again with another angioplasty or a coronary artery bypass graft. An artery with a stent also can reclose.

**Coronary Artery Bypass Graft Operation**. Also known as "bypass surgery," the procedure uses a piece of vein taken from the leg, or of an artery taken from the chest or wrist. This piece is attached to the heart artery above and below the narrowed area, thus making a bypass around the blockage. Sometimes, more than one bypass is needed.

Bypass surgery may be needed due to various reasons, such as an angioplasty that did not sufficiently widen the blood vessel, or blockages that cannot be reached by, or are too long or hard for, angioplasty. In certain cases, bypass surgery may be preferred to angioplasty. For instance, it may be used for persons who have both CHD and diabetes.

A bypass also can close again. This happens in about 10 percent of bypass surgeries, usually after 10 or more years.

Other procedures also may be used to open coronary arteries:

- *Atherectomy*. A specially equipped catheter is threaded through an artery to a blockage, where thin strips of plaque are shaved off and removed. Balloon angioplasty or insertion of a stent may be done as well.

- *Laser angioplasty*. A catheter with a laser tip is inserted into an artery to burn, vaporize, or break down plaque. The procedure may be used alone or along with balloon angioplasty.

It is important to understand that these procedures relieve the symptoms of CHD but do not cure the disease. Life-style changes must still be followed, and any necessary medications must continue to be taken.

# Section 2.2

# *Heart Attack*

Reprinted from "Heart Attack Warning Signs," National Heart, Lung, and Blood Institute, National Institutes of Health, September 2001, http://www.nhlbi.nih.gov/actintime/haws/haws.htm,; and "Frequently Asked Questions about Heart Attack," National Heart, Lung, and Blood Institute, National Institutes of Health, September 2001, http://www.nhlbi.nih.gov/actintime/faq/faq.htm.

## *Heart Attack Warning Signs*

A heart attack is a frightening event, and you probably don't want to think about it. But, if you learn the signs of a heart attack and what steps to take, you can save a life—maybe your own.

What are the signs of a heart attack? Many people think a heart attack is sudden and intense, like a "movie" heart attack, where a person clutches his or her chest and falls over.

The truth is that many heart attacks start slowly, as a mild pain or discomfort. If you feel such a symptom, you may not be sure what's wrong. Your symptoms may even come and go. Even those who have had a heart attack may not recognize their symptoms, because the next attack can have entirely different ones.

It's vital that everyone learn the warning signs of a heart attack. These are:

- *Chest discomfort.* Most heart attacks involve discomfort in the center of the chest that lasts for more than a few minutes, or goes away and comes back. The discomfort can feel like uncomfortable pressure, squeezing, fullness, or pain.

- *Discomfort in other areas of the upper body.* Can include pain or discomfort in one or both arms, the back, neck, jaw, or stomach.

- *Shortness of breath.* Often comes along with chest discomfort. But it also can occur before chest discomfort.

- *Other symptoms.* May include breaking out in a cold sweat, nausea, or light-headedness.

23

Learn the signs—but also remember: Even if you're not sure it's a heart attack, you should still have it checked out. Fast action can save lives—maybe your own.

## Frequently Asked Questions about Heart Attack

### Heart Attack Warning Signs

**How would I know if I were having a heart attack?**

Often, it is not easy to tell. But there are symptoms people may have. These are: an uncomfortable pressure, squeezing, fullness, or pain in the center of the chest that lasts more than a few minutes, or goes away and comes back; discomfort in other areas of the upper body, which may be felt in one or both arms, the back, neck, jaw, or stomach; shortness of breath, which often occurs with or before chest discomfort; and other symptoms such as breaking out in a cold sweat, nausea, or light-headedness. When in doubt, check it out! Call 911. Don't wait more than a few minutes, five at most. Call right away!

**What is angina and how is it different from a heart attack?**

An episode of angina is *not* a heart attack. However, people with angina report having a hard time telling the difference between angina symptoms and heart attack symptoms. Angina is a recurring pain or discomfort in the chest that happens when some part of the heart does not receive enough blood temporarily. A person may notice it during exertion (such as in climbing stairs). It is usually relieved within a few minutes by resting or by taking prescribed angina medicine. People who have been diagnosed with angina have a greater risk of a heart attack than do other people.

### Prehospital Delay Time

**I'd rather wait until I'm sure something's really wrong. What's the rush anyway?**

Clot-busting drugs and other artery-opening treatments work best when given within the first hour after a heart attack starts. The first hour also is the most risky time during a heart attack—it's when your heart might stop suddenly. Responding fast to your symptoms really increases your chance of surviving.

## So how quickly should I act?

If you have any heart attack symptoms, call 911 immediately. Don't wait for more than a few minutes—five at most—to call 911.

## Why should I bother? If I'm going to die, there's not much I can do about it anyway, is there?

That's not true. There is something that can be done about a heart attack. Doctors have clot-busting drugs and other artery-opening procedures that can stop or reverse a heart attack, if given quickly. These drugs can limit the damage to the heart muscle by removing the blockage and restoring blood flow. Less heart damage means a better quality of life after a heart attack.

Given that these new therapies are available, it's very sad to know that so many people cannot receive these treatments because they delay too long before seeking care. The greatest benefits of these therapies are gained when patients come in early (preferably within the first hour of the start of their symptoms).

### *The Role of Emergency Medical Personnel*

## Emergency medical personnel cause such a commotion. Can't I just have my wife/husband/friend/co-worker take me to the hospital?

Emergency medical personnel—also called EMS, for emergency medical services—bring medical care to you. For example, they bring oxygen and medications. And they can actually restart someone's heart if it stops after they arrive. Your wife/husband/friend/co-worker can't do that, or help you at all if they are driving. In the ambulance, there are enough people to give you the help you need and get you to the hospital right away.

### *Steps to Survival*

## I'm not sure I can remember all this. What can I do to make it easier for me?

You can make a plan and discuss it in advance with your family, your friends, your co-workers, and, of course, your doctor. Then you can rehearse this plan, just like a fire drill. Keep it simple. Know the warning signs. Keep information—such as what medications you're taking—in one place. If you have any symptoms of a heart attack for a few minutes (no more than five), call the EMS by dialing 911 right away.

**I carry nitroglycerin pills all the time for my heart condition. If I have heart attack symptoms, shouldn't I try them first?**

Yes, if your doctor has prescribed nitroglycerin pills, you should follow your doctor's orders. If you are not sure about how to take your nitroglycerin when you get chest pain, check with your doctor.

**What about taking an aspirin like we see on television?**

You should not delay calling 911 to take an aspirin. Studies have shown that people sometimes delay seeking help if they take an aspirin (or other medicine). Emergency department personnel will give people experiencing a heart attack an aspirin as soon as they arrive. So, the best thing to do is to call 911 immediately and let the professionals give the aspirin.

# Section 2.3

# *Smoking and Heart Disease*

Cigarette smoking is the most important preventable cause of premature death in the United States. It accounts for more than 440,000 of the more than 2.4 million annual deaths. Cigarette smokers have a higher risk of developing a number of chronic disorders. These include fatty buildups in arteries, several types of cancer, and chronic obstructive pulmonary disease (lung problems). Atherosclerosis (clogged arteries) is the chief contributor to the high number of deaths from smoking. Many studies detail the evidence that cigarette smoking is a major cause of coronary heart disease, which leads to heart attack.

## *How Does Smoking Affect Coronary Heart Disease Risk?*

Cigarette and tobacco smoke, high blood cholesterol, high blood pressure, physical inactivity, obesity, and diabetes are the six major independent risk factors for coronary heart disease that you can modify or control. Cigarette smoking is so widespread and significant as a risk factor that the surgeon general has called it "the most important of the known modifiable risk factors for coronary heart disease in the United States."

Cigarette smoking increases the risk of coronary heart disease by itself. When it acts with other factors, it greatly increases risk. Smoking increases blood pressure, decreases exercise tolerance, and increases the tendency for blood to clot.

Cigarette smoking is the most important risk factor for young men and women. It produces a greater relative risk in persons under 50 than in those over 50.

Women who smoke and use oral contraceptives greatly increase their risk of coronary heart disease and stroke compared with non-smoking women who use oral contraceptives.

Smoking increases LDL (bad) cholesterol and decreases HDL (good) cholesterol. Cigarette smoking combined with a family history of heart disease also seems to greatly increase the risk.

## What about Cigarette Smoking and Stroke?

Studies show that cigarette smoking is an important risk factor for stroke. Inhaling cigarette smoke produces several effects that damage the cardiovascular system. Women who take oral contraceptives and smoke increase their risk of stroke many times.

## What about Cigar and Pipe Smoking?

People who smoke cigars or pipes seem to have a higher risk of death from coronary heart disease (and possibly stroke), but their risk isn't as great as that of cigarette smokers. This is probably because they're less likely to inhale the smoke. Currently, there's very little scientific information on cigar and pipe smoking and cardiovascular disease.

## What about Passive or Second-hand Smoking?

The American Heart Association believes more research is needed on the effects of passive smoking (also called second-hand smoke or environmental tobacco smoke) on heart and blood vessel disease in nonsmokers. Several studies document the health hazards posed by passive smoking. About 37,000 to 40,000 people die from heart and blood vessel disease caused by other people's smoke each year. Of these, about 35,000 nonsmokers die from coronary heart disease, which includes heart attack.

# Section 2.4

# *Cholesterol and Heart Disease*

Reprinted from "High Blood Cholesterol: What You Need to Know," National Heart, Lung, and Blood Institute, National Institutes of Health (NIH), May 2001, http://www.nhlbi.nih.gov/health/public/heart/chol/wyntk. htm. Also available as NIH Pub. No. 01-3290.

## *Why Is Cholesterol Important?*

Your blood cholesterol level has a lot to do with your chances of getting heart disease. High blood cholesterol is one of the major risk factors for heart disease. A risk factor is a condition that increases your chance of getting a disease. In fact, the higher your blood cholesterol level, the greater your risk for developing heart disease or having a heart attack. Heart disease is the number-one killer of women and men in the United States. Each year, more than one million Americans have heart attacks, and about a half million people die from heart disease.

## *How Does Cholesterol Cause Heart Disease?*

When there is too much cholesterol (a fat-like substance) in your blood, it builds up in the walls of your arteries. Over time, this buildup causes "hardening of the arteries" so that arteries become narrowed and blood flow to the heart is slowed down or blocked. The blood carries oxygen to the heart, and if enough blood and oxygen cannot reach your heart, you may suffer chest pain. If the blood supply to a portion of the heart is completely cut off by a blockage, the result is a heart attack.

High blood cholesterol itself does not cause symptoms, so many people are unaware that their cholesterol level is too high. It is important to find out what your cholesterol numbers are because lowering cholesterol levels that are too high lessens the risk for developing heart disease and reduces the chance of a heart attack or dying of heart disease, even if you already have it. Cholesterol lowering is important for everyone—younger, middle age, and older adults; women and men; and people with or without heart disease.

## What Do Your Cholesterol Numbers Mean?

Everyone age 20 and older should have their cholesterol measured at least once every five years. It is best to have a blood test called a lipoprotein profile to find out your cholesterol numbers. This blood test is done after a 9- to 12-hour fast and gives information about your:

- Total cholesterol

- LDL (bad) cholesterol—the main source of cholesterol buildup and blockage in the arteries

- HDL (good) cholesterol—helps keep cholesterol from building up in the arteries

- Triglycerides—another form of fat in your blood

If it is not possible to get a lipoprotein profile done, knowing your total cholesterol and HDL cholesterol can give you a general idea about your cholesterol levels. If your total cholesterol is 200 mg/dL [milligrams (mg) of cholesterol per deciliter (dL) of blood] or more or if your HDL is less than 40 mg/dL, you will need to have a lipoprotein profile done. See how your cholesterol numbers compare to Tables 2.1 and 2.2.

**Table 2.1.** Risk Category by Total Cholesterol Level

| Total Cholesterol Level | Category |
| --- | --- |
| Less than 200 mg/dL | Desirable |
| 200–239 mg/dL | Borderline high |
| 240 mg/dL and above | High |

HDL (good) cholesterol protects against heart disease, so for HDL, higher numbers are better. A level less than 40 mg/dL is low and is considered a major risk factor because it increases your risk for developing heart disease. HDL levels of 60 mg/dL or more help to lower your risk for heart disease.

Triglycerides can also raise heart disease risk. Levels that are borderline high (150-199 mg/dL) or high (200 mg/dL or more) may need treatment in some people.

enough by reducing your saturated fat and cholesterol intakes, the amount of soluble fiber in your diet can be increased. Certain food products that contain plant stanols or plant sterols (for example, cholesterol-lowering margarines and salad dressings) can also be added to the TLC diet to boost its LDL-lowering power. Foods low in saturated fat include fat free or 1 percent dairy products, lean meats, fish, skinless poultry, whole grain foods, and fruits and vegetables. Look for soft margarines (liquid or tub varieties) that are low in saturated fat and contain little or no trans fat (another type of dietary fat that can raise your cholesterol level). Limit foods high in cholesterol such as liver and other organ meats, egg yolks, and full-fat dairy products. Good sources of soluble fiber include oats, certain fruits (such as oranges and pears) and vegetables (such as brussels sprouts and carrots), and dried peas and beans.

- *Weight management.* Losing weight if you are overweight can help lower LDL and is especially important for those with a cluster of risk factors that includes high triglyceride and/or low HDL levels and being overweight with a large waist measurement (more than 40 inches for men and more than 35 inches for women).

- *Physical activity.* Regular physical activity (30 minutes on most, if not all, days) is recommended for everyone. It can help raise HDL and lower LDL and is especially important for those with high triglyceride and/or low HDL levels who are overweight with a large waist measurement.

## Drug Treatment

Even if you begin drug treatment to lower your cholesterol, you will need to continue your treatment with life-style changes. This will keep the dose of medicine as low as possible, and lower your risk in other ways as well. There are several types of drugs available for cholesterol lowering including statins, bile acid sequestrants, nicotinic acid, and fibric acids. Your doctor can help decide which type of drug is best for you. The statin drugs are very effective in lowering LDL levels and are safe for most people. Bile acid sequestrants also lower LDL and can be used alone or in combination with statin drugs. Nicotinic acid lowers LDL and triglycerides and raises HDL. Fibric acids lower LDL somewhat but are used mainly to treat high triglyceride and low HDL levels.

Once your LDL goal has been reached, your doctor may prescribe treatment for high triglycerides and/or a low HDL level, if present. The treatment includes losing weight if needed, increasing physical activity, quitting smoking, and possibly taking a drug.

## Section 2.5

# *Congestive Heart Failure*

Reprinted from "Facts about Heart Failure," National Heart, Lung, and Blood Institute, National Institutes of Health (NIH), May 1997, http://www.nhlbi.nih.gov/health/public/heart/other/hrtfail.htm#what%20is. Also available as NIH Pub. No. 95-923. Reviewed and revised by David A. Cooke, M.D., on August 23, 2003.

### *What Is Heart Failure?*

Heart failure occurs when the heart loses its ability to pump enough blood through the body. Usually, the loss in pumping action is a symptom of an underlying heart problem, such as coronary artery disease.

The term heart failure suggests a sudden and complete stop of heart activity. But, actually, the heart does not suddenly stop. Rather, heart failure usually develops slowly, often over years, as the heart gradually loses its pumping ability and works less efficiently. Some people may not become aware of their condition until symptoms appear years after their heart began its decline.

How serious the condition is depends on how much pumping capacity the heart has lost. Nearly everyone loses some pumping capacity as he or she ages. But the loss is significantly more in heart failure and often results from a heart attack or other disease that damages the heart.

The severity of the condition determines the impact it has on a person's life. At one end of the spectrum, the mild form of heart failure may have little effect on a person's life; at the other end, severe heart failure can interfere with even simple activities and prove fatal. Between those extremes, treatment often helps people lead full lives.

But all forms of heart failure, even the mildest, are a serious health problem, which must be treated. To improve their chance of living longer, patients must take care of themselves, see their physician regularly, and closely follow treatments.

## Is There Only One Type of Heart Failure?

The term congestive heart failure is often used to describe all patients with heart failure. In reality, congestion (the buildup of fluid) is just one feature of the condition and does not occur in all patients. There are two main categories of heart failure although within each category, symptoms and effects may differ from patient to patient. The two categories are:

- *Systolic heart failure*—This occurs when the heart's ability to contract decreases. The heart cannot pump with enough force to push a sufficient amount of blood into the circulation. Blood coming into the heart from the lungs may back up and cause fluid to leak into the lungs, a condition known as pulmonary congestion.

- *Diastolic heart failure*—This occurs when the heart has a problem relaxing. The heart cannot properly fill with blood because the muscle has become stiff, losing its ability to relax. This form may lead to fluid accumulation, especially in the feet, ankles, and legs. Some patients may have lung congestion.

## How Common Is Heart Failure?

Between 2 to 3 million Americans have heart failure, and 400,000 new cases are diagnosed each year. The condition is slightly more common among men than women and is twice as common among African Americans as whites.

Heart failure causes 39,000 deaths a year and is a contributing factor in another 225,000 deaths. The death rate attributed to heart failure rose by 64 percent from 1970 to 1990, while the death rate from coronary heart disease dropped by 49 percent during the same period. Heart failure mortality is about twice as high for African Americans as whites for all age groups.

In a sense, heart failure's growing presence as a health problem reflects the nation's changing population: More people are living longer. People age 65 and older represent the fastest growing segment of the population, and the risk of heart failure increases with age. The condition affects 1 percent of people age 50, but about 5 percent of people age 75.

## What Causes Heart Failure?

As stated, the heart loses some of its blood-pumping ability as a natural consequence of aging. However, a number of other factors can lead to a potentially life-threatening loss of pumping activity.

As a symptom of underlying heart disease, heart failure is closely associated with the major risk factors for coronary heart disease: smoking, high cholesterol levels, hypertension (persistent high blood pressure), diabetes and abnormal blood sugar levels, and obesity. A person can change or eliminate those risk factors and thus lower their risk of developing or aggravating their heart disease and heart failure.

Among prominent risk factors, hypertension (high blood pressure) and diabetes are particularly important. Uncontrolled high blood pressure increases the risk of heart failure by 200 percent, compared with those who do not have hypertension. Moreover, the degree of risk appears directly related to the severity of the high blood pressure.

Persons with diabetes have about a two- to eightfold greater risk of heart failure than those without diabetes. Women with diabetes have a greater risk of heart failure than men with diabetes. Part of the risk comes from diabetes' association with other heart failure risk factors, such as high blood pressure, obesity, and high cholesterol levels. However, the disease process in diabetes also damages the heart muscle.

The presence of coronary disease is among the greatest risks for heart failure. Muscle damage and scarring caused by a heart attack greatly increase the risk of heart failure. Cardiac arrhythmias, or irregular heartbeats, also raise heart failure risk. Any disorder that causes abnormal swelling or thickening of the heart sets the stage for heart failure.

In some people, heart failure arises from problems with heart valves, the flap-like structures that help regulate blood flow through the heart. Infections in the heart are another source of increased risk for heart failure.

A single risk factor may be sufficient to cause heart failure, but a combination of factors dramatically increases the risk. Advanced age adds to the potential impact of any heart failure risk.

Finally, genetic abnormalities contribute to the risk for certain types of heart disease, which in turn may lead to heart failure. However, in most instances, a specific genetic link to heart failure has not been identified.

## What Are the Symptoms?

A number of symptoms are associated with heart failure, but none is specific for the condition. Perhaps the best known symptom is shortness of breath (dyspnea). In heart failure, this may result from excess fluid in the lungs. The breathing difficulties may occur at rest or during exercise. In some cases, congestion may be severe enough to prevent or interrupt sleep.

Fatigue or easy tiring is another common symptom. As the heart's pumping capacity decreases, muscles and other tissues receive less oxygen and nutrition, which are carried in the blood. Without proper "fuel," the body cannot perform as much work, which translates into fatigue.

Fluid accumulation, or edema, may cause swelling of the feet, ankles, legs, and occasionally the abdomen. Excess fluid retained by the body may result in weight gain, which sometimes occurs fairly quickly.

Persistent coughing is another common sign, especially coughing that regularly produces mucus or pink, blood-tinged sputum. Some people develop raspy breathing or wheezing.

Because heart failure usually develops slowly, the symptoms may not appear until the condition has progressed over years. The heart hides the underlying problem by making adjustments that delay—but do not prevent—the eventual loss in pumping capacity. The heart adjusts, or compensates, in three ways to cope with and hide the effects of heart failure:

- Enlargement (dilatation), which allows more blood into the heart

- Thickening of muscle fibers (hypertrophy) to strengthen the heart muscle, which allows the heart to contract more forcefully and pump more blood

- More frequent contraction, which increases circulation

By making these adjustments, or compensating, the heart can temporarily make up for losses in pumping ability, sometimes for years. However, compensation has its limits. Eventually, the heart cannot offset the lost ability to pump blood, and the signs of heart failure appear.

## How Do Doctors Diagnose Heart Failure?

In many cases, physicians diagnose heart failure during a physical examination. Readily identifiable signs are shortness of breath, fatigue, and swollen ankles and feet. The physician also will check for the presence of risk factors, such as hypertension, obesity, and a history of heart problems. Using a stethoscope, the physician can listen to a patient breathe and identify the sounds of lung congestion. The stethoscope also picks up the abnormal heart sounds indicative of heart failure.

If neither the symptoms nor the patient's history point to a clear-cut diagnosis, the physician may recommend any of a variety of laboratory tests, including, initially, an electrocardiogram, which uses recording devices placed on the chest to evaluate the electrical activity of a patient's heartbeat.

Echocardiography is another means of evaluating heart function from outside the body. Sound waves bounced off the heart are recorded and translated into images. The pictures can reveal abnormal heart size, shape, and movement. Echocardiography also can be used to calculate a patient's ejection fraction, a measure of the amount of blood pumped out when the heart contracts.

Another possible test is the chest x-ray, which also determines the heart's size and shape, as well as the presence of congestion in the lungs.

Tests help rule out other possible causes of symptoms. The symptoms of heart failure can result when the heart is made to work too hard, instead of from damaged muscle. Conditions that overload the heart occur rarely and include severe anemia and thyrotoxicosis (a disease resulting from an overactive thyroid gland).

## What Treatments Are Available?

Heart failure caused by an excessive workload is curable by treating the primary disease, such as anemia or thyrotoxicosis. Also curable are forms caused by anatomical problems, such as a heart valve defect. These defects can be surgically corrected.

However, for the common forms of heart failure—those due to damaged heart muscle—no known cure exists. But treatment for these forms may be quite successful. The treatment seeks to improve patients' quality of life and length of survival through lifestyle change and drug therapy.

Patients can minimize the effects of heart failure by controlling the risk factors for heart disease. Obvious steps include quitting smoking, losing weight if necessary, abstaining from alcohol, and making dietary changes to reduce the amount of salt and fat consumed. Regular, modest exercise is also helpful for many patients, though the amount and intensity should be carefully monitored by a physician.

But, even with life-style changes, most heart failure patients must take medication. Many patients receive three or more kinds of drugs.

Since the early 1990s, there has been a revolution in medication treatment for heart failure. While the disease remains a serious and potentially deadly condition, several types of drugs have proven quite useful in the treatment of heart failure:

- *Angiotensin converting enzyme inhibitors* (ACE inhibitors) have become one of two mainstays for treating systolic heart failure, and are also useful in other forms of heart failure. They have been shown in studies to sharply reduce the rate of death from heart failure and to improve heart function. Originally developed as a treatment for hypertension, ACE inhibitors help heart failure patients by, among other things, decreasing the pressure inside blood vessels. As a result, the heart does not have to work as hard to pump blood through the vessels. Patients who cannot take ACE inhibitors are usually given ARBs (see below). If they cannot take either drug, they may get a nitrate and/or a drug called hydralazine, each of which helps relax tension in blood vessels to improve blood flow.

- *Beta blockers* are the other mainstay of heart failure treatment. They have complex effects on the heart that include slowing the heart rate and preventing harmful changes in the heart muscle related to heart failure. These drugs have also been shown to have dramatic effects on the rates of death and hospitalization due to heart failure.

- *Angiotensin II receptor blockers* (ARBs) are an emerging alternative to ACE inhibitors in treating heart failure. Their effects are very similar to those of ACE inhibitors, but they are achieved in a slightly different way. Most studies so far have concluded that ARBs are as good as ACE inhibitors in treating heart failure. Trials are underway to determine if ARBs are any better than ACE inhibitors, and whether a combination of ACE inhibitors and ARBs is better than either drug alone.

- *Diuretics* help reduce the amount of fluid in the body and are useful for patients with fluid retention and hypertension. Spironolactone is an unusual diuretic that also has hormonal effects

41

on the heart. It has been shown in one large study to be very helpful in patients with severe systolic heart failure, by preventing changes in the heart muscle that worsen heart failure. Other drugs that work in a similar manner are expected to be available shortly.

• *Digitalis* increases the force of the heart's contractions, helping to improve circulation.

Sometimes, heart failure is life-threatening. Usually, this happens when drug therapy and life-style changes fail to control symptoms. In such cases, a heart transplant may be the only treatment option. However, candidates for transplantation often have to wait months or even years before a suitable donor heart is found. Recent studies indicate that some transplant candidates improve during this waiting period through drug treatment and other therapy, and can be removed from the transplant list.

Patients with advanced heart failure are prone to life-threatening disturbances of heart rhythms, known as arrhythmias. These arrhythmias may occur with no warning, and are frequently fatal. A device known as the automated implantable cardiac defibrillator (AICD) can prevent many of these cases of sudden death. An AICD is about the size of a deck of cards, and is implanted under the skin of the chest, much like a pacemaker. The AICD monitors the heart rhythm, and can deliver electrical shocks to the heart to return it to normal if a serious arrhythmia occurs. AICDs have been shown to substantially cut the risk of death in certain kinds of heart failure patients. They are usually placed in patients who have survived serious arrhythmias, and as a precautionary measure in other patients who meet certain criteria.

Transplant candidates who do not improve sometimes need mechanical pumps, which are attached to the heart. Called left ventricular assist devices (LVADs), the machines take over part or virtually all of the heart's blood-pumping activity. Current LVADs are not permanent solutions for heart failure but are considered bridges to transplantation. However, research is underway that looks at LVADs as long-term or even permanent treatments for severe heart failure.

A fully mechanical ("artificial") heart known as the Jarvik-7 was first developed and tested in several patients during the early 1980s. However, these patients developed fatal complications from the device, and the tests were stopped. In 2001, a new artificial heart with improved technology, the AbioCor™ heart, was implanted into several patients who were near death from severe heart failure. The results with the new device have been somewhat promising, but years of further testing and refinement will be necessary before this device will be available for general use.

An experimental surgical procedure for severe heart failure is available at a few U.S. medical centers. The procedure, called cardiomyoplasty, involves detaching one end of a muscle in the back, wrapping it around the heart, and then suturing the muscle to the heart. An implanted electric stimulator causes the back muscle to contract, pumping blood from the heart.

## Common Heart Failure Medications

Listed below are some of the medications prescribed for heart failure. Not all medications are suitable for all patients, and more than one drug may be needed.

Also, the list provides the full range of possible side effects for these drugs. Not all patients will develop these side effects. If you suspect that you are having a side effect, alert your physician.

### ACE Inhibitors

These prevent the production of a chemical that causes blood vessels to narrow. As a result, blood pressure drops and the heart does not have to work as hard to pump blood. Side effects may include coughing, skin rashes, fluid retention, excess potassium in the bloodstream, kidney problems, and an altered or lost sense of taste.

### ARBs

These drugs provide the same benefits as ACE inhibitors. Unlike ACE inhibitors, they don't stop production of the chemical ACE inhibitors target, but they block its effects on the heart and blood vessels. ARBs do not cause cough, but can also result in excess potassium in the bloodstream and kidney problems.

### Beta Blockers

These drugs slow the heart rate, reduce the effects of adrenaline on the heart and blood vessels, and prevent changes in the shape of the heart tissue, called remodeling. They substantially improve overall heart function. Side effects can include excessively slow heart rate, fatigue, wheezing, and occasionally initial worsening of heart failure.

## *Digitalis*

This medication increases the force of the heart's contractions. It also slows certain fast heart rhythms. As a result, the heart beats less frequently but more effectively, and more blood is pumped into the arteries. Side effects may include nausea, vomiting, loss of appetite, diarrhea, confusion, and new heartbeat irregularities.

## *Diuretics*

These medications decrease the body's retention of salt and so of water. Diuretics are commonly prescribed to reduce high blood pressure. Diuretics come in many types, with different periods of effectiveness. Side effects may include loss of too much potassium, weakness, muscle cramps, joint pains, and impotence.

## *Spironolactone*

This drug blocks the effects of a chemical called aldosterone, which is produced in abnormally high levels in patients with heart failure. High levels of aldosterone cause heart failure to worsen; by blocking this chemical, spironolactone improves heart failure. Side effects can include high levels of potassium in the blood, breast soreness or enlargement, and impotence.

## *Hydralazine*

This drug widens blood vessels, easing blood flow. Side effects may include headaches, rapid heartbeat, and joint pain.

## *Nitrates*

These drugs are used mostly for chest pain, but may also help diminish heart failure symptoms. They relax smooth muscle and widen blood vessels. They act to lower primarily systolic blood pressure. Side effects may include headaches.

## Can a Person Live with Heart Failure?

Heart failure is one of the most serious symptoms of heart disease. About two-thirds of all patients die within five years of diagnosis. However, some live beyond five years, even into old age. The outlook for an individual patient depends on the patient's age, severity of heart failure, overall health, and a number of other factors.

As heart failure progresses, the effects can become quite severe, and patients often lose the ability to perform even modest physical activity. Eventually, the heart's reduced pumping capacity may interfere with routine functions, and patients may become unable to care for themselves. The loss in functional ability can occur quickly if the heart is further weakened by heart attacks or the worsening of other conditions that affect heart failure, such as diabetes and coronary heart disease.

Heart failure patients also have an increased risk of sudden death, or cardiac arrest, caused by an irregular heartbeat.

To improve the chances of surviving with heart failure, patients must take care of themselves. Patients must:

- See their physician regularly
- Closely follow all of their physician's instructions
- Take any medication according to instructions
- Immediately inform their physician of any significant change in their condition, such as an intensified shortness of breath or swollen feet.

Patients with heart failure also should:

- Control their weight
- Watch what they eat
- Not smoke cigarettes or use other tobacco products
- Abstain from or strictly limit alcohol consumption

Even with the best care, heart failure can worsen, but patients who don't take care of themselves are almost writing themselves a prescription for poor health.

The best defense against heart failure is the prevention of heart disease. Almost all of the major coronary risk factors can be controlled or eliminated: smoking, high cholesterol, high blood pressure, diabetes, and obesity.

# Chapter 3

# *Cancer*

## *Chapter Contents*

# Section 3.1

## *Cancer: What Is It?*

Reprinted from "What You Need to Know™ About Cancer—An Overview," National Cancer Institute, updated September 16, 2002, http://www.nci. nih.gov/templates/page_print.aspx?viewid=1a5e47ea-8cdd-4efb-b05c-2988190a8b43. Also available in hard copy as NIH Pub. No. 00-1566 via https://cissecure.nci.nih.gov/ncipubs/.

### *What Is Cancer?*

Cancer is a group of many related diseases that begin in cells, the body's basic unit of life. To understand cancer, it is helpful to know what happens when normal cells become cancerous.

The body is made up of many types of cells. Normally, cells grow and divide to produce more cells only when the body needs them. This orderly process helps keep the body healthy. Sometimes, however, cells keep dividing when new cells are not needed. These extra cells form a mass of tissue, called a growth or tumor.

Tumors can be benign or malignant:

- *Benign tumors are not cancer*. They can often be removed and, in most cases, they do not come back. Cells from benign tumors do not spread to other parts of the body. Most important, benign tumors are rarely a threat to life.

- *Malignant tumors are cancer*. Cells in these tumors are abnormal and divide without control or order. They can invade and damage nearby tissues and organs. Also, cancer cells can break away from a malignant tumor and enter the bloodstream or the lymphatic system. That is how cancer spreads from the original cancer site to form new tumors in other organs. The spread of cancer is called metastasis.

Leukemia and lymphoma are cancers that arise in blood-forming cells. The abnormal cells circulate in the bloodstream and lymphatic system. They may also invade (infiltrate) body organs and form tumors.

Most cancers are named for the organ or type of cell in which they begin. For example, cancer that begins in the lung is lung cancer, and cancer that begins in cells in the skin known as melanocytes is called melanoma.

When cancer spreads (metastasizes), cancer cells are often found in nearby or regional lymph nodes (sometimes called lymph glands). If the cancer has reached these nodes, it means that cancer cells may have spread to other organs, such as the liver, bones, or brain. When cancer spreads from its original location to another part of the body, the new tumor has the same kind of abnormal cells and the same name as the primary tumor. For example, if lung cancer spreads to the brain, the cancer cells in the brain are actually lung cancer cells. The disease is called metastatic lung cancer (it is not brain cancer).

## Possible Causes and Prevention of Cancer

The more we can learn about what causes cancer, the more likely we are to find ways to prevent it. In the laboratory, scientists explore possible causes of cancer and try to determine exactly what happens in cells when they become cancerous. Researchers also study patterns of cancer in the population to look for risk factors, conditions that increase the chance that cancer might occur. They also look for protective factors, things that decrease the risk.

Even though doctors can seldom explain why one person gets cancer and another does not, it is clear that cancer is not caused by an injury, such as a bump or bruise. And although being infected with certain viruses may increase the risk of some types of cancer, cancer is not contagious; no one can "catch" cancer from another person.

Cancer develops over time. It is a result of a complex mix of factors related to life-style, heredity, and environment. A number of factors that increase a person's chance of developing cancer have been identified. Many types of cancer are related to the use of tobacco, what people eat and drink, exposure to ultraviolet (UV) radiation from the sun, and, to a lesser extent, exposure to cancer-causing agents (carcinogens) in the environment and the workplace. Some people are more sensitive than others to factors that can cause cancer.

Still, most people who get cancer have none of the known risk factors. And most people who do have risk factors do not get the disease.

Some cancer risk factors can be avoided. Others, such as inherited factors, are unavoidable, but it may be helpful to be aware of them. People can help protect themselves by avoiding known risk factors whenever possible. They can also talk with their doctor about regular checkups and about whether cancer screening tests could be of benefit.

These are some of the factors that increase the likelihood of cancer.

### Tobacco

Smoking tobacco, using smokeless tobacco, and being regularly exposed to environmental tobacco smoke are responsible for one-third of all cancer deaths in the United States each year. Tobacco use is the most preventable cause of death in this country.

Smoking accounts for more than 85 percent of all lung cancer deaths. For smokers, the risk of getting lung cancer increases with the amount of tobacco smoked each day, the number of years they have smoked, the type of tobacco product, and how deeply they inhale. Overall, for those who smoke one pack a day, the chance of getting lung cancer is about 10 times greater than for nonsmokers. Cigarette smokers are also more likely than nonsmokers to develop several other types of cancer, including oral cancer and cancers of the larynx, esophagus, pancreas, bladder, kidney, and cervix. Smoking may also increase the likelihood of developing cancers of the stomach, liver, prostate, colon, and rectum. The risk of cancer begins to decrease soon after a smoker quits, and the risk continues to decline gradually each year after quitting.

People who smoke cigars or pipes have a risk for cancers of the oral cavity that is similar to the risk for people who smoke cigarettes. Cigar smokers also have an increased chance of developing cancers of the lung, larynx, esophagus, and pancreas.

The use of smokeless tobacco (chewing tobacco and snuff) causes cancer of the mouth and throat. Precancerous conditions, tissue changes that may lead to cancer, often begin to go away after a person stops using smokeless tobacco.

Studies suggest that exposure to environmental tobacco smoke, also called second-hand smoke, increases the risk of lung cancer for nonsmokers.

People who use tobacco in any form and need help quitting may want to talk with their doctor, dentist, or other health professional, or join a smoking cessation group sponsored by a local hospital or voluntary organization. Information about finding such groups or programs is available from the Cancer Information Service (CIS) at (800) 4-CANCER. CIS information specialists can send printed materials, and also can give suggestions about quitting that are tailored to a caller's needs.

## *Diet*

Researchers are exploring how dietary factors play a role in the development of cancer. Some evidence suggests a link between a high-fat diet and certain cancers, such as cancers of the colon, uterus, and prostate. Being seriously overweight may be linked to breast cancer among older women and to cancers of the prostate, pancreas, uterus, colon, and ovary. On the other hand, some studies suggest that foods containing fiber and certain nutrients may help protect against some types of cancer.

People may be able to reduce their cancer risk by making healthy food choices. A well-balanced diet includes generous amounts of foods that are high in fiber, vitamins, and minerals, and low in fat. This includes eating lots of fruits and vegetables and more whole-grain breads and cereals every day, fewer eggs, and not as much high-fat meat, high-fat dairy products (such as whole milk, butter, and most cheeses), salad dressing, margarine, and cooking oil.

Most scientists think that making healthy food choices is more beneficial than taking vitamin and mineral supplements.

## *Ultraviolet (UV) Radiation*

UV radiation from the sun causes premature aging of the skin and skin damage that can lead to skin cancer. Artificial sources of UV radiation, such as sunlamps and tanning booths, also can cause skin damage and probably an increased risk of skin cancer.

To help reduce the risk of skin cancer caused by UV radiation, it is best to reduce exposure to the midday sun (from 10 a.m. to 3 p.m.). Another simple rule is to avoid the sun when your shadow is shorter than you are.

Wearing a broad-brimmed hat, UV-absorbing sunglasses, long pants, and long sleeves offers protection. Many doctors believe that in addition to avoiding the sun and wearing protective clothing, wearing a sunscreen (especially one that reflects, absorbs, and/or scatters both types of ultraviolet radiation) may help prevent some forms of skin cancer. Sunscreens are rated in strength according to a sun protection factor (SPF). The higher the SPF, the more sunburn protection is provided. Sunscreens with an SPF of 12 through 29 are adequate for most people, but sunscreens are not a substitute for avoiding the sun and wearing protective clothing.

## Alcohol

Heavy drinkers have an increased risk of cancers of the mouth, throat, esophagus, larynx, and liver. (People who smoke cigarettes and drink heavily have an especially high risk of getting these cancers.) Some studies suggest that even moderate drinking may slightly increase the risk of breast cancer.

## Ionizing Radiation

Cells may be damaged by ionizing radiation from x-ray procedures, radioactive substances, rays that enter the earth's atmosphere from outer space, and other sources. In very high doses, ionizing radiation may cause cancer and other diseases. Studies of survivors of the atomic bomb in Japan show that ionizing radiation increases the risk of developing leukemia and cancers of the breast, thyroid, lung, stomach, and other organs.

Before 1950, x-rays were used to treat noncancerous conditions (such as an enlarged thymus, enlarged tonsils and adenoids, ringworm of the scalp, and acne) in children and young adults. Those who have received radiation therapy to the head and neck have a higher-than-average risk of developing thyroid cancer years later. People with a history of such treatments should report it to their doctor.

Radiation that patients receive as therapy for cancer can also damage normal cells. Patients may want to talk with their doctor about the effect of radiation treatment on their risk of a second cancer. This risk can depend on the patient's age at the time of treatment as well as on the part of the body that was treated.

X-rays used for diagnosis expose people to lower levels of radiation than x-rays used for therapy. The benefits nearly always outweigh the risks. However, repeated exposure could be harmful, so it is a good idea for people to talk with their doctor about the need for each x-ray and to ask about the use of shields to protect other parts of the body.

## Chemicals and Other Substances

Being exposed to substances such as certain chemicals, metals, or pesticides can increase the risk of cancer. Asbestos, nickel, cadmium, uranium, radon, vinyl chloride, benzidine, and benzene are examples of well-known carcinogens. These may act alone or along with another carcinogen, such as cigarette smoke, to increase the risk of cancer. For example, inhaling asbestos fibers increases the risk of lung diseases, including cancer, and the cancer risk is especially high for asbestos workers who smoke. It is important to follow work and safety rules to avoid or minimize contact with dangerous materials.

### Diethylstilbestrol (DES)

DES is a synthetic form of estrogen that was used between the early 1940s and 1971. Some women took DES during pregnancy to prevent certain complications. There is evidence that DES-exposed sons may have testicular abnormalities, such as undescended or abnormally small testicles. The possible risk for testicular cancer in these men is under study.

### Close Relatives with Certain Types of Cancer

Some types of cancer (including melanoma and cancers of the breast, ovary, prostate, and colon) tend to occur more often in some families than in the rest of the population. It is often unclear whether a pattern of cancer in a family is primarily due to heredity, factors in the family's environment or life-style, or just a matter of chance.

Researchers have learned that cancer is caused by changes (called mutations or alterations) in genes that control normal cell growth and cell death. Most cancer-causing gene changes are the result of factors in life-style or the environment. However, some alterations that may lead to cancer are inherited; that is, they are passed from parent to child. But having such an inherited gene alteration does not mean that the person is certain to develop cancer; it means that the risk of cancer is increased.

## Screening and Early Detection

Sometimes, cancer can be found before the disease causes symptoms. Checking for cancer (or for conditions that may lead to cancer) in a person who does not have any symptoms of the disease is called screening.

In routine physical exams, the doctor looks for anything unusual and feels for any lumps or growths. Specific screening tests, such as lab tests, x-rays, or other procedures, are used routinely for only a few types of cancer, such as prostate and colorectal.

Although it is not certain that screening for other cancers actually saves lives, doctors also may suggest screening for cancers of the skin, lung, and oral cavity. And doctors may offer to screen men for prostate or testicular cancer, and women for ovarian cancer.

Doctors consider many factors before recommending a screening test. They weigh factors related to the individual, the test, and the cancer that the test is intended to detect. For example, doctors take into account the person's age, medical history and general health, family history, and life-style. The doctor pays special attention to a person's risk for developing specific types of cancer. In addition, the doctor will assess the accuracy and the risks of the screening test and any follow-up tests that may be necessary. Doctors also consider the effectiveness and side effects of the treatment that will be needed if cancer is found.

People may want to discuss any concerns or questions they have about screening with their doctors, so they can weigh the pros and cons and make informed decisions about having screening tests.

## Symptoms of Cancer

Cancer can cause a variety of symptoms:

- Thickening or lump in any part of the body
- Obvious change in a wart or mole
- A sore that does not heal
- Nagging cough or hoarseness
- Changes in bowel or bladder habits
- Indigestion or difficulty swallowing
- Unexplained changes in weight
- Unusual bleeding or discharge

When these or other symptoms occur, they are not always caused by cancer. They may also be caused by infections, benign tumors, or other problems. It is important to see the doctor about any of these symptoms or about other physical changes. Only a doctor can make a diagnosis. One should not wait to feel pain: Early cancer usually does not cause pain.

## Diagnosis

If symptoms are present, the doctor asks about the person's medical history and performs a physical exam. In addition to checking general signs of health, the doctor may order various tests and exams. These may include laboratory tests and imaging procedures. A biopsy is usually necessary to determine whether cancer is present.

## *Laboratory Tests*

Blood and urine tests can give the doctor important information about a person's health. In some cases, special tests are used to measure the amount of certain substances, called tumor markers, in the blood, urine, or certain tissues. Tumor marker levels may be abnormal if certain types of cancer are present. However, lab tests alone cannot be used to diagnose cancer.

## *Imaging*

Images (pictures) of areas inside the body help the doctor see whether a tumor is present. These pictures can be made in several ways.

X-rays are the most common way to view organs and bones inside the body. A computed tomography (CT or CAT) scan is a special kind of imaging that uses a computer linked to an x-ray machine to make a series of pictures.

In radionuclide scanning, the patient swallows or receives an injection of a radioactive substance. A machine (scanner) measures radioactivity levels in certain organs and prints a picture on paper or film. The doctor can detect abnormal areas by looking at the amount of radioactivity in the organs. The radioactive substance is quickly eliminated by the patient's body after the test is done.

Ultrasonography is another procedure for viewing areas inside the body. High-frequency sound waves that cannot be heard by humans enter the body and bounce back. Their echoes produce a picture called a sonogram. These pictures are shown on a monitor like a TV screen and can be printed on paper.

In MRI, a powerful magnet linked to a computer is used to make detailed pictures of areas in the body. These pictures are viewed on a monitor and can also be printed.

## *Biopsy*

A biopsy is almost always necessary to help the doctor make a diagnosis of cancer. In a biopsy, tissue is removed for examination under a microscope by a pathologist. Tissue may be removed in three ways: endoscopy, needle biopsy, or surgical biopsy.

- During an *endoscopy*, the doctor can look at areas inside the body through a thin, lighted tube. Endoscopy allows the doctor to see what's going on inside the body, take pictures, and remove tissue or cells for examination, if necessary.

- In a *needle biopsy*, the doctor takes a small tissue sample by inserting a needle into the abnormal (suspicious) area.

- A *surgical biopsy* may be excisional or incisional. In an excisional biopsy, the surgeon removes the entire tumor, often with some surrounding normal tissue. In an incisional biopsy, the doctor removes just a portion of the tumor. If cancer is present, the entire tumor may be removed immediately or during another operation.

Patients sometimes worry that having a biopsy (or any other type of surgery for cancer) will spread the disease. This is a very rare occurrence. Surgeons use special techniques and take many precautions to prevent cancer from spreading during surgery. For example, if tissue samples must be removed from more than one site, they use different instruments for each one. Also, a margin of normal tissue is often removed along with the tumor. Such efforts reduce the chance that cancer cells will spread into healthy tissue.

Some people may be concerned that exposing cancer to air during surgery will cause the disease to spread. This is not true. Exposure to air does not cause the cancer to spread.

Patients should discuss their concerns about the biopsy or other surgery with their doctor.

### Staging

When cancer is diagnosed, the doctor will want to learn the stage, or extent, of the disease. Staging is a careful attempt to find out whether the cancer has spread and, if so, to which parts of the body. Treatment decisions depend on the results of staging. The doctor may order more laboratory tests and imaging studies or additional biopsies to find out whether the cancer has spread. An operation called a laparotomy can help the doctor find out whether cancer has spread within the abdomen. During this operation, a surgeon makes an incision into the abdomen and removes samples of tissue.

## Handling the Diagnosis

It is natural for anyone facing cancer to be concerned about what the future holds. Understanding the nature of cancer and what to expect can help patients and their loved ones plan treatment, anticipate life-style changes, and make financial decisions. Cancer patients frequently ask their doctor or search on their own for statistics to answer the question, "What is my prognosis?"

Prognosis is a prediction of the future course and outcome of a disease, and an indication of the likelihood of recovery from that disease. However, it is only a prediction. When doctors discuss a patient's prognosis, they are attempting to project what is likely to occur for that individual patient. A cancer patient's prognosis can be affected by many factors, particularly the type of cancer, the stage of the disease, and its grade (how closely the cancer resembles normal tissue and how fast the cancer is likely to grow and spread). Other factors that may also affect the prognosis include the patient's age, general health, and response to treatment. As these factors change over time, a patient's prognosis is also likely to change.

Sometimes people use statistics to try to figure out their chances of being cured. However, for individual patients and their families, statistics are seldom helpful because they reflect the experience of a large group of patients. Statistics cannot predict what will happen to a particular patient because no two patients are alike; treatment and responses vary greatly.

If people want prognostic information, they should talk with the doctor. The doctor who is most familiar with a person's situation is in the best position to help interpret statistics and discuss prognosis. But even the doctor may not be able to describe exactly what to expect.

Seeking information about prognosis and statistics can help some people reduce their fears. How much information to seek and how to deal with it are personal matters.

## Treatment

Treatment for cancer depends on the type of cancer; the size, location, and stage of the disease; the person's general health; and other factors. The doctor develops a treatment plan to fit each person's situation.

People with cancer are often treated by a team of specialists, which may include a surgeon, radiation oncologist, medical oncologist, and others. Most cancers are treated with surgery, radiation therapy, chemotherapy, hormone therapy, or biological therapy. The doctors may decide to use one treatment method or a combination of methods.

Clinical trials (research studies) offer important treatment options for many people with cancer. Research studies evaluate promising new therapies and answer scientific questions. The goal of such trials is to find treatments that are more effective in controlling cancer with fewer side effects.

## *Getting a Second Opinion*

Before starting treatment, the patient may want to have a second opinion from another doctor about the diagnosis and the treatment plan. Some insurance companies require a second opinion; others may cover a second opinion if the patient requests it.

There are a number of ways to find a doctor who can give a second opinion:

- The patient's doctor may be able to suggest specialists to consult.

- The Cancer Information Service, at (800) 4-CANCER, can tell callers about cancer treatment facilities all over the country, including cancer centers and other programs supported by the National Cancer Institute.

- Patients can get the names of doctors from their local medical society, a nearby hospital, or a medical school.

- The *Official ABMS Directory of Board-Certified Medical Specialists* lists doctors names along with their specialty and their educational background. This resource, produced by the American Board of Medical Specialties (ABMS), is available in most public libraries. The ABMS also provides an online service to help people locate doctors (http://www.certifieddoctor.org).

## *Methods of Treatment and Their Side Effects*

Treatment for cancer can be either local or systemic. Local treatments affect cancer cells in the tumor and the area near it. Systemic treatments travel through the bloodstream, reaching cancer cells all over the body. Surgery and radiation therapy are types of local treatment. Chemotherapy, hormone therapy, and biological therapy are examples of systemic treatment.

It is hard to protect healthy cells from the harmful effects of cancer treatment. Because treatment does damage healthy cells and tissues, it often causes side effects. The side effects of cancer treatment depend mainly on the type and extent of the treatment. Also, the effects may not be the same for each person, and they may change for a person from one treatment to the next. A patient's reaction to treatment is closely monitored by physical exams, blood tests, and other tests. Doctors and nurses can explain the possible side effects of treatment, and they can suggest ways to reduce or eliminate problems that may occur during and after treatment.

**Surgery.** Surgery is therapy to remove the cancer; the surgeon may also remove some of the surrounding tissue and lymph nodes near the tumor. Sometimes surgery is done on an outpatient basis, or the patient may have to stay in the hospital. This decision depends mainly on the type of surgery and the type of anesthesia.

**Radiation therapy.** Radiation therapy (also called radiotherapy) uses high-energy rays to kill cancer cells. For some types of cancer, radiation therapy may be used instead of surgery as the primary treatment. Radiation therapy also may be given before surgery (neoadjuvant therapy) to shrink a tumor so that it is easier to remove. In other cases, radiation therapy is given after surgery (adjuvant therapy) to destroy any cancer cells that may remain in the area. Radiation also may be used alone, or along with other types of treatment, to relieve pain or other problems if the tumor cannot be removed.

Radiation therapy can be in either of two forms: external or internal. Some patients receive both.

External radiation comes from a machine that aims the rays at a specific area of the body. Most often, this treatment is given on an outpatient basis in a hospital or clinic. There is no radioactivity left in the body after the treatment.

With internal radiation (also called implant radiation, interstitial radiation, or brachytherapy), the radiation comes from radioactive material that is sealed in needles, seeds, wires, or catheters and placed directly in or near the tumor. Patients may stay in the hospital while the level of radiation is highest. They may not be able to have visitors during the hospital stay or may have visitors for only a short time. The implant may be permanent or temporary. The amount of radiation in a permanent implant goes down to a safe level before the person leaves the hospital. The doctor will advise the patient if any special precautions should be taken at home. With a temporary implant, there is no radioactivity left in the body after the implant is removed.

The National Cancer Institute booklet *Radiation Therapy and You* has helpful information about radiation therapy and managing its side effects.

**Chemotherapy.** Chemotherapy is the use of drugs to kill cancer cells. The doctor may use one drug or a combination of drugs. Chemotherapy may be the only kind of treatment a patient needs, or it may be combined with other forms of treatment. Neoadjuvant chemotherapy refers to drugs given before surgery to shrink a tumor;

adjuvant chemotherapy refers to drugs given after surgery to help prevent the cancer from recurring. Chemotherapy also may be used (alone or along with other forms of treatment) to relieve symptoms of the disease.

Chemotherapy is usually given in cycles: a treatment period (one or more days when treatment is given) followed by a recovery period (several days or weeks), then another treatment period, and so on. Most anticancer drugs are given by injection into a vein (IV); some are injected into a muscle or under the skin; and some are given by mouth.

The side effects of chemotherapy depend mainly on the drugs and the doses the patient receives. As with other types of treatment, side effects vary from person to person. Generally, anticancer drugs affect cells that divide rapidly. In addition to cancer cells, these include blood cells, which fight infection, help the blood to clot, and carry oxygen to all parts of the body. When blood cells are affected, patients are more likely to get infections, may bruise or bleed easily, and may feel unusually weak and very tired. Rapidly dividing cells in hair roots and cells that line the digestive tract may also be affected. As a result, side effects may include loss of hair, poor appetite, nausea and vomiting, diarrhea, or mouth and lip sores.

Hair loss is a major concern for many people with cancer. Some anticancer drugs only cause the hair to thin, while others may result in the loss of all body hair. Patients may cope better if they prepare for hair loss before starting treatment (for example, by buying a wig or hat). Most side effects go away gradually during the recovery periods between treatments, and hair grows back after treatment is over.

Some anticancer drugs can cause long-term side effects such as loss of fertility (the ability to produce children). Loss of fertility may be temporary or permanent, depending on the drugs used and the patient's age and sex. For men, sperm banking before treatment may be an option.

**Other treatments.** Hormone therapy is used against certain cancers that depend on hormones for their growth. Hormone therapy keeps cancer cells from getting or using the hormones they need. This treatment may include the use of drugs that stop the production of certain hormones or that change the way they work. Another type of hormone therapy is surgery to remove organs, such as the testicles, that make hormones.

Biological therapy (also called immunotherapy) helps the body's natural ability (immune system) to fight disease or protects the body from some of the side effects of cancer treatment. Monoclonal antibodies, interferon, interleukin-2, and colony-stimulating factors are some types of biological therapy.

Bone marrow transplantation (BMT) or peripheral stem cell transplantation (PSCT) may also be used in cancer treatment. The transplant may be autologous (the person's own cells that were saved earlier), allogeneic (cells donated by another person), or syngeneic (cells donated by an identical twin). Both BMT and PSCT provide the patient with healthy stem cells (very immature cells that mature into blood cells). These replace stem cells that have been damaged or destroyed by very high doses of chemotherapy and/or radiation treatment.

### Nutrition during Cancer Treatment

Eating well during cancer treatment means getting enough calories and protein to help prevent weight loss and maintain strength. Eating well often helps people feel better and have more energy.

Some people with cancer find it hard to eat because they lose their appetite. In addition, common side effects of treatment, such as nausea, vomiting, or mouth and lip sores, can make eating difficult. Often, foods taste different. Also, people being treated for cancer may not feel like eating when they are uncomfortable or tired.

Doctors, nurses, and dietitians can offer advice on how to get enough calories and protein during cancer treatment. Patients and their families can find many useful tips in the National Cancer Institute booklet *Eating Hints for Cancer Patients*.

### Pain Control

Pain is a common problem for people with some types of cancer, especially when the cancer grows and presses against other organs and nerves. Pain may also be a side effect of treatment. However, pain can generally be relieved or reduced with prescription medicines or over-the-counter drugs as recommended by the doctor. Other ways to reduce pain, such as relaxation exercises, may also be useful. It is important for patients to report pain so that steps can be taken to help relieve it.

### Rehabilitation

Rehabilitation is an important part of the overall cancer treatment process. The goal of rehabilitation is to improve a person's quality of life. The medical team, which may include doctors, nurses, a physical therapist, an occupational therapist, or a social worker, develops a rehabilitation plan to meet each patient's physical and emotional needs, helping the patient return to normal activities as soon as possible.

Patients and their families may need to work with an occupational therapist to overcome any difficulty in eating, dressing, bathing, using the toilet, or other activities. Physical therapy may be needed to regain strength in muscles and to prevent stiffness and swelling. Physical therapy may also be necessary if an arm or leg is weak or paralyzed, or if a patient has trouble with balance.

## *Follow-up Care*

It is important for people who have had cancer to continue to have examinations regularly after their treatment is over. Follow-up care ensures that any changes in health are identified, and if the cancer recurs, it can be treated as soon as possible. Checkups may include a careful physical exam, imaging procedures, endoscopy, or lab tests.

Between scheduled appointments, people who have had cancer should report any health problems to their doctor as soon as they appear.

# Section 3.2

# *Lung Cancer*

Adapted from "What You Need To Know About™ Lung Cancer," National Cancer Institute, updated September 16, 2002, http://www.nci.nih.gov/templates/page_print.aspx?viewid=4b129348-f3ec-4c30-9c65-b34255667eb1. Also available in hard copy as NIH Pub. No. 99-1553 via https://cissecure.nci.nih.gov/ncipubs/.

The diagnosis of lung cancer brings with it many questions and a need for clear, understandable answers. This chapter provides information about some causes and ways to prevent lung cancer, and it describes the symptoms, detection, diagnosis, and treatment of this disease. Having this important information can make it easier for patients and their families to handle the challenges they face.

Cancer research has led to progress against lung cancer—and our knowledge is increasing. Researchers continue to look for better ways to prevent, detect, diagnose, and treat lung cancer.

## The Lungs

The lungs, a pair of sponge-like, cone-shaped organs, are part of the respiratory system (see Figure 3.1). The right lung has three sections, called lobes; it is a little larger than the left lung, which has two lobes. When we breathe in, the lungs take in oxygen, which our cells need to live and carry out their normal functions. When we breathe out, the lungs get rid of carbon dioxide, which is a waste product of the body's cells.

## Understanding Lung Cancer

Cancers that begin in the lungs are divided into two major types, non–small-cell lung cancer and small-cell lung cancer, depending on how the cells look under a microscope. Each type of lung cancer grows and spreads in different ways and is treated differently.

Non–small-cell lung cancer is more common than small-cell lung cancer, and it generally grows and spreads more slowly. There are

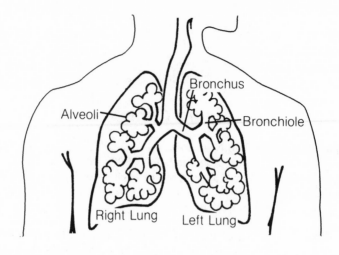

*Figure 3.1. The lungs.*

three main types of non–small-cell lung cancer. They are named for the type of cells in which the cancer develops: squamous cell carcinoma (also called epidermoid carcinoma), adenocarcinoma, and large-cell carcinoma.

Small-cell lung cancer, sometimes called oat cell cancer, is less common than non–small-cell lung cancer. This type of lung cancer grows more quickly and is more likely to spread to other organs in the body.

## Lung Cancer: Who's at Risk?

Researchers have discovered several causes of lung cancer; most are related to the use of tobacco.

### Cigarettes

Smoking cigarettes causes lung cancer. Harmful substances, called carcinogens, in tobacco damage the cells in the lungs. Over time, the damaged cells may become cancerous. The likelihood that a smoker will develop lung cancer is affected by the age at which smoking began, how long the person has smoked, the number of cigarettes smoked per day, and how deeply the smoker inhales. Stopping smoking greatly reduces a person's risk for developing lung cancer.

## Cigars and Pipes

Cigar and pipe smokers have a higher risk of lung cancer than nonsmokers. The number of years a person smokes, the number of pipes or cigars smoked per day, and how deeply the person inhales all affect the risk of developing lung cancer. Even cigar and pipe smokers who do not inhale are at increased risk for lung, mouth, and other types of cancer.

## Environmental Tobacco Smoke

The chance of developing lung cancer is increased by exposure to environmental tobacco smoke (ETS)—the smoke in the air when someone else smokes. Exposure to ETS, or second-hand smoke, is called involuntary or passive smoking.

## Radon

Radon is an invisible, odorless, and tasteless radioactive gas that occurs naturally in soil and rocks. It can cause damage to the lungs that may lead to lung cancer. People who work in mines may be exposed to radon, and, in some parts of the country, radon is found in houses. Smoking increases the risk of lung cancer even more for those already at risk because of exposure to radon. A kit available at most hardware stores allows homeowners to measure radon levels in their homes. The home radon test is relatively easy to use and inexpensive. Once a radon problem is corrected, the hazard is gone for good.

## Asbestos

Asbestos is the name of a group of minerals that occur naturally as fibers and are used in certain industries. Asbestos fibers tend to break easily into particles that can float in the air and stick to clothes. When the particles are inhaled, they can lodge in the lungs, damaging cells and increasing the risk for lung cancer. Studies have shown that workers who have been exposed to large amounts of asbestos have a risk of developing lung cancer that is three to four times greater than that for workers who have not been exposed to asbestos. This exposure has been observed in such industries as shipbuilding, asbestos mining and manufacturing, insulation work, and brake repair. The risk of lung cancer is even higher among asbestos workers who also smoke. Asbestos workers should use the protective equipment provided by their employers and follow recommended work practices and safety procedures.

## *Pollution*

Researchers have found a link between lung cancer and exposure to certain air pollutants, such as by-products of the combustion of diesel and other fossil fuels. However, this relationship has not been clearly defined, and more research is being done.

## *Lung Diseases*

Certain lung diseases, such as tuberculosis (TB), increase a person's chance of developing lung cancer. Lung cancer tends to develop in areas of the lung that are scarred from TB.

## *Personal History*

A person who has had lung cancer once is more likely to develop a second lung cancer compared with a person who has never had lung cancer. Quitting smoking after lung cancer is diagnosed may prevent the development of a second lung cancer.

Researchers continue to study the causes of lung cancer and to search for ways to prevent it. We already know that the best way to prevent lung cancer is to quit (or never start) smoking. The sooner a person quits smoking the better. Even if you have been smoking for many years, it's never too late to benefit from quitting.

The best way to prevent lung cancer is to quit, or never start, smoking.

## Recognizing Symptoms

Common signs and symptoms of lung cancer include:

- A cough that doesn't go away and gets worse over time
- Constant chest pain
- Coughing up blood
- Shortness of breath, wheezing, or hoarseness
- Repeated problems with pneumonia or bronchitis
- Swelling of the neck and face
- Loss of appetite or weight loss
- Fatigue

These symptoms may be caused by lung cancer or by other conditions. It is important to check with a doctor.

## Diagnosing Lung Cancer

To help find the cause of symptoms, the doctor evaluates a person's medical history, smoking history, exposure to environmental and occupational substances, and family history of cancer. The doctor also performs a physical exam and may order a chest x-ray and other tests. If lung cancer is suspected, sputum cytology (the microscopic examination of cells obtained from a deep-cough sample of mucus in the lungs) is a simple test that may be useful in detecting lung cancer. To confirm the presence of lung cancer, the doctor must examine tissue from the lung. A biopsy—the removal of a small sample of tissue for examination under a microscope by a pathologist—can show whether a person has cancer. A number of procedures may be used to obtain this tissue:

- *Bronchoscopy.* The doctor puts a bronchoscope (a thin, lighted tube) into the mouth or nose and down through the windpipe to look into the breathing passages. Through this tube, the doctor can collect cells or small samples of tissue.

- *Needle aspiration.* A needle is inserted through the chest into the tumor to remove a sample of tissue.

- *Thoracentesis.* Using a needle, the doctor removes a sample of the fluid that surrounds the lungs to check for cancer cells.

- *Thoracotomy.* Surgery to open the chest is sometimes needed to diagnose lung cancer. This procedure is a major operation performed in a hospital.

## Staging the Disease

If the diagnosis is cancer, the doctor will want to learn the stage (or extent) of the disease. Staging is done to find out whether the cancer has spread and, if so, to what parts of the body. Lung cancer often spreads to the brain or bones. Knowing the stage of the disease helps the doctor plan treatment. Some tests used to determine whether the cancer has spread include:

- *CAT (or CT) scan (computed tomography).* A computer linked to an x-ray machine creates a series of detailed pictures of areas inside the body.

- *MRI (magnetic resonance imaging).* A powerful magnet linked to a computer makes detailed pictures of areas inside the body.

- *Radionuclide scanning.* Scanning can show whether cancer has spread to other organs, such as the liver. The patient swallows or receives an injection of a mildly radioactive substance. A machine (scanner) measures and records the level of radioactivity in certain organs to reveal abnormal areas.

- *Bone scan.* A bone scan, one type of radionuclide scanning, can show whether cancer has spread to the bones. A small amount of radioactive substance is injected into a vein. It travels through the bloodstream and collects in areas of abnormal bone growth. An instrument called a scanner measures the radioactivity levels in these areas and records them on x-ray film.

- *Mediastinoscopy or mediastinotomy.* A mediastinoscopy can help show whether the cancer has spread to the lymph nodes in the chest. Using a lighted viewing instrument, called a scope, the doctor examines the center of the chest (mediastinum) and nearby lymph nodes. In mediastinoscopy, the scope is inserted through a small incision in the neck; in mediastinotomy, the incision is made in the chest. In either procedure, the scope is also used to remove a tissue sample. The patient receives a general anesthetic.

## Treatment for Lung Cancer

Treatment depends on a number of factors, including the type of lung cancer (non–small- or small-cell lung cancer), the size, location, and extent of the tumor, and the general health of the patient. Many different treatments and combinations of treatments may be used to control lung cancer, and/or to improve quality of life by reducing symptoms.

- *Surgery* is an operation to remove the cancer. The type of surgery a doctor performs depends on the location of the tumor in the lung. An operation to remove only a small part of the lung is called a segmental or wedge resection. When the surgeon removes an entire lobe of the lung, the procedure is called a lobectomy. Pneumonectomy is the removal of an entire lung. Some tumors are inoperable (cannot be removed by surgery) because of the size or location, and some patients cannot have surgery for other medical reasons.

- *Chemotherapy* is the use of anticancer drugs to kill cancer cells throughout the body. Even after cancer has been removed from the lung, cancer cells may still be present in nearby tissue or elsewhere in the body. Chemotherapy may be used to control cancer growth or to relieve symptoms. Most anticancer drugs are given by injection directly into a vein (IV) or by means of a catheter, a thin tube that is placed into a large vein and remains there as long as it is needed. Some anticancer drugs are given in the form of a pill.

- *Radiation therapy*, also called radiotherapy, involves the use of high-energy rays to kill cancer cells. Radiation therapy is directed to a limited area and affects the cancer cells only in that area. Radiation therapy may be used before surgery to shrink a tumor, or after surgery to destroy any cancer cells that remain in the treated area. Doctors also use radiation therapy, often combined with chemotherapy, as primary treatment instead of surgery. Radiation therapy may also be used to relieve symptoms such as shortness of breath. Radiation for the treatment of lung cancer most often comes from a machine (external radiation). The radiation can also come from an implant (a small container of radioactive material) placed directly into or near the tumor (internal radiation).

- *Photodynamic therapy* (PDT), a type of laser therapy, involves the use of a special chemical that is injected into the bloodstream and absorbed by cells all over the body. The chemical rapidly leaves normal cells but remains in cancer cells for a longer time. A laser light aimed at the cancer activates the chemical, which then kills the cancer cells that have absorbed it. Photodynamic therapy may be used to reduce symptoms of lung cancer—for example, to control bleeding or to relieve breathing problems due to blocked airways when the cancer cannot be removed through surgery. Photodynamic therapy may also be used to treat very small tumors in patients for whom the usual treatments for lung cancer are not appropriate.

Clinical trials (research studies) to evaluate new ways to treat cancer are an option for many lung cancer patients. In some studies, all patients receive the new treatment. In others, doctors compare different therapies by giving the new treatment to one group of patients and the usual (standard) therapy to another group. Through research, doctors are exploring new and possibly more effective ways to treat lung cancer.

## Treating Non–Small-Cell Lung Cancer

Patients with non–small-cell lung cancer may be treated in several ways. The choice of treatment depends mainly on the size, location, and extent of the tumor. Surgery is the most common way to treat this type of lung cancer. Cryosurgery, a treatment that freezes and destroys cancer tissue, may be used to control symptoms in the later stages of non–small-cell lung cancer. Radiation therapy and chemotherapy may also be used to slow the progress of the disease and to manage symptoms.

## Treating Small-Cell Lung Cancer

Small-cell lung cancer spreads quickly. In many cases, cancer cells have already spread to other parts of the body when the disease is diagnosed. In order to reach cancer cells throughout the body, doctors almost always use chemotherapy. Treatment may also include radiation therapy aimed at the tumor in the lung or tumors in other parts of the body (such as in the brain). Some patients have radiation therapy to the brain even though no cancer is found there. This treatment, called prophylactic cranial irradiation (PCI), is given to prevent tumors from forming in the brain. Surgery is part of the treatment plan for a small number of patients with small-cell lung cancer.

## Side Effects

The side effects of cancer treatment depend on the type of treatment and may be different for each person. Side effects are often only temporary. Doctors and nurses can explain the possible side effects of treatment, and they can suggest ways to help relieve symptoms that may occur during and after treatment.

- Surgery for lung cancer is a major operation. After lung surgery, air and fluid tend to collect in the chest. Patients often need help turning over, coughing, and breathing deeply. These activities are important for recovery because they help expand the remaining lung tissue and get rid of excess air and fluid. Pain or weakness in the chest and the arm and shortness of breath are common side effects of lung cancer surgery. Patients may need several weeks or months to regain their energy and strength.

- Chemotherapy affects normal as well as cancerous cells. Side effects depend largely on the specific drugs and the dose (amount of drug given). Common side effects of chemotherapy include nausea and vomiting, hair loss, mouth sores, and fatigue.

- Radiation therapy, like chemotherapy, affects normal as well as cancerous cells. Side effects of radiation therapy depend mainly on the part of the body that is treated and the treatment dose. Common side effects of radiation therapy are a dry, sore throat; difficulty swallowing; fatigue; skin changes at the site of treatment; and loss of appetite. Patients receiving radiation to the brain may have headaches, skin changes, fatigue, nausea and vomiting, hair loss, or problems with memory and thought processes.

- Photodynamic therapy makes the skin and eyes sensitive to light for six weeks or more after treatment. Patients are advised to avoid direct sunlight and bright indoor light for at least six weeks. If patients must go outdoors, they need to wear protective clothing, including sunglasses. Other temporary side effects of PDT may include coughing, trouble swallowing, and painful breathing or shortness of breath. Patients should talk with their doctor about what to do if the skin becomes blistered, red, or swollen.

Today, because of what has been learned in clinical trials, doctors are able to control, lessen, or avoid many of the side effects of treatment.

# Section 3.3

# *Colorectal Cancer*

Adapted from "What You Need To Know About™ Cancer of the Colon and Rectum," National Cancer Institute, updated September 16, 2002, http://www.nci.nih.gov/templates/page_print.aspx?viewid=b5ecd606-69f5-4e0b-87a7-20c8b9d8172d. Also available in hard copy NIH Pub. No. 99-1552 via https://cissecure.nci.nih.gov/ncipubs/.

## *The Colon and Rectum*

The colon and rectum are parts of the body's digestive system (see Figure 3.2), which removes nutrients from food and stores waste until it passes out of the body. Together, the colon and rectum form a long, muscular tube called the large intestine (also called the large

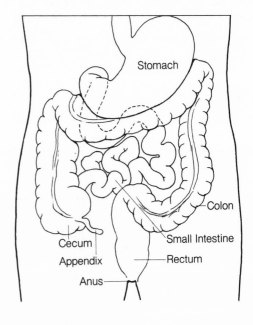

*Figure 3.2.* The colon, rectum, and other parts of the digestive system.

bowel). The colon is the first six feet of the large intestine, and the rectum is the last eight to 10 inches.

## Understanding Colorectal Cancer

Cancer that begins in the colon is called colon cancer, and cancer that begins in the rectum is called rectal cancer. Cancers affecting either of these organs may also be called colorectal cancer.

## Colorectal Cancer: Who's at Risk?

The exact causes of colorectal cancer are not known. However, studies show that the following risk factors increase a person's chances of developing colorectal cancer:

### Age

Colorectal cancer is more likely to occur as people get older. This disease is more common in people over the age of 50. However, colorectal cancer can occur at younger ages, even, in rare cases, in the teens.

### Diet

Colorectal cancer seems to be associated with diets that are high in fat and calories and low in fiber. Researchers are exploring how these and other dietary factors play a role in the development of colorectal cancer.

### Polyps

Polyps are benign growths on the inner wall of the colon and rectum. They are fairly common in people over age 50. Some types of polyps increase a person's risk of developing colorectal cancer.

A rare, inherited condition, called familial polyposis, causes hundreds of polyps to form in the colon and rectum. Unless this condition is treated, familial polyposis is almost certain to lead to colorectal cancer.

### Personal Medical History

Research shows that women with a history of cancer of the ovary, uterus, or breast have a somewhat increased chance of developing colorectal cancer. Also, a person who has already had colorectal cancer may develop this disease a second time.

### *Family Medical History*

First-degree relatives (parents, siblings, children) of a person who has had colorectal cancer are somewhat more likely to develop this type of cancer themselves, especially if the relative had the cancer at a young age. If many family members have had colorectal cancer, the chances increase even more.

### *Ulcerative Colitis*

Ulcerative colitis is a condition in which the lining of the colon becomes inflamed. Having this condition increases a person's chance of developing colorectal cancer.

## Colorectal Cancer: Reducing the Risk

The National Cancer Institute supports and conducts research on the causes and prevention of colorectal cancer. Research shows that colorectal cancer develops gradually from benign polyps. Early detection and removal of polyps may help to prevent colorectal cancer. Studies are looking at smoking cessation, use of dietary supplements, use of aspirin or similar medicines, decreased alcohol consumption, and increased physical activity to see if these approaches can prevent colorectal cancer. Some studies suggest that a diet low in fat and calories and high in fiber can help prevent colorectal cancer.

Researchers have discovered that changes in certain genes (basic units of heredity) raise the risk of colorectal cancer. Individuals in families with several cases of colorectal cancer may find it helpful to talk with a genetic counselor. The genetic counselor can discuss the availability of a special blood test to check for a genetic change that may increase the chance of developing colorectal cancer. Although having such a genetic change does not mean that a person is sure to develop colorectal cancer, those who have the change may want to talk with their doctor about what can be done to prevent the disease or detect it early.

## Detecting Cancer Early

People who have any of the risk factors described under "Colorectal Cancer: Who's at Risk?" should ask a doctor when to begin checking for colorectal cancer, what tests to have, and how often to have them. The doctor may suggest one or more of the tests listed below. These tests are used to detect polyps, cancer, or other abnormalities, even when a person does not have symptoms. Your health care provider can explain more about each test.

- A *fecal occult blood test* (FOBT) is a test used to check for hidden blood in the stool. Sometimes cancers or polyps can bleed, and FOBT is used to detect small amounts of bleeding.

- A *sigmoidoscopy* is an examination of the rectum and lower colon (sigmoid colon) with a lighted instrument called a sigmoidoscope.

- A *colonoscopy* is an examination of the rectum and entire colon with a lighted instrument called a colonoscope.

- A *double-contrast barium enema* (DCBE) is a series of x-rays of the colon and rectum. The patient is given an enema with a solution that contains barium, which outlines the colon and rectum on the x-rays.

- A *digital rectal exam* (DRE) is an exam in which the doctor inserts a lubricated, gloved finger into the rectum to feel for abnormal areas.

## Recognizing Symptoms

Common signs and symptoms of colorectal cancer include:

- A change in bowel habits
- Diarrhea, constipation, or the feeling that the bowel does not empty completely
- Blood (either bright red or very dark) in the stool
- Stools that are narrower than usual
- General abdominal discomfort (frequent gas pains, bloating, fullness, and/or cramps)
- Weight loss with no known reason
- Constant tiredness
- Vomiting

These symptoms may be caused by colorectal cancer or by other conditions. It is important to check with a doctor.

## *Diagnosing Colorectal Cancer*

To help find the cause of symptoms, the doctor evaluates a person's medical history. The doctor also performs a physical exam and may order one or more diagnostic tests.

- *X-rays* of the large intestine, such as the DCBE, can reveal polyps or other changes.

- A *sigmoidoscopy* lets the doctor see inside the rectum and the lower colon and remove polyps or other abnormal tissue for examination under a microscope.

- A *colonoscopy* lets the doctor see inside the rectum and the entire colon and remove polyps or other abnormal tissue for examination under a microscope.

- A *polypectomy* is the removal of a polyp during a sigmoidoscopy or colonoscopy.

- A *biopsy* is the removal of a tissue sample for examination under a microscope by a pathologist to make a diagnosis.

## *Stages of Colorectal Cancer*

If the diagnosis is cancer, the doctor needs to learn the stage (or extent) of disease. Staging is a careful attempt to find out whether the cancer has spread and, if so, to what parts of the body. More tests may be performed to help determine the stage. Knowing the stage of the disease helps the doctor plan treatment. The list below describes the various stages of colorectal cancer.

- *Stage 0*: The cancer is very early. It is found only in the innermost lining of the colon or rectum.

- *Stage I*: The cancer involves more of the inner wall of the colon or rectum.

- *Stage II*: The cancer has spread outside the colon or rectum to nearby tissue, but not to the lymph nodes. (Lymph nodes are small, bean-shaped structures that are part of the body's immune system.)

- *Stage III*: The cancer has spread to nearby lymph nodes, but not to other parts of the body.

- *Stage IV*: The cancer has spread to other parts of the body. Colorectal cancer tends to spread to the liver and/or lungs.

* *Recurrent*: Recurrent cancer means the cancer has come back after treatment. The disease may recur in the colon or rectum or in another part of the body.

## Treatment for Colorectal Cancer

Treatment depends mainly on the size, location, and extent of the tumor, and on the patient's general health. Patients are often treated by a team of specialists, which may include a gastroenterologist, surgeon, medical oncologist, and radiation oncologist. Several different types of treatment are used to treat colorectal cancer. Sometimes different treatments are combined.

* *Surgery* to remove the tumor is the most common treatment for colorectal cancer. Generally, the surgeon removes the tumor along with part of the healthy colon or rectum and nearby lymph nodes. In most cases, the doctor is able to reconnect the healthy portions of the colon or rectum. When the surgeon cannot reconnect the healthy portions, a temporary or permanent colostomy is necessary. Colostomy, a surgical opening (stoma) through the wall of the abdomen into the colon, provides a new path for waste material to leave the body. After a colostomy, the patient wears a special bag to collect body waste. Some patients need a temporary colostomy to allow the lower colon or rectum to heal after surgery. About 15 percent of colorectal cancer patients require a permanent colostomy.

* *Chemotherapy* is the use of anticancer drugs to kill cancer cells. Chemotherapy may be given to destroy any cancerous cells that may remain in the body after surgery, to control tumor growth, or to relieve symptoms of the disease. Chemotherapy is a systemic therapy, meaning that the drugs enter the bloodstream and travel through the body. Most anticancer drugs are given by injection directly into a vein (IV) or by means of a catheter, a thin tube that is placed into a large vein and remains there as long as it is needed. Some anticancer drugs are given in the form of a pill.

* *Radiation therapy*, also called radiotherapy, involves the use of high-energy x-rays to kill cancer cells. Radiation therapy is a local therapy, meaning that it affects the cancer cells only in the treated area. Most often it is used in patients whose cancer is in the rectum. Doctors may use radiation therapy before surgery (to shrink a tumor so that it is easier to remove) or after surgery

(to destroy any cancer cells that remain in the treated area). Radiation therapy is also used to relieve symptoms. The radiation may come from a machine (external radiation) or from an implant (a small container of radioactive material) placed directly into or near the tumor (internal radiation). Some patients have both kinds of radiation therapy.

- *Biological therapy*, also called immunotherapy, uses the body's immune system to fight cancer. The immune system finds cancer cells in the body and works to destroy them. Biological therapies are used to repair, stimulate, or enhance the immune system's natural anticancer function. Biological therapy may be given after surgery, either alone or in combination with chemotherapy or radiation treatment. Most biological treatments are given by injection into a vein (IV).

- *Clinical trials* (research studies) to evaluate new ways to treat cancer are an appropriate option for many patients with colorectal cancer. In some studies, all patients receive the new treatment. In others, doctors compare different therapies by giving the promising new treatment to one group of patients and the usual (standard) therapy to another group.

## Side Effects

The side effects of cancer treatment depend on the type of treatment and may be different for each person. Most often the side effects are temporary. Doctors and nurses can explain the possible side effects of treatment. Patients should report severe side effects to their doctor. Doctors can suggest ways to help relieve symptoms that may occur during and after treatment.

- Surgery causes short-term pain and tenderness in the area of the operation. Surgery for colorectal cancer may also cause temporary constipation or diarrhea. Patients who have a colostomy may have irritation of the skin around the stoma. The doctor, nurse, or enterostomal therapist can teach the patient how to clean the area and prevent irritation and infection.

- Chemotherapy affects normal as well as cancer cells. Side effects depend largely on the specific drugs and the dose (amount of drug given). Common side effects of chemotherapy include nausea and vomiting, hair loss, mouth sores, diarrhea, and fatigue. Less often, serious side effects may occur, such as infection or bleeding.

- Radiation therapy, like chemotherapy, affects normal as well as cancer cells. Side effects of radiation therapy depend mainly on the treatment dose and the part of the body that is treated. Common side effects of radiation therapy are fatigue, skin changes at the site where the treatment is given, loss of appetite, nausea, and diarrhea. Sometimes, radiation therapy can cause bleeding through the rectum (bloody stools).

- Biological therapy may cause side effects that vary with the specific type of treatment. Often, treatments cause flu-like symptoms, such as chills, fever, weakness, and nausea.

# Section 3.4

## *Prostate Cancer*

Adapted from "What You Need To Know About™ Prostate Cancer," National Cancer Institute, updated September 16, 2002, http://www.nci.nih.gov/templates/page_print.aspx?viewid=b94a9092-bbc1-4ba2-8c75-6793238d92a4. Also available in hard copy as NIH Pub. No. 00-1576 via https://cissecure.nci.nih.gov/ncipubs/.

### The Prostate

The prostate is a gland in a man's reproductive system (Figure 3.3). It makes and stores seminal fluid, a milky fluid that nourishes sperm. This fluid is released to form part of semen.

The prostate is about the size of a walnut. It is located below the bladder and in front of the rectum. It surrounds the upper part of the urethra, the tube that empties urine from the bladder. If the prostate grows too large, the flow of urine can be slowed or stopped.

To work properly, the prostate needs male hormones (androgens). Male hormones are responsible for male sex characteristics. The main male hormone is testosterone, which is made mainly by the testicles. Some male hormones are produced in small amounts by the adrenal glands.

Benign prostatic hyperplasia (BPH) is the abnormal growth of benign (noncancerous) prostate cells. In BPH, the prostate grows larger and presses against the urethra and bladder, interfering with the normal flow of urine. More than half of the men in the United States between the ages of 60 and 70 and as many as 90 percent between the ages of 70 and 90 have symptoms of BPH. For some men, the symptoms may be severe enough to require treatment.

Malignant tumors are cancer. Cells in these tumors are abnormal. They divide without control or order, and they do not die. They can invade and damage nearby tissues and organs. Also, cancer cells can break away from a malignant tumor and enter the bloodstream and lymphatic system. This is how cancer spreads from the original (primary) cancer site to form new (secondary) tumors in other organs. The spread of cancer is called metastasis.

When prostate cancer spreads (metastasizes) outside the prostate, cancer cells are often found in nearby lymph nodes. If the cancer has reached these nodes, it means that cancer cells may have spread to other parts of the body—other lymph nodes and other organs, such as the bones, bladder, or rectum. When cancer spreads from its original location to another part of the body, the new tumor has the same kind of abnormal cells and the same name as the primary tumor. For example, if prostate cancer spreads to the bones, the cancer cells in the new tumor are prostate cancer cells. The disease is metastatic prostate cancer; it is not bone cancer.

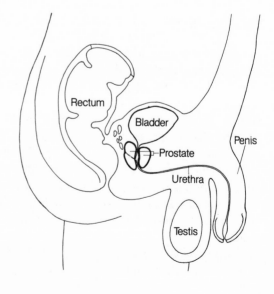

*Figure 3.3.* The prostate and the organs located close to it.

## Prostate Cancer: Who's at Risk

The causes of prostate cancer are not well understood. Doctors cannot explain why one man gets prostate cancer and another does not.

Researchers are studying factors that may increase the risk of this disease. Studies have found that the following risk factors are associated with prostate cancer:

- *Age*. In the United States, prostate cancer is found mainly in men over age 55. The average age of patients at the time of diagnosis is 70.

- *Family history of prostate cancer*. A man's risk for developing prostate cancer is higher if his father or brother has had the disease.

- *Race*. This disease is much more common in African American men than in white men. It is less common in Asian and American Indian men.

- *Diet and dietary factors*. Some evidence suggests that a diet high in animal fat may increase the risk of prostate cancer and a diet high in fruits and vegetables may decrease the risk. Studies are in progress to learn whether men can reduce their risk of prostate cancer by taking certain dietary supplements.

Although a few studies suggested that having a vasectomy might increase a man's risk for prostate cancer, most studies do not support this finding. Scientists have studied whether benign prostatic hyperplasia, obesity, lack of exercise, smoking, radiation exposure, or a sexually transmitted virus might increase the risk for prostate cancer. At this time, there is little evidence that these factors contribute to an increased risk.

## Detecting Prostate Cancer

A man who has any of the risk factors may want to ask a doctor whether to begin screening for prostate cancer (even though he does not have any symptoms), what tests to have, and how often to have them. The doctor may suggest either of the tests described below. These tests are used to detect prostate abnormalities, but they cannot show whether abnormalities are cancer or another, less serious condition. The doctor will take the results into account in deciding whether to check the patient further for signs of cancer. The doctor can explain more about each test.

- *Digital rectal exam.* The doctor inserts a lubricated, gloved finger into the rectum and feels the prostate through the rectal wall to check for hard or lumpy areas.

- *Blood test for prostate-specific antigen (PSA).* A lab measures the levels of PSA in a blood sample. The level of PSA may rise in men who have prostate cancer, BPH, or infection in the prostate.

## Recognizing Symptoms

Early prostate cancer often does not cause symptoms. But prostate cancer can cause any of these problems:

- A need to urinate frequently, especially at night
- Difficulty starting urination or holding back urine
- Inability to urinate
- Weak or interrupted flow of urine
- Painful or burning urination
- Difficulty in having an erection
- Painful ejaculation
- Blood in urine or semen
- Frequent pain or stiffness in the lower back, hips, or upper thighs

Any of these symptoms may be caused by cancer or by other, less serious health problems, such as BPH or an infection. A man who has symptoms like these should see his doctor or a urologist (a doctor who specializes in treating diseases of the genitourinary system).

## Diagnosing Prostate Cancer

If a man has symptoms or test results that suggest prostate cancer, his doctor asks about his personal and family medical history, performs a physical exam, and may order laboratory tests. The exams and tests may include a digital rectal exam, a urine test to check for blood or infection, and a blood test to measure PSA. In some cases, the doctor also may check the level of prostatic acid phosphatase (PAP) in the blood, especially if the results of the PSA indicate there might be a problem.

The doctor may order exams to learn more about the cause of the symptoms. These may include:

- *Transrectal ultrasonography*. Sound waves that cannot be heard by humans (ultrasound) are sent out by a probe inserted into the rectum. The waves bounce off the prostate, and a computer uses the echoes to create a picture called a sonogram.

- *Intravenous pyelogram*. A series of x-rays of the organs of the urinary tract.

- *Cystoscopy*. A procedure in which a doctor looks into the urethra and bladder through a thin, lighted tube.

## Biopsy

If test results suggest that cancer may be present, the man will need to have a biopsy. During a biopsy, the doctor removes tissue samples from the prostate, usually with a needle. A pathologist looks at the tissue under a microscope to check for cancer cells. If cancer is present, the pathologist usually reports the grade of the tumor. The grade tells how much the tumor tissue differs from normal prostate tissue and suggests how fast the tumor is likely to grow. One way of grading prostate cancer, called the Gleason system, uses scores of 2 to 10. Another system uses G1 through G4. Tumors with higher scores or grades are more likely to grow and spread than tumors with lower scores.

If the physical exam and test results do not suggest cancer, the doctor may recommend medicine to reduce the symptoms caused by an enlarged prostate. Surgery is another way to relieve these symptoms. The surgery most often used in such cases is called transurethral resection of the prostate (TURP or TUR). In TURP, an instrument is inserted through the urethra to remove prostate tissue that is pressing against the upper part of the urethra and restricting the flow of urine. (Patients may want to ask whether other procedures might be appropriate.)

## Stages of Prostate Cancer

If cancer is found in the prostate, the doctor needs to know the stage, or extent, of the disease. Staging is a careful attempt to find out whether the cancer has spread and, if so, what parts of the body are affected. The doctor may use various blood and imaging tests to learn the stage of the disease. Treatment decisions depend on these findings.

Prostate cancer staging is a complex process. The doctor may describe the stage using a Roman number (I-IV) or a capital letter (A-D). These are the main features of each stage:

- *Stage I* or *Stage A*. The cancer cannot be felt during a rectal exam. It may be found by accident when surgery is done for another reason, usually for BPH. There is no evidence that the cancer has spread outside the prostate.

- *Stage II* or *Stage B*. The tumor involves more tissue within the prostate, it can be felt during a rectal exam, or it is found with a biopsy that is done because of a high PSA level. There is no evidence that the cancer has spread outside the prostate.

- *Stage III* or *Stage C*. The cancer has spread outside the prostate to nearby tissues.

- *Stage IV* or *Stage D*. The cancer has spread to lymph nodes or to other parts of the body.

## Treatment for Prostate Cancer

### Preparing for Treatment

The doctor develops a treatment plan to fit each man's needs. Treatment for prostate cancer depends on the stage of the disease and the grade of the tumor (which indicates how abnormal the cells look, and how likely they are to grow or spread). Other important factors in planning treatment are the man's age and general health and his feelings about the treatments and their possible side effects.

Many men with prostate cancer want to learn all they can about their disease, their treatment choices, and the possible side effects of treatment, so they can take an active part in decisions about their medical care. Prostate cancer can be managed in a number of ways (with watchful waiting, surgery, radiation therapy, and hormonal therapy). If the doctor recommends watchful waiting, the man's health will be monitored closely, and he will be treated only if symptoms occur or worsen. Patients considering surgery, radiation therapy, or hormonal therapy may want to consult doctors who specialize in these types of treatment.

The patient and his doctor may want to consider both the benefits and possible side effects of each option, especially the effects on sexual activity and urination, and other concerns about quality of life.

## *Methods of Treatment*

Treatment for prostate cancer may involve watchful waiting, surgery, radiation therapy, or hormonal therapy. Some patients receive a combination of therapies. In addition, doctors are studying other methods of treatment to find out whether they are effective against this disease.

Watchful waiting may be suggested for some men who have prostate cancer that is found at an early stage and appears to be slow-growing. Also, watchful waiting may be advised for older men or men with other serious medical problems. For these men, the risks and possible side effects of surgery, radiation therapy, or hormonal therapy may outweigh the possible benefits. Men with early stage prostate cancer are taking part in a study to determine when or whether treatment may be necessary and effective.

Surgery is a common treatment for early stage prostate cancer. The doctor may remove all of the prostate (a type of surgery called radical prostatectomy) or only part of it. In some cases, the doctor can use a new technique known as nerve-sparing surgery. This type of surgery may save the nerves that control erection. However, men with large tumors or tumors that are very close to the nerves may not be able to have this surgery.

The doctor can describe the types of surgery and can discuss and compare their benefits and risks.

- In *radical retropubic prostatectomy*, the doctor removes the entire prostate and nearby lymph nodes through an incision in the abdomen.

- In *radical perineal prostatectomy*, the doctor removes the entire prostate through an incision between the scrotum and the anus. Nearby lymph nodes are sometimes removed through a separate incision in the abdomen.

- In *transurethral resection of the prostate (TURP)*, the doctor removes part of the prostate with an instrument that is inserted through the urethra. The cancer is cut from the prostate by electricity passing through a small wire loop on the end of the instrument. This method is used mainly to remove tissue that blocks urine flow.

If the pathologist finds cancer cells in the lymph nodes, it is likely that the disease has spread to other parts of the body. Sometimes, the doctor removes the lymph nodes before doing a prostatectomy. If the prostate cancer has not spread to the lymph nodes, the doctor then removes the prostate. But if cancer has spread to the nodes, the doctor usually does not remove the prostate, but may suggest other treatment.

Radiation therapy (also called radiotherapy) uses high-energy x-rays to kill cancer cells. Like surgery, radiation therapy is local therapy; it can affect cancer cells only in the treated area. In early stage prostate cancer, radiation can be used instead of surgery, or it may be used after surgery to destroy any cancer cells that may remain in the area. In advanced stages, it may be given to relieve pain or other problems.

Radiation may be directed at the body by a machine (external radiation), or it may come from tiny radioactive seeds placed inside or near the tumor (internal or implant radiation, or brachytherapy). Men who receive radioactive seeds alone usually have small tumors. Some men with prostate cancer receive both kinds of radiation therapy.

For external radiation therapy, patients go to the hospital or clinic, usually five days a week for several weeks. Patients may stay in the hospital for a short time for implant radiation.

Hormonal therapy keeps cancer cells from getting the male hormones they need to grow. It is called systemic therapy because it can affect cancer cells throughout the body. Systemic therapy is used to treat cancer that has spread. Sometimes this type of therapy is used to try to prevent the cancer from coming back after surgery or radiation treatment.

There are several forms of hormonal therapy:

- Orchiectomy is surgery to remove the testicles, which are the main source of male hormones.

- Drugs known as luteinizing hormone-releasing hormone (LH-RH) agonists can prevent the testicles from producing testosterone. Examples are leuprolide, goserelin, and buserelin.

- Drugs known as anti-androgens can block the action of androgens. Two examples are flutamide and bicalutamide.

- Drugs that can prevent the adrenal glands from making androgens include ketoconazole and aminoglutethimide.

After orchiectomy or treatment with an LH-RH agonist, the body no longer gets testosterone from the testicles. However, the adrenal glands still produce small amounts of male hormones. Sometimes, the patient is also given an anti-androgen, which blocks the effect of any remaining male hormones. This combination of treatments is known as total androgen blockade. Doctors do not know for sure whether total androgen blockade is more effective than orchiectomy or LH-RH agonist alone.

Prostate cancer that has spread to other parts of the body usually can be controlled with hormonal therapy for a period of time, often several years. Eventually, however, most prostate cancers are able to grow with very little or no male hormones. When this happens, hormonal therapy is no longer effective, and the doctor may suggest other forms of treatment that are under study.

## Side Effects of Treatment

It is hard to limit the effects of treatment so that only cancer cells are removed or destroyed. Because healthy cells and tissues may be damaged, treatment often causes unwanted side effects. Doctors and nurses will explain the possible side effects of treatment.

The side effects of cancer treatment depend mainly on the type and extent of the treatment. Also, each patient reacts differently.

### Watchful Waiting

Although men who choose watchful waiting avoid the side effects of surgery and radiation, there can be some negative aspects to this choice. Watchful waiting may reduce the chance of controlling the disease before it spreads. Also, older men should keep in mind that it may be harder to manage surgery and radiation therapy as they age.

Some men may decide against watchful waiting because they feel they would be uncomfortable living with an untreated cancer, even one that appears to be growing slowly or not at all. A man who chooses watchful waiting but later becomes concerned or anxious should discuss his feelings with his doctor. A different treatment approach is nearly always available.

### Surgery

Patients are often uncomfortable for the first few days after surgery. Their pain usually can be controlled with medicine, and patients should discuss pain relief with the doctor or nurse. The patient will wear a catheter (a tube inserted into the urethra) to drain urine for 10 days to three weeks. The nurse or doctor will show the man how to care for the catheter.

It is also common for patients to feel extremely tired or weak for a while. The length of time it takes to recover from an operation varies. Surgery to remove the prostate may cause long-term problems, including rectal injury or urinary incontinence. Some men may have permanent impotence. Nerve-sparing surgery is an attempt to avoid the problem of impotence. When the doctor can use nerve-sparing surgery and the operation is fully successful, impotence may be only temporary. Still, some men who have this procedure may be permanently impotent.

Men who have a prostatectomy no longer produce semen, so they have dry orgasms. Men who wish to father children may consider sperm banking or a sperm retrieval procedure.

## Radiation Therapy

Radiation therapy may cause patients to become extremely tired, especially in the later weeks of treatment. Resting is important, but doctors usually encourage men to try to stay as active as they can. Some men may have diarrhea or frequent and uncomfortable urination.

When men with prostate cancer receive external radiation therapy, it is common for the skin in the treated area to become red, dry, and tender. External radiation therapy can also cause hair loss in the treated area. The loss may be temporary or permanent, depending on the dose of radiation.

Both types of radiation therapy may cause impotence in some men, but internal radiation therapy is not as likely as external radiation therapy to damage the nerves that control erection. However, internal radiation therapy may cause temporary incontinence. Long-term side effects from internal radiation therapy are uncommon.

## Hormonal Therapy

The side effects of hormonal therapy depend largely on the type of treatment. Orchiectomy and LH-RH agonists often cause side effects such as impotence, hot flashes, and loss of sexual desire. When first taken, an LH-RH agonist may make a patient's symptoms worse for a short time. This temporary problem is called "flare." Gradually, however, the treatment causes a man's testosterone level to fall. Without testosterone, tumor growth slows down and the patient's condition improves. (To prevent flare, the doctor may give the man an anti-androgen for a while along with the LH-RH agonist.)

Anti-androgens can cause nausea, vomiting, diarrhea, or breast growth or tenderness. If used a long time, ketoconazole may cause liver problems, and aminoglutethimide can cause skin rashes. Men who receive total androgen blockade may experience more side effects than men who receive a single method of hormonal therapy. Any method of hormonal therapy that lowers androgen levels can contribute to weakening of the bones in older men.

# Section 3.5

# *Testicular Cancer*

Text in this section is reprinted from two sources: "Testicular Cancer: Questions and Answers," National Cancer Institute, updated May 2002, http://cis.nci.nih.gov/fact/6_34.htm; "Testicular Cancer: What to Look for" is excerpted and reprinted with permission from http://familydoctor.org/ handouts/387.html. Copyright © 2003 American Academy of Family Physicians. All rights reserved.

## *Testicular Cancer: Questions and Answers*

### *What is testicular cancer?*

Testicular cancer is a disease in which cells become malignant (cancerous) in one or both testicles.

The testicles (also called testes or gonads) are a pair of male sex glands. They produce and store sperm, and are also the body's main source of male hormones. These hormones control the development of the reproductive organs and male characteristics. The testicles are located under the penis in a sac-like pouch called the scrotum.

Testicular cancer can be broadly classified into two types: seminoma and nonseminoma. Seminomas make up about 30 percent of all testicular cancers. Nonseminomas are a group of cancers that include choriocarcinoma, embryonal carcinoma, teratoma, and yolk sac tumors. A testicular cancer may have a combination of both types.

An estimated 7,400 men in the United States will be diagnosed with testicular cancer in 1999. Although testicular cancer accounts for only 1 percent of all cancers in men, it is the most common form of cancer in young men between the ages of 15 and 35. Any man can get testicular cancer, but it is more common in white men than in black men.

## *What are the risk factors for testicular cancer?*

The causes of testicular cancer are not known. However, studies show that several factors increase a man's chance of developing testicular cancer.

- *Undescended testicle (cryptorchidism)*. Normally, the testicles descend into the scrotum before birth. Men who have had a testicle that did not move down into the scrotum are at greater risk for developing the disease. This is true even if surgery is performed to place the testicle in the scrotum.

- *Abnormal testicular development*. Men whose testicles did not develop normally are also at increased risk.

- *Klinefelter syndrome*. Men with Klinefelter syndrome (a sex chromosome disorder that may be characterized by low levels of male hormones, sterility, breast enlargement, and small testes) are at greater risk of developing testicular cancer.

- *History of testicular cancer*. Men who have previously had testicular cancer are at increased risk of developing cancer in the other testicle.

## *How is testicular cancer detected? What are symptoms of testicular cancer?*

Most testicular cancers are found by men themselves. Also, doctors generally examine the testicles during routine physical exams. Between regular checkups, if a man notices anything unusual about his testicles, he should talk with his doctor. When testicular cancer is found early, the treatment can often be less aggressive and may cause fewer side effects.

Men should see a doctor if they notice any of the following symptoms:

- A painless lump or swelling in either testicle

- Any enlargement of a testicle or change in the way it feels

- A feeling of heaviness in the scrotum

- A dull ache in the lower abdomen or the groin (the area where the thigh meets the abdomen)

- A sudden collection of fluid in the scrotum

- Pain or discomfort in a testicle or in the scrotum.

These symptoms can be caused by cancer or by other conditions. It is important to see a doctor to determine the cause of any symptoms.

## How is testicular cancer diagnosed?

To help find the cause of symptoms, the doctor evaluates a man's general health. The doctor also performs a physical exam and may order laboratory and diagnostic tests. If a tumor is suspected, the doctor will probably suggest a biopsy, which involves surgery to remove the testicle.

- *Blood tests* measure the levels of tumor markers. Tumor markers are substances often found in higher-than-normal amounts when cancer is present. Tumor markers such as alpha-fetoprotein (AFP), human chorionic gonadotropin (HCG), and lactase dehydrogenase (LDH) may detect a tumor that is too small to be detected during physical exams or imaging tests.

- *Ultrasound* is a diagnostic test in which high-frequency sound waves are bounced off tissues and internal organs. Their echoes produce a picture called a sonogram. Ultrasound of the scrotum can show the presence and size of a mass in the testicle. It is also helpful in ruling out other conditions, such as swelling due to infection.

- *Biopsy*. Microscopic examination of testicular tissue by a pathologist is the only sure way to know whether cancer is present. In nearly all cases of suspected cancer, the entire affected testicle is removed through an incision in the groin. This procedure is called inguinal orchiectomy. In rare cases (for example, when a man has only one testicle), the surgeon performs an inguinal biopsy, removing a sample of tissue from the testicle through an incision in the groin and proceeding with orchiectomy only if the pathologist finds cancer cells. (The surgeon does not cut through the scrotum to remove tissue, because if the problem is cancer, this procedure could cause the disease to spread.)

If testicular cancer is found, more tests are needed to find out if the cancer has spread from the testicle to other parts of the body. Determining the stage (extent) of the disease helps the doctor to plan appropriate treatment.

### How is testicular cancer treated? What are the side effects of treatment?

Most men with testicular cancer can be cured with surgery, radiation therapy, and/or chemotherapy. The side effects depend on the type of treatment and may be different for each person.

Seminomas and nonseminomas grow and spread differently, and each type may need different treatment. Treatment also depends on the stage of the cancer, the patient's age and general health, and other factors. Men are often treated by a team of specialists, which may include a surgeon, a medical oncologist, and a radiation oncologist.

*Surgery*

Surgery to remove the testicle through an incision in the groin is called a radical inguinal orchiectomy. Men may be concerned that losing a testicle will affect their ability to have sexual intercourse or make them sterile (unable to produce children). However, a man with one remaining healthy testicle can still have a normal erection and produce sperm. Therefore, an operation to remove one testicle does not make a man impotent (unable to have an erection) and seldom interferes with fertility (the ability to produce children). Men can also have an artificial testicle, called a prosthesis, placed in the scrotum. The implant has the weight and feel of a normal testicle.

Some of the lymph nodes located deep in the abdomen may also be removed (lymph node dissection). This type of surgery does not change a man's ability to have an erection or an orgasm, but it can cause sterility because it interferes with ejaculation. Patients may wish to talk with the doctor about the possibility of removing the lymph nodes using a special nerve-sparing surgical technique that may protect the ability to ejaculate normally.

*Radiation*

Radiation therapy, also called radiotherapy, uses high-energy rays to kill cancer cells and shrink tumors. Radiation therapy is a local therapy; it affects cancer cells only in the treated areas. Radiation therapy for testicular cancer comes from a machine outside the body (external beam radiation) and is usually aimed at lymph nodes in the abdomen. Seminomas are highly sensitive to radiation. Nonseminomas are less sensitive to radiation, so men with this type of cancer usually do not undergo radiation.

Radiation therapy affects normal as well as cancerous cells. The side effects of radiation therapy depend mainly on the treatment dose. Common side effects include fatigue, skin changes at the site where the treatment is given, loss of appetite, nausea, and diarrhea. Radiation therapy interferes with sperm production, but most patients regain their fertility within a matter of months.

*Chemotherapy*

Chemotherapy is the use of anticancer drugs to kill cancer cells throughout the body. Chemotherapy is given to destroy cancerous cells that may remain in the body after surgery. The use of anticancer drugs following surgery is known as adjuvant therapy. Chemotherapy may also be the initial treatment if the cancer is advanced; that is, if it has spread outside the testicle. Most anticancer drugs are given by injection into a vein (IV).

Chemotherapy is a systemic therapy, meaning that drugs travel through the bloodstream and affect normal as well as cancerous cells all over the body. The side effects depend largely on the specific drugs and the dose. Common side effects may include nausea, loss of hair, fatigue, diarrhea, vomiting, fever, chills, coughing/shortness of breath, mouth sores, or skin rash. Other common side effects are dizziness, numbness, loss of reflexes, or difficulty hearing. Some anticancer drugs interfere with sperm production. Although the reduction in sperm count is permanent for some patients, many others recover their fertility.

Men with testicular cancer should discuss their concerns about sexual function and fertility with the doctor. If a man is to have treatment that might lead to infertility, he may want to ask the doctor about sperm banking (freezing sperm before treatment for use in the future). This procedure can allow some men to produce children after loss of fertility.

### Is follow-up treatment necessary? What does it involve?

Regular follow-up exams are extremely important for men who have been treated for testicular cancer. Like all cancers, testicular cancer can recur. Men who have had testicular cancer should see their doctor regularly and should report any unusual symptoms right away.

Follow-up may vary for different types and stages of testicular cancer. Generally, patients are checked frequently by a doctor and have regular blood tests to measure tumor marker levels. They also have regular x-rays and computed tomography, also called CT scans or CAT scans (detailed pictures of areas inside the body created by a computer linked to an x-ray machine). Men who have had testicular cancer have an increased likelihood of developing cancer in the remaining testicle. They also have an increased risk of certain types of leukemia, as well as other types of cancers. Regular follow-up care ensures that any changes in health are discussed, and any recurrent cancer can be treated as soon as possible.

### Are clinical trials (research studies) available for men with testicular cancer?

Yes. Participation in clinical trials is an important treatment option for many men with testicular cancer. To develop new, more effective treatments, and better ways to use current treatments, the National Cancer Institute (NCI) is sponsoring clinical trials in many hospitals and cancer centers around the country. Clinical trials are a critical step in the development of new methods of treatment. Before any new treatment can be recommended for general use, doctors conduct clinical trials to find out whether the treatment is safe for patients and effective against the disease.

Patients who are interested in learning more about participating in clinical trials can call NCI's Cancer Information Service [(800) 4-CANCER or (800) 422-6237)] or access the clinical trials page of the NCI's Cancer.gov website at http://cancer.gov/clinical_trials on the Internet.

## Testicular Cancer: What to Look for

The best time to do the exam is during or right after a shower or a bath. The warm water relaxes the skin on your scrotum and makes the exam easier.

- Check your testicles one at a time. Use one or both hands.

- Cup your scrotum with one hand to see if there is any change from the way it feels normally.

- Place your index and middle fingers under one testicle with your thumb on top.

- Gently roll the testicle between your thumb and fingers.

- Feel for any lumps in or on the side of the testicle. Repeat with the other testicle.

- Feel along the epididymis (a soft, tubelike, comma-shaped structure behind the testicle that collects and carries sperm) for swelling.

It's normal for one testicle to be a little bit bigger than the other. The testicles should be smooth and firm. If you feel any bumps or lumps, visit your doctor right away.

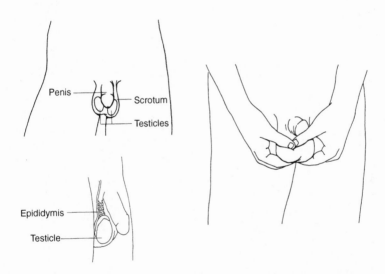

*Figure 3.4.* How to exam the testicles for cancer. Source: *National Cancer Institute Visuals Online, 1992.*

# Chapter 4

# *Stroke: Brain Attack*

## *Stroke Basics*

### *What causes a stroke?*

Stroke is a cardiovascular disease. It affects the blood vessels that supply blood to the brain.

A stroke occurs when a blood vessel that brings oxygen and nutrients to the brain bursts or is clogged by a blood clot or some other particle. Because of this rupture or blockage, part of the brain doesn't get the blood and oxygen it needs. Deprived of oxygen, nerve cells in the affected area of the brain can't work and die within minutes. And when nerve cells can't work, the part of the body they control can't work either. The devastating effects of stroke are often permanent because dead brain cells are not replaced.

There are four main types of stroke. Two are caused by blood clots or other particles, and two by bleeding (hemorrhage) (HEM'or-ij). Cerebral thrombosis (SER'eh-bral or seh-RE'bral throm-BO'sis) and cerebral embolism (EM'bo-lizm) are caused by clots or particles that plug an artery. These strokes account for about 70–80 percent of all strokes. Ruptured blood vessels cause cerebral and subarachnoid (sub-ah-RAK'noid) hemorrhages. These (bleeding) strokes have a much higher fatality rate than strokes caused by clots.

---

This chapter includes "Stroke," "Stroke Effects," "Stroke Risk Factors," and "Stroke Symptoms/Warning Signs," which are reproduced with permission from the American Heart Association world wide website, http://www.americanheart.org. © 2003. Copyright American Heart Association.

## What is a cerebral thrombosis?

Cerebral thrombosis is the most common stroke. It occurs when a blood clot (thrombus) forms and blocks blood flow in an artery bringing blood to part of the brain. Blood clots usually form in arteries damaged by fatty buildups, called atherosclerosis (ath"er-o-skleh-RO'sis).

Cerebral thrombotic strokes often occur at night or first thing in the morning. Another distinguishing feature is that very often they're preceded by a transient ischemic (is-KEM'ik) attack. This is also called a TIA or "ministroke."

## What is a cerebral embolism?

This type of stroke occurs when a wandering clot [an embolus (EM'bo-lus)] or some other particle forms away from the brain, usually in the heart. The clot is carried by the bloodstream until it lodges in an artery leading to or in the brain, blocking the flow of blood.

The most common cause of these emboli (EM'bo-li) is blood clots that form during atrial fibrillation (fib"rih-LA'shun). This is a disorder found in 2 to 3 million Americans. In atrial fibrillation the heart's two small upper chambers (the atria) quiver instead of beating effectively. Some blood isn't pumped completely out of them when the heart beats, so it pools and clots. When a blood clot enters the circulation and lodges in a narrowed artery of the brain, a stroke occurs.

## What is a hemorrhage?

A subarachnoid hemorrhage occurs when a blood vessel on the brain's surface ruptures and bleeds into the space between the brain and the skull (but not into the brain itself).

Another type of stroke occurs when a defective artery in the brain bursts, flooding the surrounding tissue with blood. This is a cerebral hemorrhage.

Hemorrhage (or bleeding) from an artery in the brain can be caused by a head injury or a burst aneurysm (AN'u-rizm). Aneurysms are blood-filled pouches that balloon out from weak spots in the artery wall. They're often caused or made worse by high blood pressure. Aneurysms aren't always dangerous, but if one bursts in the brain, they cause a hemorrhagic stroke.

When a cerebral or subarachnoid hemorrhage occurs, the loss of a constant blood supply means some brain cells no longer can work. Accumulated blood from the burst artery also may put pressure on surrounding brain tissue and interfere with how the brain works. Severe or mild symptoms can result, depending on the amount of pressure.

The amount of bleeding determines the severity of cerebral hemorrhages. In many cases, people with cerebral hemorrhages die of increased pressure on their brains. But those who live tend to recover much more than people who've had strokes caused by a clot. That's because when a blood vessel is blocked, part of the brain dies—and the brain doesn't regenerate. But when a blood vessel in the brain bursts, pressure from the blood compresses part of the brain. If the person survives, gradually the pressure goes away. Then the brain may regain some of its former function.

## Stroke Risk Factors

The American Heart Association has identified several factors that increase your risk of stroke. The more risk factors you have, the greater your chances for a stroke. You can't control some of these, such as increasing age, family health history, prior stroke, race, and gender. But you can modify, treat, or control most risk factors to lower your risk of stroke. A health care provider can help you change factors that result from life-style or environment.

### *What are the risk factors for stroke you can't change?*

- *Increasing age*—Stroke happens to people of all ages, including children. But the older you are, the greater your risk for stroke.

- *Sex (gender)*—Stroke is more common in men than in women. In most age groups, more men than women will have a stroke in a given year. However, more than half of total stroke deaths occur in women. At all ages, more women than men die of stroke. Use of birth control pills and pregnancy pose special stroke risks for women.

- *Heredity (family history) and race*—Your stroke risk is greater if a parent, grandparent, sister, or brother has had a stroke. African Americans have a much higher risk of death from a stroke than Caucasians do. In part this is because blacks have higher risks of high blood pressure, diabetes, and obesity.

- *Prior stroke or heart attack*—Someone who has had a stroke is at much higher risk of having another one. If you've had a heart attack, you're at higher risk of having a stroke, too.

## *What are the risk factors you and your health care provider can change, treat, or control?*

- *High blood pressure*—High blood pressure is defined in an adult as a systolic pressure of 140 mm Hg or higher and/or a diastolic pressure of 90 mm Hg or higher for an extended time. It's the most important risk factor for stroke.

- *Diabetes mellitus* (di"ah-BE'teez or di"ah-BE'tis meh-LI'tis)— While diabetes is treatable, having it still increases a person's risk of stroke. People with diabetes often also have high blood pressure and high blood cholesterol and are overweight. This increases their risk even more. If you have diabetes, work closely with your doctor to manage it.

- *Carotid or other artery disease*—The carotid (kah-ROT'id) arteries in your neck supply blood to your brain. A carotid artery narrowed by fatty deposits from atherosclerosis (ath"er-o-skleh-RO'sis) may become blocked by a blood clot. People with peripheral artery disease have a higher risk of carotid artery disease, which raises their risk of stroke. Peripheral artery disease is the narrowing of blood vessels carrying blood to leg and arm muscles. It's caused by atherosclerosis.

- *Atrial fibrillation*—This heart rhythm disorder raises the risk for stroke, because the heart's upper chambers quiver instead of beating effectively. This lets the blood pool and clot. If a clot breaks off, enters the bloodstream and lodges in an artery leading to the brain, a stroke results.

- *Other heart disease*—People with coronary heart disease or heart failure have more than twice the risk of stroke as those with hearts that work normally. Dilated cardiomyopathy (an enlarged heart), heart valve disease, and some types of congenital heart defects also raise the risk of stroke.

- *Transient ischemic (TRANZ'e-ent is-KEM'ik) attacks (TIAs)*— TIAs are "ministrokes" that produce stroke-like symptoms but no lasting damage. Recognizing and treating TIAs can reduce your risk of a major stroke. It's very important to recognize the warning signs of a TIA or stroke. Call 911 to get medical help immediately if they occur!

- *Certain blood disorders*—A high red blood cell count thickens the blood and makes clots more likely. This raises the risk of stroke. Doctors may treat this problem by removing blood cells or prescribing "blood thinners."

- *Sickle cell anemia*—This genetic disorder mainly affects African Americans. "Sickled" red blood cells are less able to carry oxygen to the body's tissues and organs. They also tend to stick to blood vessel walls, which can block arteries to the brain and cause a stroke.

- *High blood cholesterol*—A high level of total cholesterol in the blood (240 mg/dL or higher) is a major risk factor for heart disease, which raises your risk of stroke. Recent studies show that high levels of LDL ("bad") cholesterol (greater than 100 mg/dL) and triglycerides (blood fats) directly increase the risk of stroke in people with previous coronary heart disease, ischemic stroke, or transient ischemic attack (TIA). Low levels of HDL ("good") cholesterol (less than 40 mg/dL) also may raise stroke risk.

## *What risk factors require a life-style change?*

- *Tobacco use*—Cigarette smoking is the number-one preventable risk factor for stroke. The nicotine and carbon monoxide in tobacco smoke reduce the amount of oxygen in your blood. They also damage the walls of blood vessels, making clots more likely to form. Using some kinds of birth control pills combined with smoking cigarettes greatly increases stroke risk.

- *Physical inactivity and obesity*—Being inactive, obese, or both can increase your risk of high blood pressure, high blood cholesterol, diabetes, heart disease, and stroke. So go on a brisk walk, take the stairs, and do whatever you can to make your life more active at least 30 minutes total on most days.

- *Excessive alcohol*—An average of more than one alcoholic drink a day for women or more than two drinks a day for men raises blood pressure and can lead to stroke.

- *Illegal drug abuse*—Intravenous drug abuse carries a high risk of stroke. Cocaine use has been linked to strokes and heart attacks. Some have been fatal even in first-time users.

## *Stroke Symptoms*

*If you notice one or more of these signs, don't wait. Stroke is a medical emergency. Call 911 or your emergency medical services. Get to a hospital right away!*

The American Stroke Association wants you to learn the warning signs of stroke:

- Sudden numbness or weakness of the face, arm or leg, especially on one side of the body
- Sudden confusion, trouble speaking or understanding
- Sudden trouble seeing in one or both eyes
- Sudden trouble walking, dizziness, loss of balance or coordination
- Sudden, severe headache with no known cause

### Be Prepared for an Emergency

- Keep a list of emergency rescue service numbers next to the telephone and in your pocket, wallet, or purse.
- Find out which area hospitals are primary stroke centers that have 24-hour emergency stroke care.
- Know (in advance) which hospital or medical facility is nearest your home or office.

### Take Action in an Emergency

- Not all the warning signs occur in every stroke. Don't ignore signs of stroke, even if they go away!
- Check the time. When did the first warning sign or symptom start? You'll be asked this important question later.
- If you have one or more stroke symptoms that last more than a few minutes, don't delay! Immediately call 911 or the emergency medical service (EMS) number so an ambulance (ideally with advanced life support) can quickly be sent for you.
- If you're with someone who may be having stroke symptoms, immediately call 911 or the EMS. Expect the person to protest—denial is common. Don't take "no" for an answer. Insist on taking prompt action.

## Stroke Effects

Stroke affects different people in different ways. It depends on the type of stroke, the area of the brain affected and the extent of the brain injury. Brain injury from a stroke can affect the senses, motor activity, speech, and the ability to understand speech. It can also affect behavioral and thought patterns, memory, and emotions. Paralysis or weakness on one side of the body is common.

### How can a stroke affect emotions?

A stroke survivor may cry easily or have sudden mood swings, often for no apparent reason. This is called emotional lability (lah-BIL'ih-te). Laughing uncontrollably also may occur but isn't as common as crying. Depression is common, as stroke survivors may feel less than "whole."

### How can a stroke cause loss of awareness?

Stroke often causes people to lose mobility and/or feeling in an arm and/or leg, or suffer dimness of sight on one side. The loss of feeling or visual field results in a loss of awareness, so stroke survivors may forget or ignore their weaker side. This problem is called "neglect." As a result, they may ignore items on their affected side and have trouble reading. They also may dress only one side of their bodies and think they're fully dressed. Bumping into furniture or door jambs is also common. One-sided neglect is most common in those with injury to the brain's right hemisphere.

### How can a stroke affect perception?

A stroke can also affect seeing, touching, moving, and thinking, so a person's perception of every-day objects may be changed. Stroke survivors may not be able to recognize and understand familiar objects the way they did before. When vision is affected, objects may look closer or farther away than they really are. This causes survivors to have spills at the table or collisions when they walk.

### How can a stroke affect hearing and speech?

Stroke usually doesn't cause hearing loss, but people may have problems understanding speech. They also may have trouble saying what they're thinking. This is called aphasia (ah-FA'zhuh). Aphasia affects the ability to talk, listen, read, and write. It's most common when a stroke weakens the body's right side.

A related problem is that a stroke can affect muscles used in talking (those in the tongue, palate, and lips). Speech can be slowed, slurred, or distorted, so stroke survivors can be hard to understand. This is called dysarthria (dis-ARTH're-ah). It may require the help of a speech expert.

### *How can a stroke affect chewing and swallowing food?*

This problem, called dysphagia (dis-FA'je-ah), can occur when one side of the mouth is weak. One or both sides of the mouth can lack feeling, increasing the risk of choking.

### *How can a stroke affect the ability to think clearly?*

It may be hard to plan and carry out even simple activities. Stroke survivors may not know how to start a task, confuse the sequence of logical steps in tasks, or forget how to do tasks they've done many times before.

# Chapter 5

# *Accidents*

## *Chapter Contents*

# Section 5.1

# *Automobiles*

This section contains three sources: The first part is reprinted from "Drive Defensively," a fact sheet produced by the National Safety Council. © 2001. Permission to reprint granted by the National Safety Council, a membership organization dedicated to protecting life and promoting health. For more information visit the website of the National Safety Council at http://www.nsc.org. The second part is reprinted from "Older Drivers," National Institute on Aging, National Institutes of Health, revised 2002, http://www.nia.nih.gov/health/agepages/drivers.htm; "Pedestrian Injuries" is from the National Center for Injury Prevention and Control, *Injury Fact Book 2001–2002*. Atlanta, GA: Centers for Disease Control and Prevention, reviewed July 17, 2002, http://www.cdc.gov/ncipc/fact_book/19_ Pedestrian.htm.

## *Drive Defensively*

More than 41,000 people lose their lives in motor vehicle crashes each year, and over 2 million more suffer disabling injuries, according to the National Safety Council. The triple threat of high speeds, impaired or careless driving, and not using occupant restraints threatens every driver—regardless of how careful or how skilled.

Driving defensively means not only taking responsibility for yourself and your actions but also keeping an eye on "the other guy." The National Safety Council suggests the following guidelines to help reduce your risks on the road:

- Don't start the engine without securing each passenger in the car, including children and pets. Safety belts save thousands of lives each year! Lock all doors.

- Remember that driving too fast or too slow can increase the likelihood of collisions.

- Don't kid yourself. If you plan to drink, designate a driver who won't drink. Alcohol is a factor in almost half of all fatal motor vehicle crashes.

- Be alert! If you notice that a car is straddling the center line, weaving, making wide turns, stopping abruptly or responding slowly to traffic signals, the driver may be impaired.

- Avoid an impaired driver by turning right at the nearest corner or exiting at the nearest exit. If it appears that an oncoming car is crossing into your lane, pull over to the roadside, sound the horn, and flash your lights.

- Notify the police immediately after seeing a motorist who is driving suspiciously.

- Follow the rules of the road. Don't contest the "right of way" or try to race another car during a merge. Be respectful of other motorists.

- While driving, be cautious, aware, and responsible.

## *Older Drivers*

Almost any adult with a driver's license can remember that first trip alone in the family car, feeling completely free and independent. Those same emotions complicate the decision faced daily by many older Americans. They must decide whether to keep driving or give up their car.

Maybe driving is not fun any more. Some people may not drive at night because they have trouble seeing. Others might avoid driving on interstate highways. For many older drivers, these are the first signs that driving is becoming a problem.

But driving is necessary for many. Gone are the days when most could walk a few blocks to the grocer or doctor. Getting around is a problem for the millions of older people who live in the suburbs or rural areas. In cities there are plenty of taxis and public transportation like buses and subways. However, buses and subways may be hard for someone suffering from arthritis or using a cane. Taxis may seem to cost too much.

In 1983 one out of every 15 licensed drivers in America was over the age of 70. By 1995 this had risen to one out of every 11 drivers. By 2020 one out of every five Americans will be over 65 years of age, and most of them will probably be licensed to drive.

As a group, older drivers are some of the country's safest drivers. Fewer speed or drive after drinking alcohol than at any other age. However, compared to young and middle-age adults, people over 70 are more likely to be involved in a crash while driving and more likely to die in that crash. There are many reasons for this—some can be changed, but others cannot.

### How Does Age Affect Driving?

As we grow older, we do not turn into bad drivers. Some of us stay good drivers. Others simply have changes in their ability to handle a car safely. These include:

- Changes in our bodies
- Changes in the way we think
- Health problems
- Medications

**Changes in Our Bodies.** As you age, your joints may stiffen, and muscles weaken. Turning your head to look back or steering and braking the car may become hard to do. Movements are slower and may not be as accurate. Your senses of smell, hearing, sight, touch, and taste might grow weaker.

Vision, being able to see, is a vital part of driving, but age brings changes in the lens of the eye. Eyes need more light in order to see and are more sensitive to glare. Your ability to see things on the edge of the viewing area, peripheral vision, narrows. Vision problems include cataracts, macular degeneration, and glaucoma.

- In cataracts the lens of the eye becomes cloudy, causing problems with the ability to see.

- Macular degeneration is a breakdown of material inside the eye that leads to a loss of vision in the central part of the viewing area.

- The rise in pressure inside the eye that develops in glaucoma may limit the ability to see things on the edge of the viewing area.

**Changes in the Way We Think**. You probably know your body may change with age. You may not be aware of changes in the way your mind works as you age. Some of you find your reflexes are slower. Or, you may have trouble keeping your attention fixed on one situation. You may have a hard time doing two things at once—something you have to do to drive safely. When you drive, you have to take in new information from many sources and then react. Some of you react more slowly when you find yourself in a new situation.

These are all normal changes in how your brain works as you age. There are, however, two forms of mental problems that can also affect your ability to drive:

- Depression, being "down in the dumps" for a long time, may happen to many older people, but it is not normal. It can, and should, be treated. The attention and sleep problems depressed people of any age sometimes suffer can interfere with safe driving. So can the medicine sometimes used to treat depression.

- Dementia causes serious memory, personality, and behavioral problems that the person cannot recognize. Someone with dementia may at first remember how to operate an automobile and how to travel to familiar places. However, at some point as the disease progresses, their driving abilities do become impaired. Unfortunately, people with dementia often cannot recognize when they should no longer drive.

**Health Problems**. Other illnesses common among older people can affect your ability to drive safely. For example, having arthritis, Parkinson's disease, or stroke makes it harder to handle a car safely. Sleep problems or fainting make you less alert at an age when you may already have a hard time focusing your attention. If you have an automatic defibrillator or pacemaker, your doctor might suggest that you stop driving. There is a chance that the device might cause an irregular heartbeat or dizziness while driving. Diabetes may cause nerve damage in your hands, legs, or eyes. The eye damage in diabetes is known as diabetic retinopathy. If you also have trouble controlling your blood sugar level and might be in danger of losing consciousness, you should think about giving up your license.

**Medications**. Older Americans take more prescription medicines than any other age group. They often have one or more long-term illnesses such as arthritis, diabetes, high blood pressure, and heart disease and may be taking several different drugs. Their bodies may be more sensitive to the effects of medicine on their central nervous systems. The older body may not use up a drug as quickly as a younger body does, so the drug can be active for a longer time. Sometimes a combination of medicines increases the effects of each drug on the body.

Several types of medication can make driving harder because they affect the central nervous system. Drugs that might interfere with your driving include sleep aids, medicine to treat depression, antihistamines for allergies and colds, strong painkillers, and diabetes medications. If you are taking one or more of them, talk to your doctor. Perhaps he or she could change your prescription, or help you decide if the medicine is affecting your driving.

### *Can I Be a Better Driver?*

Perhaps you already know some driving situations that are hard—night, highways, rush hour, and bad weather. You might avoid these types of driving and limit your trips to shopping and visits to the doctor. This lowers your chance of having an accident.

While driving, older drivers are most at risk while yielding right of way, turning, especially left turns, lane changing, passing, and using expressway ramps. Pay extra attention at those times. If there is no left-turn light, look for alternate routes that do provide such lights.

Most of the advice for older drivers is helpful for all drivers. Plan your trips ahead of time. Stick to streets you know. Don't drive under stress. Keep distractions, such as the fan, radio, or talking, to a minimum. Leave a big space between your car and the one in front of you. Don't drive when you are tired.

Think about taking a driving refresher class. Some car insurance companies reduce your payment if you pass such a class. The AARP (American Association of Retired Persons) sponsors the "55 ALIVE/ Driver Safety Program." Call (888) 227-7669 [(888) AARP NOW] for details about courses in your area. The American Automobile Association (AAA) has a similar class called "Safe Driving for Mature Operators." Contact your local AAA office for class information. These are eight-hour classroom courses that talk about the aging process and help drivers adjust. You might also check with a local private driving school. Ask if they have an instructor who teaches older drivers. You might want to take such a review every few years.

Certain features on your car can make driving easier. Power steering, power brakes, automatic transmission, and larger mirrors are all helpful. Keeping the headlights on at all times and having a light-colored car helps other drivers see you. Hand controls for the accelerator and brakes might be of use to someone with leg problems. Keep the headlights clean and aligned, and check the windshield wiper blades often. A rear-window defroster is a good way to keep that window clear at all times.

Air bags have saved many lives. Advanced age is not a reason for disconnecting an air bag. However, the National Highway Traffic Safety Administration suggests that air bags may not be as effective in preventing serious injury or death in people over 70 years of age as they are in younger people. Older people are more likely to be injured in a traffic accident. Their bones and blood vessels may be rigid. They might break easily. If the accident is minor, emergency personnel may not realize the possibility of internal bleeding in time. People of any age should push their seats as far back as possible from the air bags in both the steering wheel and the passenger side. Of course, everyone in the car should always wear seat belts.

## *Should I Stop Driving?*

What if you are doing all you can to be a safe driver and still wonder if you should stop driving. This is a difficult decision. There are questions to ask yourself. Do other drivers often honk at you? Have you had some accidents, even "fender benders"? Are you getting lost, even on well-known roads? Do cars or pedestrians seem to appear out of nowhere? Have family, friends, or your doctor said they were worried about your driving? Do you drive less because you are not as confident about your ability as you once were? If you answered yes to any of these, you probably should think seriously about whether or not you are still a safe driver.

There are resources that may help you make this decision. Single copies of the AARP guide, "The Older Driver Skill Assessment and Resource Guide: Creating Mobility Choices," are available free by writing AARP Fulfillment, 601 E Street, NW, Washington, DC 20049, and asking for publication D14957. The AAA Foundation for Traffic Safety has several free books, including "Drivers 55-Plus: Test Your Own Performance," that may be viewed and ordered on their website. The Hartford company offers "At The Crossroads: A Guide to Alzheimer's Disease, Dementia & Driving

There are currently no upper age limits for driving. Because people age at different rates, it is not possible to choose one age as the limit. Setting an age limit would leave some drivers on the road too long, while others would be stopped too soon. Heredity, general health, your way of life, and surroundings all influence how you age.

The hard question is whether older drivers should be tested differently and more often. A second question is what would those tests be. The usual road and written tests do not look at the problem areas for older drivers. The useful-field-of-view test is being studied as one possibility. This looks at the amount of viewing area in which someone can absorb information from two different sources and how quickly they respond to it. This area becomes smaller as we age. The

111

smaller the area, the more likely one is to crash. Fortunately, this is a problem that can be improved by training. A doctor who could then certify the driver to the Department of Motor Vehicles would best perform this test.

The Mini Mental Status Exam is also a possible test used to decide if a person is no longer able to drive. This test looks at your ability to perform certain mental tasks. These tasks test those mental skills involved in driving, although they might seem different. You might be asked to copy a particular design or to count backwards from 100 by sevens. Like the useful-field-of-view test, this is not now used for testing drivers.

The aim of these tests is not to get every older driver off the road. Instead, if problem drivers can be identified, some of them could then receive training to improve their driving skills. Unfortunately, others cannot be helped by training and will have to stop driving.

### How Will I Get Around?

When planning for retirement, you should think about how you'd get around if you were no longer able to drive. Some communities provide low-cost bus or taxi service for older people. Some offer carpools or transportation on request. Religious groups sometimes have volunteers who take seniors where they need to go.

If such services are not available in your community, taxis may seem too expensive to use often. Remember that you won't have a car to maintain any longer. In fact, the AAA estimates that the cost of owning and running the average car is over $6,500 a year. By giving up your car, you might have as much as $125 a week that could be used for taxis, public transportation, or buying gas for friends and relatives who can drive you places.

You can contact your local Agency on Aging to learn about transportation services available in your area.

## Pedestrian Injuries

### The Problem

In 1999, nearly 5,000 pedestrians died from traffic-related injuries and another 85,000 sustained nonfatal injuries:

- Children 15 and younger accounted for 12 percent of all pedestrian fatalities and 32 percent of all nonfatal pedestrian injuries.

- People 65 and older accounted for 22 percent of all pedestrian deaths and approximately 8 percent of nonfatal pedestrian injuries. The pedestrian death rate for this age group is higher than for any other age group.

- The pedestrian fatality rate is more than twice as high for men as for women.

- Hit-and-run incidents account for one out of five pedestrian deaths.

- In 1999, approximately one-third of pedestrians 14 and older who were killed by a motor vehicle were intoxicated, with blood alcohol concentrations of 0.10 percent or more.

## *Just the Facts: Different People, Different Risks*

Certain racial and ethnic groups are at increased risk for pedestrian injuries. Compared with the pedestrian fatality rate for whites:

- The fatality rate for Hispanics is 1.8 times higher.

- The rate for African Americans is nearly twice as high.

- The rate for American Indians and Alaska Natives is close to three times as high.

Researchers believe that the differences in rates are due, in part, to differences in walking patterns and frequency of walking. For example, the Nationwide Personal Transportation Survey, conducted in 1995 by the Department of Transportation, found that African Americans walk 82 percent more than whites. Environmental and socioeconomic factors are also likely to contribute to these rate differences.

# Section 5.2

# *Home Safety*

Reprinted with permission from *Safe at Home: Everyday Tips on How to Make Your Home More Safe*, a brochure produced by Magee Rehabilitation Hospital, Philadelphia PA. © 2003 Magee Rehabilitation. For additional information, visit http://www.mageerehab.org.

Sometimes the very place you count on for comfort and relaxation can also be filled with hidden dangers. Our Safe at Home program points out some common risks that can lead to injury in the home.

Whether you are young or old, able-bodied or physically challenged, you should feel safe at home. Here are some easy tips to help you improve the safety and accessibility of your home.

## *Safe in Your Bathroom*

Tubs/shower equipment can be adapted to improve both safety and independence. Use hand-held shower heads, long-handled sponges, simple tub benches and skid-proof rubber mats. Shower curtains are safer than shower doors.

Toilets can be installed with a wide variety of enhancements to improve safety such as simple grab bars or specially designed commode chairs.

Pipes that are exposed should be insulated to prevent burns and scrapes. This is important if you have toddlers who can squeeze into small places.

Faucets can be converted to a single lever handle. Some even operate with a sensor eye so you don't need to use your hands at all.

Skid-proof rugs or rubber mats are recommended for the floor in front of the sink to avoid slipping on wet spots.

Never lock the bathroom door in case someone needs to reach you in an emergency.

To improve accessibility:

• Widen doorways by removing moldings

• Remove vanities

• Install long-levered door handles

## Safe in Your Kitchen

Cabinets often have shelves that are too high to reach safely. Store frequently used items on the lowest shelf, at waist level, or on the counter. Avoid using step stools and never stand on a chair to reach high items.

Drawers that contain knives or other sharp tools should be neatly arranged and in an area where there's lots of light. Never reach into a drawer without looking.

Skid-proof rugs or rubber mats are recommended for the floor in front of the sink to avoid slipping on wet spots.

To improve accessibility:

• Remove cabinetry underneath counters

• Hang cabinets no higher than 4½ feet from the floor

• Set electric switches or outlets in kitchen counters

• Consider a side-by-side refrigerator

## Safe Outside

Gutters/windows need to be cleaned; but if this requires a step ladder, make sure someone is bracing it for you, and don't overextend your reach.

Porch and stair railings should be checked regularly. Make certain that they're securely anchored. If they're loose, have them repaired immediately.

Cracks in cement walks or stairways need to be patched before they spread and become even more hazardous.

## Safe from Falls

Falls in the home are a leading cause of serious injury, especially among the elderly. Have a doctor check hearing, vision, or foot problems. Many of these problems increase your danger of falling.

Stairs and halls must be well lit at all times. Illuminated light switch plates make it easier to find light switches; they are inexpensive and easy to install. Use sturdy handrails when walking down steps; consider installing handrails for hallways. Tack down loose carpeting everywhere in your home, especially on steps. Consider removing loose throw rugs from your home because they can easily cause you to fall.

Furniture should be carefully arranged to provide plenty of walking room. Use chairs with strong backs and sturdy armrests and tables with four legs (not tripod or pedestal tables).

To improve accessibility:

- Make sure that light switches are easy to reach
- Carefully arrange furniture to provide plenty of space for a wheelchair or walker

## *Every Home Is Different*

Use a common-sense approach to your own home, and you will be able to do a lot to make it more secure. If you keep tripping over the same chair, move it. If you've ever slipped in the bathroom, don't automatically assume it was clumsiness. Think about the source of the problem and try to correct it. Most of all, be conscious of your surroundings. Walking down cellar steps without proper lighting or feeling your way to a bedroom in the dark can be invitations to disaster. Remember, accidents in the home are a leading cause of serious injury.

You need to take action to correct any household problems. Some modifications may cost nothing, like rearranging furniture. Some changes may require modest purchases like brighter light bulbs and rubber mats.

If you cannot fix these household problems yourself, enlist a family member or friend, or contact us for the name of a qualified contractor. The suggestions made in this brochure offer a range of options. If you're disabled, call us for a qualified rehabilitation professional who can help evaluate your individual needs.

If you take some simple steps to correct the problems you have in your home, it can be as safe as every home should be.

# Section 5.3

## *Workplace Fatalities*

Reprinted from "National Census of Fatal Occupational Injuries in 2001," Bureau of Labor Statistics, U.S. Department of Labor, September 25, 2002, http://www.bls.gov/iif/oshwc/cfoi/cfnr0008.pdf,.

A total of 8,786 fatal work injuries were reported in 2001, including fatalities related to the September 11 terrorist attacks, according to the Census of Fatal Occupational Injuries, Bureau of Labor Statistics, U.S. Department of Labor. A total of 2,886 work-related fatalities resulted from the events of September 11. Excluding these fatalities, the overall workplace fatality count was 5,900 for 2001.

## *Profile of Fatal Work Injuries Resulting from the September 11 Attacks*

Most of the more than 3,000 people killed were at work (as defined by the fatality census) in the World Trade Center or the Pentagon, were on business travel, or were crew aboard the commercial airliners that crashed in Pennsylvania, New York City, and Virginia, or were involved in rescue duties. The events of that day killed 2,886 workers from a wide range of backgrounds—janitors to managers, native and foreign-born workers, and the young and the old.

### *Industry*

Seventy-eight percent of the 2,198 nonrescue workers killed in the World Trade Center were working in the finance, insurance, and real estate industry. All of the 412 fatally injured rescue workers were killed at the World Trade Center; 99 percent worked for state and local government. Of the 125 workers killed at the Pentagon, 91 percent were civilian or military federal government employees. Of the 151 workers who were killed on the planes that crashed in Pennsylvania, Virginia, and New York City, 39 percent were employed in the services industry.

117

## *Occupation*

Of the rescue workers fatally injured, 335 were firefighters and 61 were police or detectives. Fifty percent of the other workers fatally injured in the World Trade Center were employed as managerial or professional specialty workers. Forty-three percent of the workers fatally injured at the Pentagon were working in military occupations and slightly less than half, 47 percent, were working in civilian managerial and professional specialty occupations. Twenty-five of the workers killed on the passenger airliners were flight attendants; eight were pilots. The majority of the workers killed on the airliners, 69 percent, were in managerial and professional specialty occupations.

## *Worker Characteristics*

Of the fatally injured workers in the World Trade Center, 66 percent were between the ages of 25 and 44, 9 percent were black, 10 percent were Hispanic, and 26 percent were women. Of those working in the Pentagon office building, 54 percent were between the ages of 25 and 44, 33 percent were black, 4 percent were Hispanic, and 37 percent were women. Of the workers involved in the rescue efforts, 70 percent were between the ages of 25 and 44. Ninety-nine percent were male. Of the workers on the passenger airliners, 62 percent were men, 7 percent were black, and 5 percent were Hispanic.

Overall, two-thirds of the workers fatally injured on September 11 were over 34 years old and 23 percent were women. Almost 20 percent of the workers were foreign-born.

## *Profiles of 2001 Fatal Work Injuries Excluding Fatalities Resulting from the September 11 Attacks*

Excluding the fatalities on September 11, the overall workplace fatality count of 5,900 for 2001 was down slightly, less than 1 percent from 2000. Total employment also declined slightly in 2001. As a result, the occupational fatality rate was the same in 2001 as in 2000, 4.3 fatalities per 100,000 employed.

The construction industry, with fatalities at their highest level since the fatality census was first conducted in 1992, continued to report the largest number of fatal work injuries of any industry. From 2000 to 2001, decreases in fatalities from transportation incidents and job-related homicides were offset by increases in fatalities from falls and from electrocutions.

## Profile of 2001 Fatal Work Injuries (Excluding September 11) by Type of Incident

Fatalities resulting from transportation incidents decreased for the third year in a row, from 2,573 in 2000 to 2,517 in 2001. Highway incidents, however, increased about 3 percent from 2000 and continued to be the leading cause of on-the-job fatalities. Fatal work injuries resulting from workers being struck by vehicles or mobile equipment also increased slightly in 2001. In contrast, the number of workers killed in nonhighway incidents, aircraft incidents, and railway incidents decreased. Nonhighway fatal incidents, which include tractor and forklift overturns, were at their lowest levels since the census began in 1992 (see Figure 5.1).

Work-related homicides, at 639 (excluding fatalities resulting from September 11), fell to their lowest levels since the census began; the record high was 1,080 in 1994. Homicides among technical, sales, and administrative support workers decreased 14 percent to 203 fatalities. However, homicides increased sharply among workers in service

**Number of fatalities**

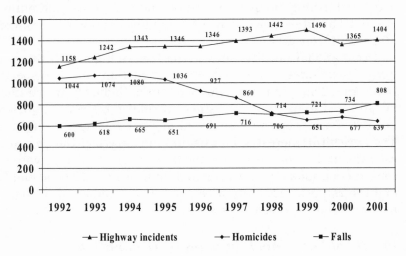

SOURCE: US Department of Labor, Bureau of Labor Statistics, Census of Fatal Occupational Injuries, 2001

**Figure 5.1.** The three most frequent work-related fatal events, 1992–2001.

occupations, which include police and detectives, food preparation workers, barbers, and hairdressers. The number of workplace suicides and fatal assaults by animals increased slightly.

Fatalities resulting from falls increased to 808 in 2001, a 10 percent rise over 2000 levels. This was the highest total since the fatality census began in 1992. Falls to lower levels increased by 39 to 698 in 2001. Falls on the same level increased by 28 to a 10-year high of 84 in 2001.

Fatal falls in the construction industry increased 13 percent from 2000 levels and accounted for over half of all fatal falls. Worker deaths resulting from electrocutions and from fires and explosions increased to levels of the late 1990s after falling to a near 10-year low in 2000.

## *Profile of Fatal Work Injuries by Industry*

While fatalities in the construction industry increased 6 percent in 2001 to a record high, fatalities in manufacturing decreased 10 percent from 2000 to their lowest recorded level since the census began in 1992. Other industries showing decreases in work-related fatalities were transportation and public utilities, wholesale trade, and retail trade. The decrease in retail trade fatalities was largely a result of the decline in workplace homicides. Fatalities to workers in services remained relatively unchanged, while fatalities in agriculture, forestry, and fishing; finance, insurance, and real estate; and mining increased. Fatalities in government (excluding September 11) increased 10 percent from 2000.

Occupational fatality rates in 2001 were highest in the mining; agriculture; forestry and fishing; construction; and transportation industries. The fatality rate for the mining industry, which includes oil and gas extraction, remained at 30.0 fatal work injuries per 100,000 workers for the second year in a row, the highest fatality rate. The agriculture, forestry, and fishing industry had the second highest rate, at 22.8 fatalities per 100,000 employed. The private sector construction industry reported 13.3 fatalities per 100,000 employed, and the rate was 11.2 fatalities per 100,000 employed in the transportation industry (see Figure 5.2).

## *Profile of Fatal Work Injuries by Occupation*

Operators, fabricators, and laborers again recorded the largest number of fatal work injuries of any occupational group, accounting for more than one out of every three fatalities in 2001 (see Figure 5.3).

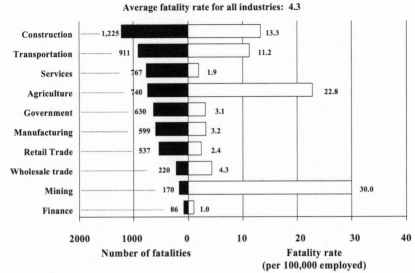

**Average fatality rate for all industries: 4.3**

SOURCE: US Department of Labor, Bureau of Labor Statistics, Census of Fatal Occupational Injuries, 2001

Rate = (Fatal work injuries/Employment) x 100,000 workers. Employment data extracted from the 2001 Current Population Survey (CPS).

**Figure 5.2.** Numbers and rates of fatal occupational injuries by industry type, 2001.

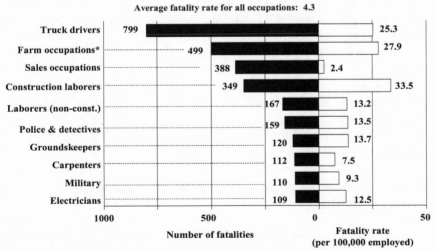

**Average fatality rate for all occupations: 4.3**

*Farm occupations include the following: Non-horticultural farmers, Non-horticultural farm managers, Farm workers, and Farm worker supervisors.

Rate = (Fatal work injuries/Employment) x 100,000 workers. Employment data extracted from the 2001 Current Population Survey (CPS). The fatality rates were calculated using employment as the denominator; employment-based rates measure the risk for those employed during a given period of time, regardless of exposure hours.

**Figure 5.3.** Numbers and rates of fatal occupational injuries for selected occupations, 2001.

However, the number of fatalities in this occupational group dropped 4 percent for the second year in a row. Most of this decrease resulted from fewer fatalities among motor vehicle operators, particularly truck drivers. There also were fewer fatalities among material moving equipment operators, machine operators, and workers in railroad transportation and water transportation. Fatalities among handlers, equipment cleaners, helpers, and laborers increased, mainly due to an increase in fatalities to construction laborers; fatalities to nonconstruction laborers decreased.

Service occupations showed an increase of 18 percent in fatalities, the highest percentage increase among the major occupation categories. Within this occupation group, police and detectives, including supervisors, had the highest number of fatalities. Fatalities in personal service occupations increased from 37 in 2000 to 59 in 2001. Precision production, craft, and repair occupations showed a small increase in the number of fatalities (3 percent). However, within this occupation group, fatalities in the extractive occupations (drillers and mining machine operators) increased from a low of 47 in 1999 to match its 10-year high of 97 fatalities in 1993.

While fatalities to truck drivers declined by 6 percent, they continued to incur more workplace fatalities than any other individual occupation. Truck drivers reported a rate of 25.3 workplace fatalities per 100,000 employed. Farm occupations had the second highest number of fatalities with 499 and rate of 27.9 fatalities, which increased from the previous year. Other occupations that typically have large numbers of worker fatalities but showed decreasing fatalities in 2001 included timber cutters, groundskeepers and gardeners, and aircraft pilots.

Fatalities to workers in military occupations increased over 25 percent from 87 in 2000 to 110 in 2001 (excluding September 11). Almost half of these fatalities resulted from aircraft crashes. The occupational fatality rate for military occupations increased in 2001 to 9.3 fatalities per 100,000 employed.

### Profile of Fatal Work Injuries by Demographic Characteristics

Fatal injuries to Hispanic or Latino workers were up 9 percent, from 815 in 2000 to 891 in 2001 (excluding September 11). This resulted from a rise in Hispanic worker fatalities in the services and agriculture industries, rather than in construction as in prior years. Fatalities to white (non-Hispanic) workers fell for the sixth year in a row; fatalities among black (non-Hispanic) workers fell for the second year in a row. Fatal work injuries to men were down slightly, although fatalities to women increased by 5 percent over 2000. The number of occupational fatalities to workers aged 17 years and younger decreased to 53 in 2001 from 73 in 2000. In 2001 fatalities to the self-employed were down by 5 percent to their lowest level recorded since 1992.

On average, about 16 workers were fatally injured each day during 2001. The total number of multiple fatality incidents (incidents that resulted in two or more worker deaths) decreased from 214 in 2000 to 197 in 2001. However, the total number of job-related deaths in multiple-fatality incidents increased from 531 in 2000 to 563 in 2001 (excluding September 11).

## *Profile of Fatal Work Injuries by State and Region*

Twenty-six states and the District of Columbia reported fewer fatal work injuries in 2001 than in 2000. The number of work injuries also declined in two of the four census regions in 2001.

# Section 5.4

## *Preventing Firearm Accidents*

"Preventing Firearm Injuries and Fatalities," by Richard L. Withers, J.D., associate director, Emergency Medicine, and co-director, Firearm Injury Center, Medical College of Wisconsin, July 2003. © 2003 Medical College of Wisconsin. Reprinted with permission of Medical College of Wisconsin HealthLink, http://www.healthlink.mcw.edu.

Current firearm injury research, involving three large American cities, concludes that a handgun in your home is 22 times more likely to be used to injure or kill a family member or acquaintance than an intruder. Up to 40 percent of American homes have firearms. In many homes with children, firearms are left unlocked and loaded. Preventing access to firearms by children and criminals is an important strategy to reduce the continuing toll of gun injury and death.

Nationwide, there have been nearly 30,000 firearm fatalities in each of the last four years for which data is available. According to the American Academy of Pediatrics, about one of every eight firearm deaths was a person under age 20. Suicides comprise 55 percent of all gun-related fatalities. Typical gun safety measures may not therefore be successful with this group. However, better locking mechanisms may prevent access to guns or make impulsive suicides more difficult to commit.

Physicians and medical organizations including the American Medical Association and the American Academy of Pediatrics have developed recommendations for reducing the risk of firearm injuries in the home. These strategies—for those who choose to keep a gun in the home—include safe storage practices, the use of gun locks, and the selection of firearms that have built-in safety features.

The Firearm Injury Center at the Medical College of Wisconsin provided a review of handgun safety features in the July 1999 issue of the *Journal of Trauma: Injury, Infection, and Critical Care*. The article described safety devices to prevent unauthorized use, such as trigger locks, built-in locks, lockboxes, and "personalized" handguns and also described safety devices that are designed to prevent unintended discharge of a handgun, such as thumb safeties, grip safeties, magazine disconnectors, drop safeties, and loaded chamber indicators.

The Firearm Injury Center also contributed to the 1998 publication by the American Medical Association (AMA) entitled *Physician Firearm Safety Guide*. The AMA guide includes 12 key educational points such as assuring that gun owners are fully informed about handling, storing, securing, cleaning, carrying, and firing their weapons. Some of these points may appear obvious but, given the potential consequences, they bear repeating.

The mission of the Firearm Injury Center at the Medical College of Wisconsin is to reduce firearm injuries and deaths. This is a mission on which gun owners and non–gun owners find agreement. The Center conducts objective and comprehensive research into firearm injuries to inform policy makers and the public. The Center does not advocate for or against gun policies, but it does evaluate the effectiveness of policies, programs, and strategies for reducing firearm injuries. The Center's programs are based on a public health approach that better data can lead to safer guns and fewer injuries.

## Gathering Data

Gathering better information about gun-related events is essential to developing effective prevention efforts. Currently, such data is not collected in a uniform manner. Firearms and tobacco are the only consumer products not subject to national product safety oversight. *Toy guns and BB guns have safety oversight, but not firearms.*

The Firearm Injury Center has established a model firearm injury reporting system (FIRS) that links law enforcement, medical examiners, coroners, and health care providers. The goal is to develop a national data system like the one used in vehicle crashes. Two additional linkages with federal firearms tracing data and with criminal background information have recently been added to the reporting system. The Center, which includes members of the National Rifle Association on its board of advisors, has provided advice and consultation to the U.S. Department of the Treasury, as well as to the United Nations, which continues to address illicit trafficking of firearms around the world.

In Milwaukee, Wisconsin, the center has examined the city's gun buyback programs, in which residents are paid for turning in guns. It found that the types of guns taken out of circulation were usually not the kind associated with firearm fatalities. Thus, the Center recommends that buyback programs consider a focus on handguns with barrels shorter than four inches because they are more highly associated with firearm fatalities.

The Center also examined the effect of the 1994 federal assault weapon ban in Milwaukee County. It found that few of the firearm fatalities involved assault weapons and there was no statistical difference before and after the ban. However, after the ban, there was a significant increase in the number of assault weapons found at the scene of the crime that were not associated with a killing. Assault weapons may have become more popular after the ban as a gun that perpetrators carry for show but not necessarily to use.

## Better Design

The Firearm Injury Center takes the position that firearms, like other consumer products, can be more safely designed. For example, a number of makes and models of pistols, as well as long guns, will fire if they are dropped. Devices such as loaded chamber indicators can be inexpensively incorporated into the manufacture of a firearm. And there are other design features such as grip safeties that gun manufacturers have known about for over a century that can make firearms safer. But most firearms do not incorporate grip safeties.

In the 1800s, a pistol was produced by Smith & Wesson and marketed as being safer, particularly in homes with young children, because it had a built-in grip safety. Known as a "lemon squeezer," the safety lever had to be pressed at the same time as the trigger for the gun to fire. Some of today's firearms have the same feature. Another safety feature available today is a loaded chamber indicator that lets the user know the gun is loaded and ready to fire. In the case of a semi-automatic pistol, a round of ammunition may remain in the firing chamber even when the magazine is removed. Some firearms today can't be fired at all if the magazine is removed—even if there's a round in the chamber.

From the early 1900s to post–World War II, the U.S. Army equipped soldiers with pistols produced by Colt's Manufacturing Company that had grip safeties, magazine disconnectors and a number of other safety features. This model, the Colt 1911A, now out of production, has been widely copied, but not uniformly with the same safety features.

In addition to the design changes described above, there are a variety of devices that can be used to better secure firearms from unauthorized users.

Trigger locks can be purchased in a variety of styles designed to secure the handgun by immobilizing the trigger. The most common design covers the trigger mechanism on either side with two steel or plastic blocks that lock together. Not all firearm designs permit the use of trigger locks. Some locks are so poorly made that they can be removed with a hammer. And there have been reports of unintended firearm discharges when a trigger lock has been applied to a loaded gun. Caution is urged in the appropriate selection and use of trigger-locking mechanisms.

There are also devices that insert into the barrel or chamber and provide a physical barrier against loading a handgun. They are available in locking and nonlocking styles. Available in both keyed and combination styles, built-in, grip-mounted locks prevent the handgun from being fired by someone other than the person who has the key or combination. Few handguns come equipped with built-in locks, but such locks can be added.

Personalized guns have a built-in magnetic or electronic locking device. The owner of the weapon wears an identifying magnetic ring or radio transmitter bracelet, which unlocks the trigger. The grip is customized to perfectly fit the owner's hand, allowing for easy alignment of the ring or bracelet. Personalized guns are not yet available in the consumer market. Several manufacturers have, however, announced plans to provide personalized guns to law enforcement agencies in the near future, and several states are considering legislation that will require personalization.

Finally, lockboxes are small, portable, safe-like boxes or cases specifically designed for the storage and/or transport of handguns. The lockbox is the device most often used by police to prevent unauthorized access to a handgun.

# Chapter 6

# COPD: Chronic Obstructive Pulmonary Disease

## Breathless in America: Background on COPD

### What Is COPD?

Chronic obstructive pulmonary disease (COPD) is an umbrella term used to describe airflow obstruction that is associated mainly with emphysema and chronic bronchitis.

- Emphysema causes irreversible lung damage by weakening and breaking the air sacs within the lungs. As a result, elasticity of the lung tissue is lost, causing airways to collapse and obstruction of airflow to occur.

- Chronic bronchitis is an inflammatory disease that begins in the smaller airways within the lungs and gradually advances to larger airways. It increases mucus in the airways and increases bacterial infections in the bronchial tubes, which, in turn, impedes airflow.

---

"Breathless in America: Background on COPD" and "American Lung Association® Fact Sheet: Chronic Obstructive Pulmonary Disease (COPD)" are reprinted with permission. © 2003 American Lung Association. For more information on how you can support the fight against lung disease, the third leading cause of death in the United States, please contact the American Lung Association at (800) LUNG-USA [(800) 586-4872], or visit the website at http:// www.lungusa.org.

## How Prevalent Is COPD?

The exact prevalence of COPD is not well defined, yet it affects tens of millions of Americans and is a serious health problem in the U.S.:

- In 1994, it was estimated that 16 million patients have been diagnosed with some form of COPD and as many as 16 million more are undiagnosed.[1]

- New government data based on a 1998 prevalence survey suggest that 3 million Americans have been diagnosed with emphysema and 9 million are affected by chronic bronchitis.[2]

- COPD was the fourth leading cause of death in the U.S. in 1998.[3]

- COPD accounted for 112,584 deaths in 1998.[3]

- COPD accounted for an estimated 668,362 hospital discharges in 1998.[4]

## What Are the Risk Factors for COPD?

Long-term smoking is the most frequent cause of COPD. It accounts for 80 to 90 percent of all cases. A smoker is 10 times more likely than a nonsmoker to die of COPD.

Other risk factors include:

- Heredity
- Second-hand smoke
- Exposure to air pollution at work and in the environment
- A history of childhood respiratory infections

## What Are the Symptoms of COPD?

The symptoms of COPD include: chronic cough, chest tightness, shortness of breath, an increased effort to breathe, increased mucus production, and frequent clearing of the throat.[5]

## How Does COPD Have an Impact on a Patient's Life?

COPD decreases the lungs' ability to take in oxygen and remove carbon dioxide. As the disease progresses, the walls of the lungs' small airways and alveoli lose their elasticity. The airway walls collapse, closing off some of the smaller air passages and narrowing larger ones. The passageways become clogged with mucus. Air continues to reach the alveoli when the lungs expand during inhalation; however, it is often unable to escape during exhalation because the air passages tend to collapse during exhalation, trapping the "stale" air in the lungs.

A typical course of COPD might begin after a person has been smoking for 10 years, during which symptoms are usually not very noticeable. Then the patient begins developing a productive, chronic cough. Usually, after age 40, the patient may begin developing shortness of breath during exertion, which continues and worsens over time.[5]

Though the severity may vary, COPD patients have some degree of airway obstruction. While symptoms may vary over time, the patient will notice a gradual deterioration over the course of four to five years. Repeated and increased productive coughing begins to disable patients, who over time take longer to recover from these attacks.[5]

Many patients with severe COPD-related lung damage have so much difficulty breathing when lying down that they sleep in a semi-sitting up position. For COPD patients, the combination of too little oxygen and too much carbon dioxide in the blood may also have an impact on the brain, and can cause a variety of other health problems, including headache, sleeplessness, impaired mental ability, and irritability.[5]

The clinical development of COPD is typically described in three stages, as defined by the American Thoracic Society:

- Stage 1: Lung function (as measured by FEV1 or forced expiratory volume in one second) is greater than or equal to 50 percent of predicted normal lung function. There is minimal impact on health-related quality of life. Symptoms may progress during this stage, and patients may begin to experience severe breathlessness, requiring evaluation by a pulmonologist.[5]

- Stage 2: FEV1 lung function is 35 to 49 percent of predicted normal lung function, and there is a significant impact on health-related quality of life.[5]

- Stage 3: FEV1 lung function is less than 35 percent of predicted normal lung function, and there is a profound impact on health-related quality of life.[5]

## What Can COPD Patients Do to Help Themselves Live As Normal a Life As Possible?

The best weapon against COPD is prevention: avoiding or ceasing smoking. Avoiding smoking almost always prevents COPD from developing, and ceasing smoking slows the disease process.

Pulmonary rehabilitation programs and medical treatment can be useful for certain patients with COPD. The key goal should be to improve physical endurance in order to overcome the conditions that cause shortness of breath and limit capacity for physical exercise and daily activities.[5]

## What Are the Goals of COPD Care?

It is important to identify and treat COPD at the earliest time possible in its natural history. Unfortunately, the diagnosis of COPD is frequently made when patients are in their late fifties or sixties, when FEV1 has declined to a symptomatic range, and when quality of life is rapidly deteriorating. Therefore, the goal of any physician treating patients with COPD is to help relieve their patients' symptoms, to help patients better manage the effects of their disease and to live as full and active lives as possible.

If patients work closely with physicians to develop a complete respiratory care program, they can:

- Improve lung function
- Reduce hospitalizations
- Prevent acute episodes
- Minimize disability
- Delay early death[5]

## What Are the Key Components of COPD Care?

In addition to smoking cessation, depending upon the severity of the disease, treatments may include bronchodilators that open up air passages in the lungs, antibiotics, and exercise to strengthen muscles. People with COPD may eventually require supplemental oxygen and, in the end stages of the disease, may have to rely on mechanical respiratory assistance.

*1. Medications that are prescribed for people with COPD may include:*

- Fast-acting beta2-agonists, such as albuterol, which can help to open narrowed airways.[5]

- Anticholinergic bronchodilators, such as ipratropium bromide, and theophylline derivatives, all of which help to open narrowed airways.[5]

- Long-acting bronchodilators, which help relieve constriction of the airways and help to prevent bronchospasm associated with COPD.

- Inhaled or oral corticosteroids, which help reduce inflammation.[6] Currently, the role of these anti-inflammatory medications in COPD therapy is not well defined, and they are not yet indicated for COPD in the U.S. However, clinical trials are under way.

- Antibiotics, which are often given at the first sign of a respiratory infection to prevent further damage and infection in diseased lungs.[5]

- Expectorants, which help loosen and expel mucus secretions from the airways and may help make breathing easier.

In addition, other medications may be prescribed to manage conditions associated with COPD. These may include:

- Diuretics, which are given as therapy to avoid excess water retention associated with right-heart failure, which may occur in some COPD patients.[5]

- Digitalis (usually in the form of digoxin), which strengthens the force of the heartbeat. It is used with caution in COPD patients, especially if their blood oxygen tensions are low, since they become vulnerable to arrhythmia when taking this drug.[5]

- Painkillers, cough suppressants, and sleeping pills, which should be used only with caution, because they depress breathing to some extent.[5]

*2. People with COPD can better manage their disease by:*

- *Avoiding*:
  - Cigarettes, dust, air pollution, cigarette smoke, and work-related fumes
  - Contact with people who have respiratory infections, such as colds and flu
  - Excessive heat, cold, or high altitudes[5]
- *Maintaining*:
  - A healthy diet and an exercise program supervised by a health care provider.

- Regular contact and visits with a health care provider so that he or she can carefully monitor the disease; this includes having regular spirometry tests.[5]

*3. Additional treatment options for patients with COPD may include:*

- Regular immunizations, such as for flu and pneumococcal pneumonia

- Pulmonary rehabilitation, which can improve exercise tolerance

- The use of supplemental oxygen, especially in patients in the later stages of COPD

- Bullectomy, or surgical removal of large air spaces in the lungs

- Lung volume reduction surgery, which is currently considered experimental

- Lung transplantation, which also has proven effective in some end-stage COPD patients

## *Sources*

1. Petty TL, "A new national strategy for COPD." *J. Resp. Dis.* 1997;18(4):365–369.

2. National Center for Health Statistics, National Health Interview Survey, 1982–1989, 1997–1998. Information cited in: American Lung Association, Epidemiology and Statistics Unit, *Trends in Chronic Bronchitis and Emphysema: Morbidity and Mortality,* December, 2000.

3. National Center for Health Statistics, Report of Final Morbidity Statistics, 1998. Information cited in: American Lung Association, *Trends in Chronic Bronchitis and Emphysema: Morbidity and Mortality*, December, 2000.

4. National Center for Health Statistics, National Hospital Discharge Survey, 1998. Information cited in: American Lung Association, *Trends in Chronic Bronchitis and Emphysema: Morbidity and Mortality*, December, 2000.

5. National Institutes of Health, "COPD Questions and Answers." Available at www.nih.gov., p. 4–7.

6. *Physicians' Desk Reference.* 1998; 52:705–6. Medical Economics Company, Inc., Montvale, NJ.

## Chronic Pulmonary Obstructive Disease

Chronic obstructive pulmonary disease (COPD) includes emphysema and chronic bronchitis—diseases that are characterized by obstruction to air flow. Emphysema and chronic bronchitis frequently coexist. Thus physicians prefer the term COPD. It does not include other obstructive diseases such as asthma. COPD, which is the fourth leading cause of death, claims the lives of 119,524 Americans annually.

- The annual cost to the nation for COPD is approximately $30.4 billion, including health care expenditures of $14.7 billion and indirect costs of $15.7 billion.

- Approximately 80 to 90 percent of COPD cases are caused by smoking; a smoker is 10 times more likely than a nonsmoker to die of COPD. Other known causes are frequent lung infections and exposure to certain industrial pollutants.

- Chronic bronchitis is an inflammation and eventual scarring of the lining of the bronchial tubes. An estimated 8.8 million people were diagnosed with chronic bronchitis in 1999.

- Females tend to have higher rates of chronic bronchitis than males.

- Symptoms of chronic bronchitis include chronic cough, increased mucus, frequent clearing of the throat, and shortness of breath.

- Emphysema causes irreversible lung damage. The walls between the air sacs within the lungs lose their ability to stretch and recoil. They become weakened and break. Elasticity of the lung tissue is lost, causing air to be trapped in the air sacs and impairing the exchange of oxygen and carbon dioxide. Also, the support of the airways is lost, allowing for obstruction of airflow.

- An estimated 2.8 million Americans have been diagnosed with emphysema sometime in their life. Of the emphysema sufferers, 58 percent are male and 42 percent are female. While more men suffer from the disease than women, the condition is increasing among women.

- Symptoms of emphysema include cough, shortness of breath, and a limited exercise tolerance. Diagnosis is made by pulmonary function tests, along with the patient's history, examination, and other tests.

- Alpha1 antitrypsin deficiency-related (AAT) emphysema is caused by the inherited deficiency of a protein called alpha1-antitrypsin (AAT) or alpha1-protease inhibitor. AAT, produced by the liver, is a "lung protector." In the absence of AAT, emphysema is almost inevitable. It is responsible for 5 percent or less of the emphysema in the United States.

- An estimated 50,000 to 100,000 Americans, primarily of northern European descent, have AAT deficiency emphysema.

- The onset of AAT deficiency emphysema, between the twenties and forties, is characterized by shortness of breath and decreased exercise capacity. Blood screening is used if the trait is suspected and can determine if a person is a carrier or AAT-deficient. If children are diagnosed as AAT-deficient through blood screening, they may undergo a liver transplant.

- Smoking significantly increases the severity of emphysema in AAT-deficient individuals.

## COPD Treatment

- The quality of life for a person suffering from COPD diminishes as the disease progresses. At the onset, there is minimal shortness of breath. People with COPD may eventually require supplemental oxygen and may have to rely on mechanical respiratory assistance.

- A recent American Lung Association (ALA) survey revealed that half of all COPD patients (51 percent) say their condition limits their ability to work. It also limits them in normal physical exertion (70 percent), household chores (56 percent), social activities (53 percent), sleeping (50 percent), and family activities (46 percent).

- None of the existing medications for COPD has been shown to modify the long-term decline in lung function that is the hallmark of this disease. Therefore, pharmacotherapy for COPD is used to decrease symptoms and/or complications.

- Bronchodilator medications are central to the symptomatic management of COPD.

- Additional treatment includes antibodies, oxygen therapy, and systemic glucocorticosteroids. The efficacy of inhaled glucocorticosteroids is under study. Chronic treatment with steroids should be avoided because of unfavorable benefit-to-risk ratio.

- Pneumonia and influenza vaccines should be given to COPD patients.

- To reduce and control symptoms of chronic bronchitis, sufferers should live a healthy lifestyle by exercising, avoiding cigarette smoke and other air pollutants, and eating well.

- Pulmonary rehabilitation is a preventive health-care program provided by a team of health professionals to help people cope physically, psychologically, and socially with COPD.

- Lung transplantation is being performed in increasing numbers and may be an option for people who suffer from severe emphysema. Additionally, lung volume reduction surgery has shown promise and is being performed with increasing frequency. However, a recent study found that emphysema patients who have severe lung obstruction with either limited ability to exchange gas when breathing or damage that is evenly distributed throughout their lungs are at high risk of death from this procedure.

- Treatments for AAT deficiency emphysema including AAT replacement therapy (a lifelong process) and gene therapy are currently being evaluated. It is hoped that a clinical trial on gene therapy will take place within the decade.

- For help with treatment decisions online, click through the COPD Lung Profiler™ (http://www.lungusa.org/diseases/index_profilerc.html).

- For more information call the American Lung Association at 1-800-LUNG-USA [(800) 586-4872], or visit our website at http://www.lungusa.org.

# Chapter 7

# *Diabetes*

## *Chapter Contents*

# Section 7.1

# *Diabetes Overview*

Excerpted from "Diabetes Overview," National Diabetes Information Clearinghouse, May 2002, http://www.niddk.nih.gov/health/diabetes/ pubs/dmover/dmover.htm. Also available as NIH Pub. No. 01-3873.

Almost everyone knows someone who has diabetes. An estimated 17 million people—6.2 percent of the population—in the United States have diabetes mellitus—a serious, lifelong condition. About 5.9 million people have not yet been diagnosed. Each year, about one million people age 20 or older are diagnosed with diabetes.

## What Is Diabetes?

Diabetes is a disorder of metabolism—the way our bodies use digested food for growth and energy. Most of the food we eat is broken

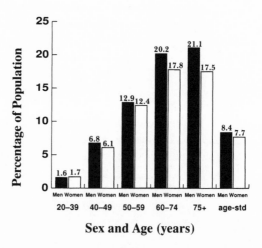

*Figure 7.1*. Prevalence of diabetes in men and women in the U.S. population age 20 years or older. More men than women suffer from the disease.

down into glucose, the form of sugar in the blood. Glucose is the main source of fuel for the body.

After digestion, glucose passes into the bloodstream, where it is used by cells for growth and energy. For glucose to get into cells, insulin must be present. Insulin is a hormone produced by the pancreas, a large gland behind the stomach.

When we eat, the pancreas is supposed to automatically produce the right amount of insulin to move glucose from blood into our cells. In people with diabetes, however, the pancreas either produces little or no insulin, or the cells do not respond appropriately to the insulin that is produced. Glucose builds up in the blood, overflows into the urine, and passes out of the body. Thus, the body loses its main source of fuel even though the blood contains large amounts of glucose.

## What Are the Types of Diabetes?

The three main types of diabetes are:

- Type 1 diabetes
- Type 2 diabetes
- Gestational diabetes

### Type 1 Diabetes

Type 1 diabetes is an autoimmune disease. An autoimmune disease results when the body's system for fighting infection (the immune system) turns against a part of the body. In diabetes, the immune system attacks the insulin-producing beta cells in the pancreas and destroys them. The pancreas then produces little or no insulin. Someone with type 1 diabetes needs to take insulin daily to live.

At present, scientists do not know exactly what causes the body's immune system to attack the beta cells, but they believe that autoimmune, genetic, and environmental factors, possibly viruses, are involved. Type 1 diabetes accounts for about 5 to 10 percent of diagnosed diabetes in the United States.

Type 1 diabetes develops most often in children and young adults, but the disorder can appear at any age. Symptoms of type 1 diabetes usually develop over a short period, although beta cell destruction can begin years earlier.

Symptoms include increased thirst and urination, constant hunger, weight loss, blurred vision, and extreme fatigue. If not diagnosed and treated with insulin, a person can lapse into a life-threatening diabetic coma, also known as diabetic ketoacidosis.

### Type 2 Diabetes

The most common form of diabetes is type 2 diabetes. About 90 to 95 percent of people with diabetes have type 2. This form of diabetes usually develops in adults age 40 and older and is most common in adults over age 55. About 80 percent of people with type 2 diabetes are overweight. Type 2 diabetes is often part of a metabolic syndrome that includes obesity, elevated blood pressure, and high levels of blood lipids. Unfortunately, as more children and adolescents become overweight, type 2 diabetes is becoming more common in young people.

When type 2 diabetes is diagnosed, the pancreas is usually producing enough insulin, but, for unknown reasons, the body cannot use the insulin effectively, a condition called insulin resistance. After several years, insulin production decreases. The result is the same as for type 1 diabetes—glucose builds up in the blood, and the body cannot make efficient use of its main source of fuel.

The symptoms of type 2 diabetes develop gradually. They are not as sudden in onset as in type 1 diabetes. Some people have no symptoms. Symptoms may include fatigue or nausea, frequent urination, unusual thirst, weight loss, blurred vision, frequent infections, and slow healing of wounds or sores.

### Gestational Diabetes

Gestational diabetes develops only during pregnancy. Like type 2 diabetes, it occurs more often in African Americans, American Indians, Hispanic Americans, and people with a family history of diabetes. Though it usually disappears after delivery, the mother is at increased risk of getting type 2 diabetes later in life.

## What Tests Are Recommended for Diagnosing Diabetes?

The fasting plasma glucose test is the preferred test for diagnosing type 1 or type 2 diabetes. However, a diagnosis of diabetes is made for any one of three positive tests, with a second positive test on a different day:

- A random plasma glucose value (taken any time of day) of 200 mg/dL (milligrams per deciliter) or more, along with the presence of diabetes symptoms.

142

- A plasma glucose value of 126 mg/dL or more, after a person has fasted for eight hours.

- An oral glucose tolerance test (OGTT) plasma glucose value of 200 mg/dL or more in the blood sample, taken two hours after a person has consumed a drink containing 75 grams of glucose dissolved in water. This test, taken in a laboratory or the doctor's office, measures plasma glucose at timed intervals over a three-hour period.

## What Are the Other Forms of Impaired Glucose Metabolism, Also Called Prediabetes?

People with prediabetes, a state between "normal" and "diabetes," are at risk for developing diabetes, heart attacks, and strokes. About 16 million people ages 40 to 74 in the United States have prediabetes. There are two forms of prediabetes.

### *Impaired Fasting Glucose*

A person has impaired fasting glucose (IFG) when fasting plasma glucose is 110 to 125 mg/dL. This level is higher than normal but less than the level indicating a diagnosis of diabetes.

### *Impaired Glucose Tolerance*

Impaired glucose tolerance (IGT) means that blood glucose during the oral glucose tolerance test is higher than normal but not high enough for a diagnosis of diabetes. IGT is diagnosed when the glucose level is 141 to 199 mg/dL two hours after a person is given a drink containing 75 grams of glucose.

## How Is Diabetes Managed?

Before the discovery of insulin in 1921, everyone with type 1 diabetes died within a few years after diagnosis. Although insulin is not considered a cure, its discovery was the first major breakthrough in diabetes treatment.

Today, healthy eating, physical activity, and insulin via injection or an insulin pump are the basic therapies for type 1 diabetes. The amount of insulin must be balanced with food intake and daily activities. Blood glucose levels must be closely monitored through frequent blood glucose checking.

Healthy eating, physical activity, and blood glucose testing are the basic management tools for type 2 diabetes. In addition, many people with type 2 diabetes require oral medication and insulin to control their blood glucose levels.

People with diabetes must take responsibility for their day-to-day care. Much of the daily care involves keeping blood glucose levels from going too low or too high. When blood glucose levels drop too low from certain diabetes medicines—a condition known as hypoglycemia—a person can become nervous, shaky, and confused. Judgment can be impaired. If blood glucose falls too low, a person can faint.

A person can also become ill if blood glucose levels rise too high, a condition known as hyperglycemia.

People with diabetes should see a doctor who helps them learn to manage their diabetes and monitors their diabetes control. An endocrinologist is one type of doctor who may specialize in diabetes care. In addition, people with diabetes often see ophthalmologists for eye examinations, podiatrists for routine foot care, and dietitians and diabetes educators to help teach the skills of day-to-day diabetes management.

The goal of diabetes management is to keep blood glucose levels as close to the normal range as safely possible. A major study, the Diabetes Control and Complications Trial (DCCT), sponsored by the National Institute of Diabetes and Digestive and Kidney Diseases (NIDDK), showed that keeping blood glucose levels as close to normal as safely possible reduces the risk of developing major complications of type 1 diabetes.

The 10-year study, completed in 1993, included 1,441 people with type 1 diabetes. The study compared the effect of two treatment approaches—intensive management and standard management—on the development and progression of eye, kidney, and nerve complications of diabetes. Intensive treatment aimed at keeping hemoglobin A-1-c as close to normal (6 percent) as possible. Hemoglobin A-1-c reflects average blood sugar over a two- to three-month period. Researchers found that study participants who maintained lower levels of blood glucose through intensive management had significantly lower rates of these complications. More recently, a follow-up study of DCCT participants showed that the ability of intensive control to lower the complications of diabetes persists up to four years after the trial ended.

The United Kingdom Prospective Diabetes Study, a European study completed in 1998, showed that intensive control of blood glucose and blood pressure reduced the risk of blindness, kidney disease, stroke, and heart attack in people with type 2 diabetes.

# Section 7.2

# *Lowering the Risk of Type 2 Diabetes*

Excerpted from "Am I at Risk for Type 2 Diabetes?," National Diabetes Information Clearinghouse, June 2002, http://www.niddk.nih.gov/health/ diabetes/pubs/risk/risk.htm. Also available as NIH Pub. No. 02-4805.

## *How Can Type 2 Diabetes Be Prevented?*

Although people with diabetes can prevent or delay complications by keeping blood glucose levels close to normal, preventing or delaying the development of type 2 diabetes in the first place is even better. The results of a major federally funded study, the Diabetes Prevention Program (DPP), show how to do so.

This study of 3,234 people at high risk for diabetes showed that moderate diet and exercise resulting in a 5 to 7 percent weight loss can delay and possibly prevent type 2 diabetes.

Study participants were overweight and had higher than normal levels of blood glucose, a condition called prediabetes (impaired glucose tolerance). Both pre-diabetes and obesity are strong risk factors for type 2 diabetes. Because of the high risk among some minority groups, about half of the DPP participants were African American, American Indian, Asian American, Pacific Islander, or Hispanic American/ Latino.

The DPP tested two approaches to preventing diabetes: a healthy eating and exercise program (lifestyle changes), and the diabetes drug metformin. People in the lifestyle modification group exercised about 30 minutes a day five days a week (usually by walking) and lowered their intake of fat and calories. Those who took the diabetes drug metformin received standard information on exercise and diet. A third group received only standard information on exercise and diet.

The results showed that people in the lifestyle modification group reduced their risk of getting type 2 diabetes by 58 percent. Average weight loss in the first year of the study was 15 pounds. Lifestyle modification was even more effective in those 60 and older. They reduced their risk by 71 percent. People receiving metformin reduced their risk by 31 percent.

## What Are the Signs and Symptoms of Type 2 Diabetes?

Many people have no signs or symptoms. Symptoms can also be so mild that you might not even notice them. Nearly 6 million people in the United States have type 2 diabetes and do not know it.

Here is what to look for:

- Increased thirst
- Increased hunger
- Fatigue
- Increased urination, especially at night
- Weight loss
- Blurred vision
- Sores that do not heal

Sometimes people have symptoms but do not suspect diabetes. They delay scheduling a checkup because they do not feel sick. Many people do not find out they have the disease until they have diabetes complications, such as blurry vision or heart trouble. It is important to find out early if you have diabetes because treatment can prevent damage to the body from diabetes.

## Should I Be Tested for Diabetes?

Anyone 45 years old or older should consider getting tested for diabetes. If you are 45 or older and overweight, it is strongly recommended that you get tested. If you are younger than 45, overweight, and have one or more of the risk factors, you should consider testing. Ask your doctor for a fasting blood glucose test or an oral glucose tolerance test.

Even if your blood glucose level is normal and you have no risk factors, if you are over 45, you may need to remind your doctor to check your blood glucose again in three years. If your blood glucose is higher than normal but lower than the diabetes range (what we now call prediabetes), have your blood glucose checked in one to two years. As you get older, your chances of getting type 2 diabetes rise. You are also more likely to get type 2 diabetes if you have one or more of the risk factors.

# Besides Age and Overweight, What Other Factors Increase My Risk for Type 2 Diabetes?

To find out your risk for type 2 diabetes, check each item that applies to you:

- I have a parent, brother, or sister with diabetes.
- My family background is African American, American Indian, Asian American, Pacific Islander, or Hispanic American/Latino.
- My blood pressure is 140/90 or higher, or I have been told that I have high blood pressure.
- My cholesterol levels are not normal. My HDL cholesterol ("good" cholesterol) is 35 or lower, or my triglyceride level is 250 or higher.
- I am fairly inactive. I exercise fewer than three times a week.

## What Can I Do about My Risk?

You can do a lot to lower your chances of getting diabetes. Exercising regularly, reducing fat and calorie intake, and losing weight can all help you reduce your risk of developing type 2 diabetes. Lowering blood pressure and cholesterol levels also help you stay healthy.

### *If You Are Overweight*

Then take these steps:

- Reach and maintain a reasonable body weight.
- Make wise food choices most of the time.
- Be physically active every day.

### *If You Are Fairly Inactive*

Then take this step:

- Be physically active every day.

### *If You Have Blood Pressure of 140/90 or Higher*

Then take these steps:

- Reach and maintain a reasonable body weight.

- Make wise food choices most of the time.
- Reduce your intake of salt and alcohol.
- Be physically active every day.
- Talk to your doctor about whether you need medicine to control your blood pressure.

### *If Your Cholesterol Levels Are Not Normal*

Then take these steps:

- Make wise food choices most of the time.
- Be physically active every day.
- Talk to your doctor about whether you need medicine to control your cholesterol levels.

## Doing My Part: Getting Started

Making big changes in your life is hard, especially if you are faced with more than one change. You can make it easier by taking these steps:

- Make a plan to change behavior.
- Decide exactly what you will do and when you will do it.
- Plan what you need to get ready.
- Think about what might prevent you from reaching your goals.
- Find family and friends who will support and encourage you.
- Decide how you will reward yourself when you do what you have planned.

Your doctor, a dietitian, or a counselor can help you make a plan. Here are some of the areas you may wish to change to reduce your risk of diabetes.

### *Reach and Maintain a Reasonable Body Weight*

Your weight affects your health in many ways. Being overweight can keep your body from making and using insulin properly. It can also cause high blood pressure. The DPP showed that losing even a few pounds can help reduce your risk of developing type 2 diabetes because it helps your body use insulin more effectively. In the DPP, people who lost between 5 and 7 percent of their body weight significantly reduced their risk of type 2 diabetes. For example, if you weigh 200 pounds, losing only 10 pounds could make a difference.

Body mass index (BMI) is a measure of body weight relative to height. You can use BMI to see whether you are underweight, normal weight, overweight, or obese. Use the body mass index table in Figure 7.2 to find your BMI.

- Find your height in the left-hand column.

- Move across in the same row to the number closest to your weight.

- The number at the top of that column is your BMI. Check the word above your BMI to see whether you are normal weight, overweight, or obese.

If you are overweight or obese, choose sensible ways to get in shape:

- Avoid crash diets. Instead, eat less of the foods you usually have. Limit the amount of fat you eat.

- Increase your physical activity. Aim for at least 30 minutes of exercise most days of the week.

- Set a reasonable weight-loss goal, such as losing one pound a week. Aim for a long-term goal of losing 5 to 7 percent of your total body weight.

## *Make Wise Food Choices Most of the Time*

What you eat has a big impact on your health. By making wise food choices, you can help control your body weight, blood pressure, and cholesterol.

- Take a hard look at the serving sizes of the foods you eat. Reduce serving sizes of main courses (such as meat), desserts, and foods high in fat. Increase the amount of fruits and vegetables.

- Limit your fat intake to about 25 percent of your total calories. For example, if your food choices add up to about 2,000 calories a day, try to eat no more than 56 grams of fat. Your doctor or a dietitian can help you figure out how much fat to have. You can check food labels for fat content too.

- You may also wish to reduce the number of calories you have each day. People in the DPP lifestyle modification group lowered

## Body Mass Index Table

| | Normal | | | | | | Overweight | | | | | Obese | | | | | | | | | | Extreme Obesity | | | | | | | | | | | | | | |
|---|---|---|---|---|---|---|---|---|---|---|---|---|---|---|---|---|---|---|---|---|---|---|---|---|---|---|---|---|---|---|---|---|---|---|---|---|
| BMI | 19 | 20 | 21 | 22 | 23 | 24 | 25 | 26 | 27 | 28 | 29 | 30 | 31 | 32 | 33 | 34 | 35 | 36 | 37 | 38 | 39 | 40 | 41 | 42 | 43 | 44 | 45 | 46 | 47 | 48 | 49 | 50 | 51 | 52 | 53 | 54 |
| Height (inches) | | | | | | | | | | | | Body Weight (pounds) | | | | | | | | | | | | | | | | | | | | | | | | |
| 58 | 91 | 96 | 100 | 105 | 110 | 115 | 119 | 124 | 129 | 134 | 138 | 143 | 148 | 153 | 158 | 162 | 167 | 172 | 177 | 181 | 186 | 191 | 196 | 201 | 205 | 210 | 215 | 220 | 224 | 229 | 234 | 239 | 244 | 248 | 253 | 258 |
| 59 | 94 | 99 | 104 | 109 | 114 | 119 | 124 | 128 | 133 | 138 | 143 | 148 | 153 | 158 | 163 | 168 | 173 | 178 | 183 | 188 | 193 | 198 | 203 | 208 | 212 | 217 | 222 | 227 | 232 | 237 | 242 | 247 | 252 | 257 | 262 | 267 |
| 60 | 97 | 102 | 107 | 112 | 118 | 123 | 128 | 133 | 138 | 143 | 148 | 153 | 158 | 163 | 168 | 174 | 179 | 184 | 189 | 194 | 199 | 204 | 209 | 215 | 220 | 225 | 230 | 235 | 240 | 245 | 250 | 255 | 261 | 266 | 271 | 276 |
| 61 | 100 | 106 | 111 | 116 | 122 | 127 | 132 | 137 | 143 | 148 | 153 | 158 | 164 | 169 | 174 | 180 | 185 | 190 | 195 | 201 | 206 | 211 | 217 | 222 | 227 | 232 | 238 | 243 | 248 | 254 | 259 | 264 | 269 | 275 | 280 | 285 |
| 62 | 104 | 109 | 115 | 120 | 126 | 131 | 136 | 142 | 147 | 153 | 158 | 164 | 169 | 175 | 180 | 186 | 191 | 196 | 202 | 207 | 213 | 218 | 224 | 229 | 235 | 240 | 246 | 251 | 256 | 262 | 267 | 273 | 278 | 284 | 289 | 295 |
| 63 | 107 | 113 | 118 | 124 | 130 | 135 | 141 | 146 | 152 | 158 | 163 | 169 | 175 | 180 | 186 | 191 | 197 | 203 | 208 | 214 | 220 | 225 | 231 | 237 | 242 | 248 | 254 | 259 | 265 | 270 | 278 | 282 | 287 | 293 | 299 | 304 |
| 64 | 110 | 116 | 122 | 128 | 134 | 140 | 145 | 151 | 157 | 163 | 169 | 174 | 180 | 186 | 192 | 197 | 204 | 209 | 215 | 221 | 227 | 232 | 238 | 244 | 250 | 256 | 262 | 267 | 273 | 279 | 285 | 291 | 296 | 302 | 308 | 314 |
| 65 | 114 | 120 | 126 | 132 | 138 | 144 | 150 | 156 | 162 | 168 | 174 | 180 | 186 | 192 | 198 | 204 | 210 | 216 | 222 | 228 | 234 | 240 | 246 | 252 | 258 | 264 | 270 | 276 | 282 | 288 | 294 | 300 | 306 | 312 | 318 | 324 |
| 66 | 118 | 124 | 130 | 136 | 142 | 148 | 155 | 161 | 167 | 173 | 179 | 186 | 192 | 198 | 204 | 210 | 216 | 223 | 229 | 235 | 241 | 247 | 253 | 260 | 266 | 272 | 278 | 284 | 291 | 297 | 303 | 309 | 315 | 322 | 328 | 334 |
| 67 | 121 | 127 | 134 | 140 | 146 | 153 | 159 | 166 | 172 | 178 | 185 | 191 | 198 | 204 | 211 | 217 | 223 | 230 | 236 | 242 | 249 | 255 | 261 | 268 | 274 | 280 | 287 | 293 | 299 | 306 | 312 | 319 | 325 | 331 | 338 | 344 |
| 68 | 125 | 131 | 138 | 144 | 151 | 158 | 164 | 171 | 177 | 184 | 190 | 197 | 203 | 210 | 216 | 223 | 230 | 236 | 243 | 249 | 256 | 262 | 269 | 276 | 282 | 289 | 295 | 302 | 308 | 315 | 322 | 328 | 335 | 341 | 348 | 354 |
| 69 | 128 | 135 | 142 | 149 | 155 | 162 | 169 | 176 | 182 | 189 | 196 | 203 | 209 | 216 | 223 | 230 | 236 | 243 | 250 | 257 | 263 | 270 | 277 | 284 | 291 | 297 | 304 | 311 | 318 | 324 | 331 | 338 | 345 | 351 | 358 | 365 |
| 70 | 132 | 139 | 146 | 153 | 160 | 167 | 174 | 181 | 188 | 195 | 202 | 209 | 216 | 222 | 229 | 236 | 243 | 250 | 257 | 264 | 271 | 278 | 285 | 292 | 299 | 306 | 313 | 320 | 327 | 334 | 341 | 348 | 355 | 362 | 369 | 376 |
| 71 | 136 | 143 | 150 | 157 | 165 | 172 | 179 | 186 | 193 | 200 | 208 | 215 | 222 | 229 | 236 | 243 | 250 | 257 | 265 | 272 | 279 | 286 | 293 | 301 | 308 | 315 | 322 | 329 | 338 | 343 | 351 | 358 | 365 | 372 | 379 | 386 |
| 72 | 140 | 147 | 154 | 162 | 169 | 177 | 184 | 191 | 199 | 206 | 213 | 221 | 228 | 235 | 242 | 250 | 258 | 265 | 272 | 279 | 287 | 294 | 302 | 309 | 316 | 324 | 331 | 338 | 346 | 353 | 361 | 368 | 375 | 383 | 390 | 397 |
| 73 | 144 | 151 | 159 | 166 | 174 | 182 | 189 | 197 | 204 | 212 | 219 | 227 | 235 | 242 | 250 | 257 | 265 | 272 | 280 | 288 | 295 | 302 | 310 | 318 | 325 | 333 | 340 | 348 | 355 | 363 | 371 | 378 | 386 | 393 | 401 | 408 |
| 74 | 148 | 155 | 163 | 171 | 179 | 186 | 194 | 202 | 210 | 218 | 225 | 233 | 241 | 249 | 256 | 264 | 272 | 280 | 287 | 295 | 303 | 311 | 319 | 326 | 334 | 342 | 350 | 358 | 365 | 373 | 381 | 389 | 396 | 404 | 412 | 420 |
| 75 | 152 | 160 | 168 | 176 | 184 | 192 | 200 | 208 | 216 | 224 | 232 | 240 | 248 | 256 | 264 | 272 | 279 | 287 | 295 | 303 | 311 | 319 | 327 | 335 | 343 | 351 | 359 | 367 | 375 | 383 | 391 | 399 | 407 | 415 | 423 | 431 |
| 76 | 156 | 164 | 172 | 180 | 189 | 197 | 205 | 213 | 221 | 230 | 238 | 246 | 254 | 263 | 271 | 279 | 287 | 295 | 304 | 312 | 320 | 328 | 336 | 344 | 353 | 361 | 369 | 377 | 385 | 394 | 402 | 410 | 418 | 426 | 435 | 443 |

Source: Adapted from *Clinical Guidelines on the Identification, Evaluation, and Treatment of Overweight and Obesity in Adults: The Evidence Report.*

*Figure 7.2. The body mass index (BMI) tells you at a glance whether you are normal in weight, overweight, or obese.*

their daily calorie total by an average of about 450 calories. Your doctor or dietitian can help you with a meal plan that emphasizes weight loss.

- Keep a food and exercise log. Write down what you eat, how much you exercise—anything that helps keep you on track.

- When you meet your goal, reward yourself with a nonfood item or activity, like watching a movie.

### *Be Physically Active Every Day*

Regular exercise tackles several risk factors at once. It helps you lose weight, keeps your cholesterol and blood pressure under control, and helps your body use insulin. People in the DPP who were physically active for 30 minutes a day five days a week reduced their risk of type 2 diabetes. Many chose brisk walking for exercise.

If you are not very active, you should start slowly, talking with your doctor first about what kinds of exercise would be safe for you. Make a plan to increase your activity level toward the goal of being active for at least 30 minutes a day most days of the week.

Choose activities you enjoy. Here are some ways to work extra activity into your daily routine:

- Take the stairs rather than an elevator or escalator.

- Park at the far end of the lot and walk.

- Get off the bus a few stops early and walk the rest of the way.

- Walk or bicycle instead of drive whenever you can.

### *Take Your Prescribed Medications*

Some people need medication to help control their blood pressure or cholesterol levels. If you do, take your medicines as directed. Ask your doctor whether there are any medicines you can take to prevent type 2 diabetes.

Chapter 8

# *Pneumonia and Influenza*

## *Chapter Contents*

# Section 8.1

## *Pneumococcal Pneumonia*

Reprinted from " Pneumococcal Pneumonia," National Institute of
Allergy and Infectious Diseases, August 2001, http://www.niaid.nih.gov/
factsheets/pneumonia.htm.

### *What is pneumonia?*

Pneumonia is a lung disease that can be caused by a variety of viruses, bacteria, and sometimes fungi. The U.S. Centers for Diseases Control and Prevention (CDC) estimate nearly 90,000 people in the United States died from one of several kinds of pneumonia in 1999. In the United States, pneumonia is the fifth leading cause of death. Rates of infection are three times higher in African Americans than in whites and are five to 10 times higher in Native American adults and 10 times higher in Native American children.

On an international scale, acute respiratory infection ranks as the third most frequent cause of death among children less than five years old and was responsible for approximately 3.5 million deaths in 1998.

### *What is pneumococcal pneumonia?*

Pneumococcal pneumonia is an infection in the lungs caused by bacteria called *Streptococcus pneumoniae. S. pneumoniae*, also called pneumococcus, can infect the upper respiratory tracts of adults and children and can spread to the blood, lungs, middle ear, or nervous system. CDC estimates *S. pneumoniae* causes 40,000 deaths and 500,000 cases of pneumonia annually in the United States. The yearly incidence of pneumococcal pneumonia is twice as high in African Americans as in whites and is responsible for 3,000 cases of meningitis (inflammation of spinal cord membranes), 50,000 cases of bacteremia (bacteria in the blood), and 7 million cases of otitis media (inner ear infection).

According to the World Health Organization, *S. pneumoniae* is the leading cause of severe pneumonia worldwide in children younger than five years old, causing more than one million deaths in children each year.

Pneumococcal pneumonia primarily causes illness in children younger than two years old and adults 65 years of age or older. The elderly are especially vulnerable to getting seriously ill and dying from this disease. In addition, people with certain medical conditions such as chronic heart, lung, or liver diseases or sickle cell anemia are also at increased risk for getting pneumococcal pneumonia as are people with HIV infection or AIDS or people who have had organ transplants and are taking medicines that lower their resistance to infection.

## How is pneumococcus spread?

The noses and throats of up to 70 percent of healthy people contain pneumococcus at any given time. It is spread from person to person by coughing, sneezing, or close contact. Researchers don't know why it suddenly invades the lungs and the bloodstream to cause disease.

## What are the symptoms of pneumococcal pneumonia?

Pneumococcal pneumonia may begin suddenly, with a severe shaking chill usually followed by:

- High fever
- Cough
- Shortness of breath
- Rapid breathing
- Chest pains

There may be other symptoms as well:

- Nausea
- Vomiting
- Headache
- Tiredness
- Muscle aches

In an otherwise healthy adult, pneumococcal pneumonia usually involves one or more parts of the lungs, known as lobes. Thus, it is sometimes called lobar pneumonia. The remainder of the respiratory system is comparatively not affected. In contrast, infants, young children, and elderly people more commonly develop a relatively mild infection in other parts of the lungs, such as around the air vessels (bronchi), causing bronchopneumonia.

## *How is pneumococcal pneumonia diagnosed?*

A doctor or other health care provider diagnoses pneumonia based on:

- Symptoms
- Physical examination
- Laboratory tests
- Chest x-ray

Because a number of bacteria, viruses, and other infectious agents can cause pneumonia, you should get diagnosed early and start taking the right medicine if you have any of the symptoms. The presence of *S. pneumoniae* in the blood, saliva, or lung fluid helps lead to a diagnosis of pneumococcal pneumonia.

## *How is pneumococcal pneumonia treated?*

Health care providers usually prescribe antibiotics, such as penicillin, to treat this bacterial disease. The symptoms of pneumococcal pneumonia usually subside within 12 to 36 hours after treatment has begun. Bacteria such as *S. pneumoniae*, however, are resisting and fighting off the powers of antibiotics to destroy them. Such antibiotic resistance is increasing worldwide because these medicines have been overused or misused. Therefore, if you are at risk of getting pneumococcal pneumonia, you should talk with your doctor about taking steps to prevent it.

## *Can pneumococcal pneumonia be prevented?*

The pneumococcal vaccine is the only way to prevent getting pneumococcal pneumonia. Vaccines are available for children and adults.

The CDC National Immunization Program (NIP) recommends that you get immunized against pneumococcal pneumonia if you are in any of the following groups.

- You are 65 years old or older.
- You have a serious long-term health problem such as heart disease, sickle cell disease, alcoholism, leaks of cerebrospinal fluid, lung disease (not including asthma), diabetes, or liver cirrhosis.

- Your resistance to infection is lowered due to HIV infection or AIDS; lymphoma, leukemia, or other cancers; cancer treatment with x-rays or drugs; treatment with long-term steroids; bone marrow or organ transplant; kidney failure; nephrotic (kidney) syndrome; damaged spleen or no spleen.

- You are an Alaskan Native or from certain Native American populations.

In February 2000, the U.S. Food and Drug Administration approved a pneumococcal vaccine for use in toddlers and children. It is the first pneumococcal vaccine approved for children younger than two years old. NIP recommends that all children ages two to 23 months old get this vaccine.

### Does pneumococcal pneumonia cause complications?

In about 30 percent of people with pneumococcal pneumonia, the bacteria invade the bloodstream from the lungs. This causes bacteremia, a very serious disease. Pneumococcal pneumonia also can cause other lung problems and certain heart problems.

### What research is going on?

The National Institute of Allergy and Infectious Diseases (NIAID) supports research on more effective prevention and treatment approaches to control pneumonia and its causes. These include:

- Developing and licensing vaccines and treatments for the disease-causing microbes (pathogens) that cause pneumonia

- Stimulating research on the structure and function of these pathogens

- Developing better and more rapid diagnostic tools

- Understanding the long-term health impact respiratory pathogens have in various populations

- Examining the effect of vaccines in high-risk populations

- Determining how pneumococcus becomes resistant to antibiotics

The recently approved pneumococcal conjugate vaccine for children is partially the result of crucial NIAID research in the early development of the vaccine. This vaccine helps prevent pneumococcal diseases in babies and toddlers and is the latest advance in developing vaccines against common bacterial infections. This effort was led in large part by NIAID for more than 30 years.

NIAID supports studies to develop improved pneumococcal conjugate vaccines for children worldwide. In one such study, NIAID researchers are working with The Gambia government and scientists from several international research institutions to test a pneumococcal conjugate vaccine in The Gambia, West Africa. Health care experts have consistently identified pneumococcus as the most common cause of bacterial pneumonia in The Gambia. In a pattern typical of many developing areas, infant and child mortality rates in The Gambia are high, acute respiratory infections are a leading cause of death, and pneumococcus is the most common cause of these infections.

## Section 8.2

# *What to Do about the Flu*

Reprinted from "What to Do about the Flu," National Institute on Aging, 2000, http://www.nia.nih.gov/health/agepages/flu.htm.

Each winter, millions of people suffer from the flu, a highly contagious infection. It spreads easily from person to person mainly when an infected person coughs or sneezes. Flu—the short name for influenza—is caused by viruses that infect the nose, throat, and lungs. It usually is a mild disease in healthy children, young adults, and middle-aged people. However, flu can be life-threatening in older adults and in people of any age who have chronic illnesses such as diabetes or heart, lung, or kidney diseases.

### *Can flu be prevented?*

A flu shot can greatly lower your chances of getting the flu. Much of the illness and death caused by flu can be prevented by a yearly flu shot.

The cost of the flu shot is covered by Medicare. Many private health insurance plans also pay for the flu shot. You can get a flu shot at your doctor's office. You also may be able to get a flu shot from your local health department or from other health care providers.

No vaccine gives complete protection, and the flu shot is no exception. In older people and those with certain chronic illnesses, the flu shot often is less effective in preventing flu than in reducing symptoms and the risk of serious illness and death. Studies have shown that the flu shot reduces hospitalization by about 70 percent and death by about 85 percent among older people who are not in nursing homes. Among nursing home residents, the flu shot reduces the risk of hospitalization by about 50 percent, the risk of pneumonia by about 60 percent, and the risk of death by 75 to 80 percent.

### Who should get the flu shot?

According to the federal government's Centers for Disease Control and Prevention, the following people are at risk for serious illness from the flu and should get a flu shot every year:

- People 65 years of age and older
- Residents of nursing homes and other long-term care facilities
- Adults and children who have chronic heart or lung diseases
- Adults and children with diabetes, kidney disease, or severe forms of anemia
- Health care workers in contact with people in high-risk groups
- Caregivers or people who live with someone in a high-risk group

### When is the best time to get the flu shot?

In the United States, flu season usually occurs from November until April. Most people get the flu between late December and early March. The best time to get your flu shot is between September and mid-November. It takes about one to two weeks after you get the shot to develop protection.

### Does the shot cause side effects?

The flu shot does not cause side effects in most people. Fewer than one-third of those who get the shot have some soreness, redness, or swelling on the arm where the shot is given. These side effects, which can last up to two days, rarely interfere with a person's daily activities. About 5 to 10 percent of people have mild side effects such as headache or low-grade fever for about a day after vaccination.

The flu shot is made from killed flu viruses, which cannot cause the flu. With very rare exceptions, the danger from getting flu—and possibly—is far greater than the danger from the side effects of the shot.

One of these rare exceptions is people who have a severe allergy to eggs. The viruses for flu vaccines are grown in eggs and may cause serious reactions in people who are severely allergic to eggs. People who have a severe allergy to eggs should not get the flu shot.

### Why do you need a flu shot every year?

Preventing flu is hard because flu viruses change all the time. This year's flu virus usually is slightly different from last year's virus. Every year the flu shot is updated to include the most current flu virus strains. That's one reason why flu shots will protect you for only one year.

### What are the symptoms of the flu?

Flu can cause fever, chills, dry cough, sore throat, runny or stuffy nose as well as headache, muscle aches, and often extreme fatigue. Although nausea, vomiting, and diarrhea can sometimes accompany the flu, especially in children, gastrointestinal symptoms rarely occur. The illness that people call "stomach flu" is not influenza.

It's easy to confuse a common cold with the flu. Overall, cold symptoms are milder and don't last as long as the flu.

### How serious is flu?

Most people who get the flu recover completely in one to two weeks, but some people develop serious and possibly life-threatening complications. While your body is busy fighting off the flu, you may be less able to resist a second infection. Older people and people with chronic illnesses run the greatest risk of getting secondary infections, especially pneumonia. In an average year, flu leads to about 20,000 deaths nationwide and many more hospitalizations.

### How is flu treated?

If you get the flu, rest in bed, drink plenty of fluids, and take medication such as aspirin or acetaminophen to relieve fever and discomfort.

Call your doctor if you have any signs of flu and:

- Your fever lasts; you may have a more serious infection.
- You have breathing or heart problems or other serious health problems.
- You are taking drugs to fight cancer or other drugs that weaken your body's natural defenses against illness.
- You feel sick and don't seem to be getting better.
- You have a cough that begins to produce phlegm.
- You are worried about your health.

Antibiotics are not effective against flu viruses. However, four drugs have been approved to treat people who get the flu:

- amantadine (Symmetrel®)
- rimantadine (Flumadine®)
- zanamivir (Relenza®)
- oseltamivir (Tamiflu®)

When taken within 48 hours after the onset of illness, these drugs reduce the duration of fever and other symptoms. These drugs are only available by prescription.

### What are the basic facts about flu?

- The flu can be very dangerous for people 65 and older.
- The flu can be prevented.
- A flu shot is necessary each fall for people in high-risk groups.
- The flu shot is covered by Medicare.
- The flu shot is safe. It can't cause the flu.
- The flu shot and the pneumococcal vaccine can be given at the same time.

# Chapter 9

# *Suicide*

## *In Harm's Way: Suicide in America*

Suicide is a tragic and potentially preventable public health problem. In 1997, suicide was the eighth leading cause of death in the U.S. Specifically, 10.6 out of every 100,000 persons died by suicide. The total number of suicides was approximately 31,000, or 1.3 percent of all deaths. Approximately 500,000 people received emergency room treatment as a result of attempted suicide in 1996. Taken together, the numbers of suicide deaths and attempts show the need for carefully designed prevention efforts.

Suicidal behavior is complex. Some risk factors vary with age, gender, and ethnic group and may even change over time. The risk factors for suicide frequently occur in combination. Research has shown that more than 90 percent of people who kill themselves have depression or another diagnosable mental or substance abuse disorder. In addition, research indicates that alterations in neurotransmitters such as serotonin are associated with the risk for suicide. Diminished levels of this brain chemical have been found in patients with depression, impulsive disorders, and a history of violent suicide attempts and also in postmortem brains of suicide victims.

---

Excerpted and compiled from three publications of the National Institute of Mental Health: "In Harm's Way: Suicide in America," January 1, 2001, http://www.nimh.nih.gov/publicat/harmaway.cfm, (also available as NIH Pub. No. 01-4594); "Suicide Facts," April 2003, http://www.nimh.nih.gov/research/suifact htm; and "Frequently Asked Questions about Suicide," January 3, 2000, http://www.nimh.nih.gov/research/suicidefaq.cfm.

Adverse life events in combination with other risk factors such as depression may lead to suicide. However, suicide and suicidal behavior are not normal responses to stress. Many people have one or more risk factors and are not suicidal. Other risk factors include: prior suicide attempt; family history of mental disorder or substance abuse; family history of suicide; family violence, including physical or sexual abuse; firearms in the home; incarceration; and exposure to the suicidal behavior of others, including family members, peers, and even in the media.

## Gender Differences

More than four times as many men than women die by suicide; however, women report attempting suicide about two to three times as often as men. Suicide by firearm is the most common method for both men and women, accounting for 58 percent of all suicides in 1997. Seventy-two percent of all suicides were committed by white men, and 79 percent of all firearm suicides were committed by white men. The highest suicide rate was for white men over 85 years of age—65 per 100,000 persons (see Figure 9.1).

## Attempted Suicides

There may be as many as eight attempted suicides to one completion; the ratio is higher in women and youth and lower in men and the elderly. Risk factors for attempted suicide in adults include depression, alcohol abuse, cocaine use, and separation or divorce. Risk factors for attempted suicide in youth include depression, alcohol or other drug use disorder, physical or sexual abuse, and aggressive or disruptive behaviors. The majority of suicide attempts are expressions of extreme distress and not just harmless bids for attention. A suicidal person should not be left alone and needs immediate mental health treatment.

## Prevention

All suicide prevention programs need to be scientifically evaluated to demonstrate whether or not they work. Preventive interventions for suicide must also be complex and intensive if they are to have lasting effects. Most school-based, information-only prevention programs focused solely on suicide have not been evaluated to see if they are effective, and research suggests that such programs may actually increase distress in the young people who are most vulnerable. School and community prevention programs designed to address suicide and suicidal behavior as part of a broader focus on mental health, coping skills in response to stress, substance abuse, aggressive behaviors, and so forth are more likely to be successful in the long run.

Recognition and appropriate treatment of mental and substance abuse disorders also hold great suicide prevention value. For example, because most elderly suicide victims—70 percent—have visited their primary care physician in the month prior to their suicides, improving the recognition and treatment of depression in medical settings is a promising way to prevent suicide in older adults. Toward this goal, National Institute of Mental Health–funded researchers are currently investigating the effectiveness of a depression education intervention delivered to primary care physicians and their elderly patients.

*If someone is suicidal, he or she must not be left alone. You may need to take emergency steps to get help, such as calling 911. It is also*

## U.S. Suicide Rates by Age, Gender, and Racial Group

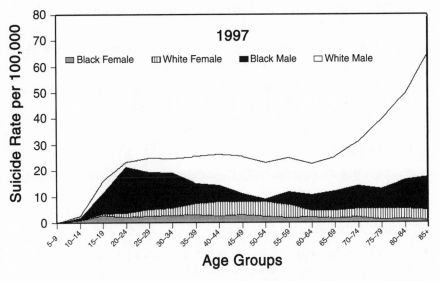

Source: National Institute of Mental Health
Data: Centers for Disease Control and Prevention; National Center for Health Statistics

*Figure 9.1. Fatal suicides are far more common among men—particularly elderly white males—than among women.*

*important to limit the person's access to firearms, large amounts of medication, or other lethal means of committing suicide.*

## Suicide Facts

### *Completed Suicides, U.S., 1999*

- Suicide was the eighth leading cause of death in the United States.

- It was the eighth leading cause of death for males, and nineteenth leading cause of death for females.

- The total number of suicide deaths was 29,199.

- The 1999 age-adjusted rate was 10.7/100,000, or 0.01 percent.

  - Of total deaths, 1.3 percent were from suicide. By contrast, 30.3 percent were from diseases of the heart, 23 percent from malignant neoplasms (cancer), and 7 percent from cerebrovascular disease (stroke), the three leading causes.

  - Suicide outnumbered homicides (16,899) by five to three.

  - There were twice as many deaths due to suicide as to HIV/AIDS (14,802).

  - There were almost exactly the same number of suicides by firearm (16,889) as homicides (16,599).

- Suicide by firearms was the most common method for both men and women, accounting for 57 percent of all suicides.

- More men than women die by suicide.

  - The gender ratio is 4:1.

  - Seventy-two percent of all suicides are committed by white men.

  - Seventy-nine percent of all firearm suicides are committed by white men.

- Among the highest rates (when categorized by gender and race) are suicide deaths for white men over 85, who had a rate of 59/100,000.

- Suicide was the third leading cause of death among young people 15 to 24 years of age, following unintentional injuries and homicide. The rate was 10.3/100,000, or .01 percent.

- The suicide rate among children ages 10–14 was 1.2/ 100,000, or 192 deaths among 19,608,000 children in this age group.
  - The 1999 gender ratio for this age group was 4:1 (males:females).
- The suicide rate among adolescents aged 15–19 was 8.2/ 100,000, or 1,615 deaths among 19,594,000 adolescents in this age group.
  - The 1999 gender ratio for this age group was 5:1 (males:females).
  - Among young people 20 to 24 years of age the suicide rate was 12.7/100,000, or 2,285 deaths among 17,594,000 people in this age group.
  - The 1999 gender ratio for this age group was 6:1 (males:females).

## Attempted Suicides

No annual national data on attempted suicide are available; reliable scientific research, however, has found that:

- There are an estimated eight to 25 attempted suicides to one completion; the ratio is higher in women and youth and lower in men and the elderly.
- More women than men report a history of attempted suicide, with a gender ratio of 3:1.
- The strongest risk factors for attempted suicide in adults are depression, alcohol abuse, cocaine use, and separation or divorce.
- The strongest risk factors for attempted suicide in youth are depression, alcohol or other drug use disorder, and aggressive or disruptive behaviors.

## Frequently Asked Questions about Suicide

### What Should You Do If Someone Tells You They Are Thinking about Suicide?

If someone tells you they are thinking about suicide, you should take their distress seriously, listen nonjudgmentally, and help them get to a professional for evaluation and treatment. People consider suicide when they are hopeless and unable to see alternative solutions to problems. Suicidal behavior is most often related to a mental disorder (depression) or to alcohol or other substance abuse. Suicidal behavior is also more likely to occur when people experience stressful events (major losses, incarceration). If someone is in imminent danger of harming himself or herself, do not leave the person alone. You may need to take emergency steps to get help, such as calling 911. When someone is in a suicidal crisis, it is important to limit access to firearms or other lethal means of committing suicide.

## What Are the Most Common Methods of Suicide?

Firearms are the most commonly used method of suicide for men and women, accounting for 60 percent of all suicides. Nearly 80 percent of all firearm suicides are committed by white males. The second most common method for men is hanging; for women, the second most common method is self-poisoning including drug overdose. The presence of a firearm in the home has been found to be an independent, additional risk factor for suicide. Thus, when a family member or health care provider is faced with an individual at risk for suicide, they should make sure that firearms are removed from the home.

## Why Do Men Commit Suicide More Often Than Women Do?

More than four times as many men as women die by suicide; but women attempt suicide more often during their lives than do men, and women report higher rates of depression. Several explanations have been offered:

- Completed suicide is associated with aggressive behavior that is more common in men and that may in turn be related to some of the biological differences identified in suicidality.

- Men and women use different suicide methods. Women in all countries are more likely to ingest poisons than men. In countries where the poisons are highly lethal and/or where treatment resources scarce, rescue is rare and hence female suicides outnumber males.

More research is needed on the social-cultural factors that may protect women from completing suicide, and on how to encourage men to recognize and seek treatment for their distress, instead of resorting to suicide.

### Who Is at Highest Risk for Suicide in the U.S.?

There is a common perception that suicide rates are highest among the young. However, it is the elderly, particularly older white males, that have the highest rates. And among white males 65 and older, risk goes up with age. White men 85 and older have a suicide rate that is six times that of the overall national rate.

Why are rates so high for this group? White males are more deliberate in their suicide intentions; they use more lethal methods (firearms), and are less likely to talk about their plans. It may also be that older persons are less likely to survive attempts because they are less likely to recuperate. Over 70 percent of older suicide victims have been to their primary care physician within the month of their death, many with a depressive illness that was not detected. This has led to research efforts to determine how to best improve physicians' abilities to detect and treat depression in older adults.

### Is Suicide Related to Impulsiveness?

Impulsiveness is the tendency to act without thinking through a plan or its consequences. It is a symptom of a number of mental disorders, and, therefore, it has been linked to suicidal behavior usually through its association with mental disorders and/or substance abuse. The mental disorders with impulsiveness most linked to suicide include borderline personality disorder among young females, conduct disorder among young males and antisocial behavior in adult males, and alcohol and substance abuse among young and middle-aged males. Impulsiveness appears to have a lesser role in older adult suicides. Attention deficit hyperactivity disorder that has impulsiveness as a characteristic is not a strong risk factor for suicide by itself. Impulsiveness has been linked with aggressive and violent behaviors including homicide and suicide. However, impulsiveness without aggression or violence present has also been found to contribute to risk for suicide.

### Is There Such a Thing As "Rational" Suicide?

Some right-to-die advocacy groups promote the idea that suicide, including assisted suicide, can be a rational decision. Others have argued that suicide is never a rational decision and that it is the result of depression, anxiety, and fear of being dependent or a burden. Surveys of terminally ill persons indicate that very few consider taking their own life, and when they do, it is in the context of depression. Attitude surveys suggest that assisted suicide is more acceptable by the public and health providers for the old who are ill or disabled, compared to the young who are ill or disabled. At this time, there is limited research on the frequency with which persons with terminal illness have depression and suicidal ideation, whether they would consider assisted suicide, the characteristics of such persons, and the context of their depression and suicidal thoughts, such as family stress or availability of palliative care. Neither is it yet clear what effect other factors such as the availability of social support, access to care, and pain relief may have on end-of-life preferences. This public debate will be better informed after such research is conducted.

### What Biological Factors Increase Risk for Suicide?

Researchers believe that both depression and suicidal behavior can be linked to decreased serotonin in the brain. Low levels of a serotonin metabolite, 5-HIAA, have been detected in cerebrospinal fluid in persons who have attempted suicide, as well as by postmortem studies examining certain brain regions of suicide victims. One of the goals of understanding the biology of suicidal behavior is to improve treatments. Scientists have learned that serotonin receptors in the brain increase their activity in persons with major depression and suicidality, which explains why medications that desensitize or down-regulate these receptors (such as the serotonin reuptake inhibitors, or SSRIs) have been found effective in treating depression. Currently, studies are under way to examine to what extent medications like SSRIs can reduce suicidal behavior.

### Can the Risk for Suicide Be Inherited?

There is growing evidence that familial and genetic factors contribute to the risk for suicidal behavior. Major psychiatric illnesses, including bipolar disorder, major depression, schizophrenia, alcoholism and substance abuse, and certain personality disorders, which run in families, increase the risk for suicidal behavior. This does not mean that suicidal behavior is inevitable for individuals with this family history; it simply means that such persons may be more vulnerable and should take steps to reduce their risk, such as getting evaluation and treatment at the first sign of mental illness.

### Does Depression Increase the Risk for Suicide?

Although the majority of people who have depression do not die by suicide, having major depression does increase suicide risk compared to people without depression. The risk of death by suicide may, in part, be related to the severity of the depression. New data on depression that has followed people over long periods of time suggests that about 2 percent of those people ever treated for depression in an outpatient setting will die by suicide. Among those ever treated for depression in an inpatient hospital setting, the rate of death by suicide is twice as high (4 percent). Those treated for depression as inpatients following suicide ideation or suicide attempts are about three times as likely to die by suicide (6 percent) as those who were only treated as outpatients. There are also dramatic gender differences in lifetime risk of suicide in depression. Whereas about 7 percent of men with a lifetime history of depression will die by suicide, only one percent of women with a lifetime history of depression will die by suicide.

Another way about thinking of suicide risk and depression is to examine the lives of people who have died by suicide and see what proportion of them were depressed. From that perspective, it is estimated that about 60 percent of people who commit suicide have had a mood disorder (e.g., major depression, bipolar disorder, dysthymia). Younger persons who kill themselves often have a substance abuse disorder in addition to being depressed.

## *Does Alcohol and Other Drug Abuse Increase the Risk for Suicide?*

A number of recent national surveys have helped shed light on the relationship between alcohol and other drug use and suicidal behavior. A review of minimum-age drinking laws and suicides among youths age 18 to 20 found that lower minimum-age drinking laws were associated with higher youth suicide rates. In a large study following adults who drink alcohol, suicide ideation was reported among persons with depression. In another survey, persons who reported that they had made a suicide attempt during their lifetime were more likely to have had a depressive disorder, and many also had an alcohol and/or substance abuse disorder. In a study of all non-traffic injury deaths associated with alcohol intoxication, over 20 percent were suicides.

In studies that examine risk factors among people who have completed suicide, substance use and abuse occurs more frequently among youth and adults, compared to older persons. For particular groups at risk, such as American Indians and Alaskan Natives, depression and alcohol use and abuse are the most common risk factors for completed suicide. Alcohol and substance abuse problems contribute to suicidal behavior in several ways. Persons who are dependent on substances often have a number of other risk factors for suicide. In addition to being depressed, they are also likely to have social and financial problems. Substance use and abuse can be common among persons prone to be impulsive, and among persons who engage in many types of high risk behaviors that result in self-harm. Fortunately, there are a number of effective prevention efforts that reduce risk for substance abuse in youth, and there are effective treatments for alcohol and substance use problems. Researchers are currently testing treatments specifically for persons with substance abuse problems who are also suicidal or have attempted suicide in the past.

### What Does "Suicide Contagion" Mean, and What Can Be Done to Prevent It?

Suicide contagion is the exposure to suicide or suicidal behaviors within one's family, one's peer group, or through media reports of suicide and can result in an increase in suicide and suicidal behaviors. Direct and indirect exposure to suicidal behavior has been shown to precede an increase in suicidal behavior in persons at risk for suicide, especially in adolescents and young adults.

The risk for suicide contagion as a result of media reporting can be minimized by factual and concise media reports of suicide. Reports of suicide should not be repetitive, as prolonged exposure can increase the likelihood of suicide contagion. Suicide is the result of many complex factors; therefore, media coverage should not report oversimplified explanations such as recent negative life events or acute stressors. Reports should not divulge detailed descriptions of the method used to avoid possible duplication. Reports should not glorify the victim and should not imply that suicide was effective in achieving a personal goal such as gaining media attention. In addition, information such as hotlines or emergency contacts should be provided for those at risk for suicide.

Following exposure to suicide or suicidal behaviors within one's family or peer group, suicide risk can be minimized by having family members, friends, peers, and colleagues of the victim evaluated by a mental health professional. Persons deemed at risk for suicide should then be referred for additional mental health services.

### Is It Possible to Predict Suicide?

At the current time there is no definitive measure to predict suicide or suicidal behavior. Researchers have identified factors that place individuals at higher risk for suicide, but very few persons with these risk factors will actually commit suicide. Risk factors include mental illness, substance abuse, previous suicide attempts, family history of suicide, history of being sexually abused, and impulsive or aggressive tendencies. Suicide is a relatively rare event, and it is therefore difficult to predict which persons with these risk factors will ultimately commit suicide.

# Chapter 10

# *Chronic Kidney Disease*

Many diseases affect kidney function by attacking the glomeruli, the tiny units within the kidney where blood is cleaned. Glomerular diseases include many conditions with a variety of genetic and environmental causes, but they fall into two major categories:

- Glomerulonephritis (gloh-MAIR-yoo-loh-neh-FRY-tis) describes the inflammation of the membrane tissue in the kidney that serves as a filter, separating wastes and extra fluid from the blood.

- Glomerulosclerosis (gloh-MAIR-yoo-loh-skleh-ROH-sis) describes the scarring or hardening of the tiny blood vessels within the kidney.

Although glomerulonephritis and glomerulosclerosis have different causes, they can both lead to end-stage renal disease (ESRD).

## *What Are the Kidneys and What Do They Do?*

The two kidneys are bean-shaped organs located near the middle of the back, just below the rib cage to the left and right of the spine. Each about the size of a fist, these organs act as sophisticated filters for the body. They process about 400 quarts of blood a day to sift out

Adapted from "Glomerular Diseases," National Kidney and Urologic Diseases Information Clearinghouse (NKUDIC), March 2003, http://www.niddk.nih.gov/health/kidney/pubs/glomer/glomer.htm.

about two quarts of waste products and extra water that eventually leave the body as urine.

Blood enters the kidneys through arteries that branch inside the kidneys into tiny clusters of looping blood vessels. Each cluster is called a glomerulus, which comes from the Latin word meaning filter. The plural form of the word is glomeruli. There are approximately one million glomeruli, or filters, in each kidney. The glomerulus is attached to the opening of a small fluid-collecting tube called a tubule. Blood is filtered in the glomerulus, and extra water and wastes pass into the tubule and become urine. Eventually, the urine drains from the kidneys into the bladder through larger tubes called ureters.

Each glomerulus-and-tubule unit is called a nephron. Each kidney is composed of about one million nephrons. In healthy nephrons, the glomerular membrane that separates the blood vessel from the tubule allows waste products and extra water to pass into the tubule while keeping blood cells and protein in the bloodstream (see Figure 10.1).

## How Do Glomerular Diseases Interfere with Kidney Function?

Glomerular diseases damage the glomeruli, letting protein and sometimes red blood cells leak into the urine. Sometimes a glomerular disease also interferes with the clearance of waste products by the kidney, so they begin to build up in the blood. Furthermore, loss of blood proteins like albumin in the urine can result in a fall in their level in the bloodstream. In normal blood, albumin acts like a sponge, drawing extra fluid from the body into the bloodstream, where it remains until the kidneys remove it. But when albumin leaks into the urine, the blood loses its capacity to absorb extra fluid from the body. Fluid can accumulate outside the circulatory system in the face, hands, feet, or ankles and cause swelling.

## What Are the Symptoms of Glomerular Disease?

The signs and symptoms of glomerular disease include:

- Proteinuria: large amounts of protein in the urine

- Hematuria: blood in the urine

- Reduced glomerular filtration rate: inefficient filtering of wastes from the blood

- Hypoproteinemia: low blood protein
- Edema: swelling in parts of the body

One or more of these symptoms can be the first sign of kidney disease. But how would you know, for example, whether you have proteinuria? Before seeing a doctor, you may not. But some of these symptoms have signs, or visible manifestations:

- Proteinuria may cause foamy urine.
- Blood may cause the urine to be pink or cola-colored.
- Edema may be obvious in hands and ankles, especially at the end of the day, or around the eyes when awakening in the morning, for example.

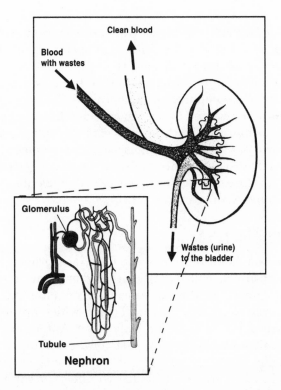

**Figure 10.1.** *In the nephron (left), tiny blood vessels intertwine with fluid-collecting tubules. Each kidney contains about one million nephrons.*

## How Is Glomerular Disease Diagnosed?

Urinalysis provides information about kidney damage by indicating levels of protein and red blood cells in the urine. Blood tests measure the levels of waste products such as creatinine and urea nitrogen to determine whether the filtering capacity of the kidneys is impaired. If these lab tests indicate kidney damage, the doctor may recommend ultrasound or x-ray to see whether the shape or size of the kidneys is abnormal. These tests are called renal imaging. But since glomerular disease causes problems at the cellular level, the doctor will probably also recommend a kidney biopsy—a procedure in which a needle is used to extract small pieces of tissue for examination under different types of microscopes, each of which shows a different aspect of the tissue. A biopsy may be helpful in confirming glomerular disease and identifying the cause.

## What Causes Glomerular Disease?

A number of different diseases can result in glomerular disease. It may be the direct result of an infection or a drug toxic to the kidneys, or it may result from a disease that affects the entire body, like diabetes or lupus. Many different kinds of diseases can cause swelling or scarring of the nephron or glomerulus.

The categories presented below can overlap: that is, a disease might belong to two or more of the categories. For example, diabetic nephropathy is a form of glomerular disease that can be placed in two categories: systemic diseases, since diabetes itself is a systemic disease; and sclerotic diseases, because the specific damage done to the kidneys is associated with scarring.

### Autoimmune Diseases

When the body's immune system functions properly, it creates protein-like substances called antibodies and immunoglobulins to protect the body against invading organisms. In an autoimmune disease, the immune system creates autoantibodies, which are antibodies or immunoglobulins that attack the body itself. Autoimmune diseases may be systemic and affect many parts of the body, or they may affect only specific organs or regions.

Systemic lupus erythematosus (SLE) affects many parts of the body: primarily the skin and joints, but also the kidneys. Because women are more likely to develop SLE than men, some researchers believe that a sex-linked genetic factor may play a part in making a person susceptible, although viral infection has also been implicated as a triggering factor. Lupus nephritis is the name given to the kidney disease caused by SLE, and it occurs when autoantibodies form or are deposited in the glomeruli, causing inflammation. Ultimately, the inflammation may create scars that keep the kidneys from functioning properly.

Goodpasture's syndrome involves an autoantibody that specifically targets the kidneys and the lungs. Often, the first indication that patients have the autoantibody comes when they cough up blood. But lung damage in Goodpasture's syndrome is usually superficial compared with progressive and permanent damage to the kidneys. Goodpasture's syndrome is a rare condition that affects mostly young men but also occurs in women, children, and older adults. Treatments include immunosuppressive drugs and a blood-cleaning therapy called plasmapheresis that removes the autoantibodies.

IgA nephropathy is a form of glomerular disease that results when immunoglobulin A (IgA) forms deposits in the glomeruli, where it creates inflammation. Researchers funded by the National Institute of Diabetes and Digestive and Kidney Diseases (NIDDK) are trying to discover why these deposits in the glomeruli are formed and whether dietary supplements of fish oil can inhibit IgA-induced inflammation and scarring in the kidney. A study is being conducted to compare the effectiveness of therapy involving daily fish oil supplements with that of a therapy involving prednisone, a drug that blocks the body's immune system. The study includes a placebo group. All three groups of patients in the study are receiving medication to control blood pressure. IgA nephropathy was not recognized as a cause of glomerular disease until the late 1960s, when sophisticated biopsy techniques were developed that could identify IgA deposits in kidney tissue.

The most common symptom of IgA nephropathy is blood in the urine, but it is often a silent disease that may go undetected for many years. The silent nature of the disease makes it difficult to determine how many people are in the early stages of IgA nephropathy, when specific medical tests are the only way to detect it. This disease is estimated to be the most common cause of primary glomerulonephritis—that is, glomerular disease not caused by a systemic disease like lupus or diabetes mellitus. It appears to affect men more than women. Although IgA nephropathy is found in all age groups, young people rarely display signs of kidney failure because the disease usually takes several years to progress to the stage where it causes detectable complications.

## Hereditary Nephritis—Alport Syndrome

The primary indicator of Alport syndrome is a family history of chronic glomerular disease, although it may also involve hearing or vision impairment. This syndrome affects both men and women, but men are more likely to experience chronic renal failure and sensory loss. Men with Alport syndrome usually first show evidence of renal insufficiency while in their twenties and reach ESRD by age 40. Women rarely have significant renal impairment, and hearing loss may be so slight that it can be detected only through testing with special equipment. Usually men can pass the disease only to their daughters. Women can transmit the disease to either their sons or their daughters.

## Infection-Related Glomerular Disease

Glomerular disease sometimes develops rapidly after an infection in other parts of the body. Acute post-streptococcal glomerulonephritis (PSGN) can occur after an episode of strep throat or, in rare cases, impetigo (a skin infection). The *Streptococcus* bacteria do not attack the kidney directly, but an infection may stimulate the immune system to overproduce antibodies, which are circulated in the blood and finally deposited in the glomeruli, causing damage. PSGN can bring on sudden symptoms of swelling (edema), reduced urine output (oliguria), and blood in the urine (hematuria). Tests will show large amounts of protein in the urine and elevated levels of creatinine and urea nitrogen in the blood, thus indicating reduced kidney function. High blood pressure frequently accompanies reduced kidney function in this disease.

PSGN is most common in children between the ages of three and seven, although it can strike at any age, and it most often affects boys. It lasts only a brief time and usually allows the kidneys to recover. In a few cases, however, kidney damage may be permanent, requiring dialysis or transplantation to replace renal function.

Bacterial endocarditis, infection of the tissues inside the heart, is also associated with subsequent glomerular disease. Researchers are not sure whether the renal lesions that form after a heart infection are caused entirely by the immune response or whether some other disease mechanism contributes to kidney damage. Treating the heart infection is the most effective way of minimizing kidney damage. Chronic renal failure can result from endocarditis, but is not inevitable.

HIV, the virus that leads to AIDS, can also cause glomerular disease. Between 5 and 10 percent of people with HIV experience kidney failure, even before developing full-blown AIDS. HIV-associated nephropathy usually begins with heavy proteinuria and progresses rapidly (within a year of detection) to ESRD. Researchers are looking for therapies that can slow down or reverse this rapid deterioration of renal function, but some possible solutions involving immunosuppression are risky because of the patients' already compromised immune system.

## Sclerotic Diseases

Glomerulosclerosis is scarring (sclerosis) of the glomeruli. In several sclerotic conditions, a systemic disease like lupus or diabetes is responsible. Glomerulosclerosis is caused by the activation of glomerular cells to produce scar material. This may be stimulated by molecules called growth factors, which may be made by glomerular cells themselves or may be brought to the glomerulus by the circulating blood that enters the glomerular filter.

Diabetic nephropathy is the leading cause of ESRD in the United States. Kidney disease is one of several problems caused by elevated levels of blood glucose, the central feature of diabetes. In addition to scarring the kidney, elevated glucose levels appear to increase the speed of blood flow into the kidney, putting a strain on the filtering glomeruli and raising blood pressure.

Diabetic nephropathy usually takes many years to develop. People with diabetes can slow down damage to their kidneys by controlling their blood glucose through healthy eating with moderate protein intake, physical activity, and medications. People with diabetes should also be careful to keep their blood pressure at a level below 130/85 mm Hg, if possible. A class of blood pressure medications called angiotensin-converting enzyme (ACE) inhibitors is particularly effective at minimizing kidney damage and is now frequently prescribed to control blood pressure in patients with diabetes.

Focal segmental glomerulosclerosis (FSGS) describes scarring in scattered regions of the kidney, typically limited to one part of the glomerulus and to a minority of glomeruli in the affected region. FSGS may result from a systemic disorder, or it may develop as an idiopathic kidney disease, without a known cause. Proteinuria is the most common symptom of FSGS, but, since proteinuria is associated with several other kidney conditions, the doctor cannot diagnose FSGS on the basis of proteinuria alone. Biopsy may confirm the presence of glomerular scarring if the tissue is taken from the affected section of the kidney. But finding the affected section is a matter of chance, especially early in the disease process, when lesions may be scattered.

Confirming a diagnosis of FSGS may require repeat kidney biopsies. Arriving at a diagnosis of idiopathic FSGS requires the identification of focal scarring and the elimination of possible systemic causes such as diabetes or an immune response to infection. Since idiopathic FSGS is, by definition, of unknown cause, it is difficult to treat. No universal remedy has been found, and most patients with FSGS progress to ESRD over five to 20 years. Some patients with an aggressive form of FSGS proceed to ESRD in two to three years. Treatments involving steroids or other immunosuppressive drugs appear to help some patients by decreasing proteinuria and improving kidney function. But these treatments are beneficial only to a minority of those in whom they are tried, and some patients experience even poorer kidney function as a result of therapy. ACE inhibitors may also be used in FSGS to decrease proteinuria. Treatment should focus on controlling blood pressure and blood cholesterol levels, factors that may contribute to kidney scarring.

### Idiopathic Nephrotic Syndrome—Minimal Change Disease

Minimal change disease (MCD) is the diagnosis given when a patient has the nephrotic syndrome and the kidney biopsy reveals little or no change to the structure of glomeruli or surrounding tissues when examined by a light microscope. Tiny drops of a fatty substance called a lipid may be present, but no scarring has taken place within the kidney. MCD may occur at any age, but it is most common in childhood. A small percentage of patients with idiopathic nephrotic syndrome do not respond to steroid therapy. For these patients, the doctor may recommend a low-sodium diet and prescribe a diuretic to control edema. The doctor may recommend the use of nonsteroidal anti-inflammatory drugs to reduce proteinuria. ACE inhibitors have also been used to reduce proteinuria in patients with steroid-resistant MCD. These patients may respond to larger doses of steroids, more prolonged use of steroids, or steroids in combination with immunosuppressant drugs, such as chlorambucil, cyclophosphamide, or cyclosporine.

### What Are Renal Failure and End-Stage Renal Disease?

Renal failure is any acute or chronic loss of kidney function and is the term used when some kidney function remains. ESRD is total, or nearly total, and permanent kidney failure. Depending on the form of glomerular disease, renal function may be lost in a matter of days or weeks or may deteriorate slowly and gradually over the course of decades.

### *Acute Renal Failure*

A few forms of glomerular disease cause very rapid deterioration of kidney function. For example, PSGN can cause severe symptoms (hematuria, proteinuria, edema) within two to three weeks after a sore throat or skin infection develops. The patient may temporarily require dialysis to replace renal function. This rapid loss of kidney function is called acute renal failure (ARF). Although ARF can be life-threatening while it lasts, kidney function usually returns after the cause of the kidney failure has been treated. In many patients, ARF is not associated with any permanent damage. However, some patients may recover from ARF and subsequently develop chronic renal failure (CRF).

### *Chronic Renal Failure*

Most forms of glomerular disease develop gradually, often causing no symptoms for many years. CRF is the slow, gradual loss of kidney function. Some forms of CRF can be controlled or slowed down. For example, diabetic nephropathy can be delayed by tightly controlling blood glucose levels and using ACE inhibitors to reduce proteinuria and control blood pressure. But CRF cannot be cured. Partial loss of renal function means that some portion of the patient's nephrons have been scarred, and scarred nephrons cannot be repaired. In most cases, CRF leads to ESRD.

### *End-Stage Renal Disease*

To stay alive, a patient with ESRD must go on dialysis—hemodialysis or peritoneal dialysis—or receive a new kidney through transplantation. Patients with CRF who are approaching ESRD should learn as much about their treatment options as possible so they can make an informed decision when the time comes. With the help of dialysis or transplantation, many people continue to lead full, productive lives after reaching ESRD.

## *The Nephrotic Syndrome*

- The nephrotic syndrome is a condition marked by very high levels of protein in the urine; low levels of protein in the blood;

swelling, especially around the eyes, feet, and hands; and high cholesterol.

- The nephrotic syndrome is a set of symptoms, not a disease in itself. It can occur with many diseases, so prevention relies on controlling the diseases that cause it.

- Treatment of the nephrotic syndrome focuses on identifying and treating the underlying cause, if possible, and reducing high cholesterol, blood pressure, and protein in the urine through diet, medication, or both.

- The nephrotic syndrome may go away once the underlying cause, if known, is treated. However, often a kidney disease is the underlying cause and cannot be cured. In these cases, the kidneys may gradually lose their ability to filter wastes and excess water from the blood. If kidney failure occurs, the patient will need to be on dialysis or have a kidney transplant.

## Points to Remember

- The kidneys filter waste and extra fluid from the blood.

- The filtering process takes place in the nephron, where microscopic blood vessel filters, called glomeruli, are attached to fluid-collecting tubules.

- A number of different disease processes can damage the glomeruli and thereby cause kidney failure. Glomerulonephritis and glomerulosclerosis are broad terms that include many forms of damage to the glomeruli.

- Some forms of kidney failure can be slowed down, but scarred glomeruli can never be repaired.

- Treatment for the early stages of kidney failure depends on the disease causing the damage.

- Early signs of kidney failure include blood or protein in the urine and swelling in the hands, feet, abdomen, or face. Kidney failure may be silent for many years.

Chapter 11

# Cirrhosis and Chronic Liver Disease

## Cirrhosis of the Liver

The liver, the largest organ in the body, is essential in keeping the body functioning properly. It removes or neutralizes poisons from the blood, produces immune agents to control infection, and removes germs and bacteria from the blood. It makes proteins that regulate blood clotting and produces bile to help absorb fats and fat-soluble vitamins. You cannot live without a functioning liver.

In cirrhosis of the liver, scar tissue replaces normal, healthy tissue, blocking the flow of blood through the organ and preventing it from working as it should. Cirrhosis is the eighth leading cause of death by disease, killing about 25,000 people each year. Also, the cost of cirrhosis in terms of human suffering, hospital costs, and lost productivity is high.

### Causes

Cirrhosis has many causes. In the United States, chronic alcoholism and hepatitis C are the most common causes.

**Alcoholic liver disease**. To many people, cirrhosis of the liver is synonymous with chronic alcoholism, but in fact, alcoholism is only

Reprinted from two publications by the National Digestive Diseases Information Clearinghouse: "Cirrhosis of the Liver," NIH Pub. No. 00-1134, April 2000, http://www.niddk.nih.gov/health/digest/pubs/cirrhosi/cirrhosi.htm,; and "Viral Hepatitis A to E and Beyond," NIH Pub. No. 00-4762, October 2000, http://www.niddk.nih.gov/health/digest/pubs/hep/hepa-e/hepa-e.htm.

one of the causes. Alcoholic cirrhosis usually develops after more than a decade of heavy drinking. The amount of alcohol that can injure the liver varies greatly from person to person. In women, as few as two to three drinks per day have been linked with cirrhosis, and in men, as few as three to four drinks per day. Alcohol seems to injure the liver by blocking the normal metabolism of protein, fats, and carbohydrates.

**Chronic hepatitis C.** The hepatitis C virus ranks with alcohol as the major cause of chronic liver disease and cirrhosis in the United States. Infection with this virus causes inflammation of, and low-grade damage to, the liver that over several decades can lead to cirrhosis.

**Chronic hepatitis B and D.** The hepatitis B virus is probably the most common cause of cirrhosis worldwide, but in the United States and the Western world it is less common. Hepatitis B, like hepatitis C, causes liver inflammation and injury that over several decades can lead to cirrhosis. The hepatitis D virus is another virus that infects the liver, but only in people who already have hepatitis B.

**Autoimmune hepatitis.** This type of hepatitis is caused by a problem with the immune system.

**Inherited diseases.** Alpha-1 antitrypsin deficiency, hemochromatosis, Wilson's disease, galactosemia, and glycogen storage diseases are among the inherited diseases that interfere with the way the liver produces, processes, and stores enzymes, proteins, metals, and other substances the body needs to function properly.

**Nonalcoholic steatohepatitis (NASH).** In NASH, fat builds up in the liver and eventually causes scar tissue. This type of hepatitis appears to be associated with diabetes, protein malnutrition, obesity, coronary artery disease, and corticosteroid treatment.

**Blocked bile ducts.** When the ducts that carry bile out of the liver are blocked, bile backs up and damages liver tissue. In babies, blocked bile ducts are most commonly caused by biliary atresia, a disease in which the bile ducts are absent or injured. In adults, the most common cause is primary biliary cirrhosis, a disease in which the ducts become inflamed, blocked, and scarred. Secondary biliary cirrhosis can happen after gallbladder surgery, if the ducts are inadvertently tied off or injured.

**Drugs, toxins, and infections.** Severe reactions to prescription drugs, prolonged exposure to environmental toxins, the parasitic infection schistosomiasis, and repeated bouts of heart failure with liver congestion can each lead to cirrhosis.

### *Symptoms*

Many people with cirrhosis have no symptoms in the early stages of the disease. However, as scar tissue replaces healthy cells, liver function starts to fail and a person may experience the following symptoms:

- Exhaustion
- Loss of appetite
- Weakness
- Fatigue
- Nausea
- Weight loss

As the disease progresses, complications may develop. In some people, these may be the first signs of the disease.

### *Complications of Cirrhosis*

Loss of liver function affects the body in many ways. Following are common problems, or complications, caused by cirrhosis.

**Edema and ascites.** When the liver loses its ability to make the protein albumin, water accumulates in the leg (edema) and abdomen (ascites).

**Bruising and bleeding.** When the liver slows or stops production of the proteins needed for blood clotting, a person will bruise or bleed easily.

**Jaundice.** Jaundice is a yellowing of the skin and eyes that occurs when the diseased liver does not absorb enough bilirubin.

**Itching.** Bile products deposited in the skin may cause intense itching.

**Gallstones.** If cirrhosis prevents bile from reaching the gallbladder, a person may develop gallstones.

**Toxins in the blood or brain.** A damaged liver cannot remove toxins from the blood, causing them to accumulate in the blood and eventually the brain. There, toxins can dull mental functioning and cause personality changes, coma, and even death. Signs of the buildup of toxins in the brain include neglect of personal appearance, unresponsiveness, forgetfulness, trouble concentrating, or changes in sleep habits.

**Sensitivity to medication.** Cirrhosis slows the liver's ability to filter medications from the blood. Because the liver does not remove drugs from the blood at the usual rate, they act longer than expected and build up in the body. This causes a person to be more sensitive to medications and their side effects.

**Portal hypertension.** Normally, blood from the intestines and spleen is carried to the liver through the portal vein. But cirrhosis slows the normal flow of blood through the portal vein, which increases the pressure inside it. This condition is called portal hypertension.

**Varices.** When blood flow through the portal vein slows, blood from the intestines and spleen backs up into blood vessels in the stomach and esophagus. These blood vessels may become enlarged because they are not meant to carry this much blood. The enlarged blood vessels, called varices, have thin walls and carry high pressure, and thus are more likely to burst. If they do burst, the result is a serious bleeding problem in the upper stomach or esophagus that requires immediate medical attention.

**Problems in other organs.** Cirrhosis can cause immune system dysfunction, leading to infection. Ascites (fluid in the abdomen) may become infected with bacteria normally present in the intestines, and cirrhosis can also lead to kidney dysfunction and failure.

### Diagnosis

The doctor may diagnose cirrhosis on the basis of symptoms, laboratory tests, the patient's medical history, and a physical examination. For example, during a physical examination, the doctor may notice that the liver feels harder or larger than usual and order blood tests that can show whether liver disease is present.

If looking at the liver is necessary to check for signs of disease, the doctor might order a computerized axial tomography (CAT) scan, ultrasound, or a scan of the liver with a radioisotope (a harmless radioactive substance that highlights the liver). Or the doctor might look at the liver using a laparoscope, an instrument inserted through the abdomen that relays pictures back to a computer screen.

A liver biopsy will confirm the diagnosis. For a biopsy, the doctor uses a needle to take a small sample of tissue from the liver, then examines it for scarring or other signs of disease.

## *Treatment*

Liver damage from cirrhosis cannot be reversed, but treatment can stop or delay further progression and reduce complications. Treatment depends on the cause of cirrhosis and any complications a person is experiencing. For example, cirrhosis caused by alcohol abuse is treated by abstaining from alcohol. Treatment for hepatitis-related cirrhosis involves medications used to treat the different types of hepatitis, such as interferon for viral hepatitis and corticosteroids for autoimmune hepatitis. Cirrhosis caused by Wilson's disease, in which copper builds up in organs, is treated with medications to remove the copper. These are just a few examples; treatment for cirrhosis resulting from other diseases will depend on the underlying cause. In all cases, regardless of the cause, following a healthy diet and avoiding alcohol are essential because the body needs all the nutrients it can get, and alcohol will only lead to more liver damage.

Treatment will also include remedies for complications. For example, for ascites and edema, the doctor may recommend a low-sodium diet or the use of diuretics, which are drugs that remove fluid from the body. Antibiotics will be prescribed for infections, and various medications can help with itching. Protein causes toxins to form in the digestive tract, so eating less protein will help decrease the buildup of toxins in the blood and brain. The doctor may also prescribe laxatives to help absorb the toxins and remove them from the intestines.

For portal hypertension, the doctor may prescribe blood pressure medication such as a beta blocker. If varices bleed, the doctor may either inject them with a clotting agent or perform a rubber-band ligation, which uses a special device to compress the varices and stop the bleeding.

When complications cannot be controlled or when the liver becomes so damaged from scarring that it completely stops functioning, a liver transplant is necessary. In liver transplantation surgery, a diseased liver is removed and replaced with a healthy one from an organ donor. About 80 to 90 percent of people survive liver transplantation. Survival rates have improved over the past several years because of drugs such as cyclosporine and tacrolimus, which suppress the immune system and keep it from attacking and damaging the new liver.

## Hepatitis

Hepatitis is inflammation of the liver. Several different viruses cause viral hepatitis. They are named the hepatitis A, B, C, D, and E viruses.

All of these viruses cause acute, or short-term, viral hepatitis. The hepatitis B, C, and D viruses can also cause chronic hepatitis, in which the infection is prolonged, sometimes lifelong.

Other viruses may also cause hepatitis, but they have yet to be discovered and they are obviously rare causes of the disease.

### Symptoms of Viral Hepatitis

Symptoms include:

- Jaundice (yellowing of the skin and eyes)
- Fatigue
- Abdominal pain
- Loss of appetite
- Nausea
- Diarrhea
- Vomiting

However, some people do not have symptoms until the disease is advanced.

### Hepatitis A

**Disease spread**. Primarily through food or water contaminated by feces from an infected person. Rarely, it spreads through contact with infected blood.

**People at risk.** International travelers; people living in areas where hepatitis A outbreaks are common; people who live with or have sex with an infected person; and, during outbreaks, day-care children and employees, sexually active gay men, and injection drug users.

**Prevention.** The hepatitis A vaccine; also, avoiding tap water when traveling internationally and practicing good hygiene and sanitation.

**Treatment.** Hepatitis A usually resolves on its own over several weeks.

## *Hepatitis B*

**Disease spread.** Through contact with infected blood, through sex with an infected person, and from mother to child during childbirth.

**People at risk.** Injection drug users, people who have sex with an infected person, men who have sex with men, children of immigrants from disease-endemic areas, people who live with an infected person, infants born to infected mothers, health care workers, and hemodialysis patients.

**Prevention.** The hepatitis B vaccine.

**Treatment.** Drug treatment with alpha interferon or lamivudine.

## *Hepatitis C*

**Disease spread.** Primarily through contact with infected blood; less commonly, through sexual contact and childbirth.

**People at risk.** Injection drug users, hemodialysis patients, health care workers, people who have sex with an infected person, people who have multiple sex partners, infants born to infected women, and people who received a transfusion of blood or blood products before July 1992 or clotting factors made before 1987.

**Prevention.** There is no vaccine for hepatitis C; the only way to prevent the disease is to reduce the risk of exposure to the virus. This means avoiding behaviors like sharing drug needles or sharing personal items like toothbrushes, razors, and nail clippers with an infected person.

**Treatment.** Drug treatment with alpha interferon or combination treatment with interferon and the drug ribavirin.

## *Hepatitis D*

**Disease spread.** Through contact with infected blood. This disease occurs only in people who are already infected with hepatitis B.

**People at risk.** Anyone infected with hepatitis B. Injection drug users who have hepatitis B have the highest risk. People who have hepatitis B are also at risk if they have sex with a person infected with hepatitis D or if they live with an infected person.

**Prevention.** Immunization against hepatitis B for those not already infected; also, avoiding exposure to infected blood, contaminated needles, and an infected person's personal items (toothbrush, razor, nail clippers).

**Treatment.** Drug treatment with alpha interferon.

### Hepatitis E

**Disease spread.** Through food or water contaminated by feces from an infected person. This disease is uncommon in the United States.

**People at risk.** International travelers; people living in areas where hepatitis E outbreaks are common; and people who live or have sex with an infected person.

**Prevention.** There is no vaccine for hepatitis E; the only way to prevent the disease is to reduce the risk of exposure to the virus. This means avoiding tap water when traveling internationally and practicing good hygiene and sanitation.

**Treatment.** Hepatitis E usually resolves on its own over several weeks to months.

### Other Causes of Viral Hepatitis

Some cases of viral hepatitis cannot be attributed to the hepatitis A, B, C, D, or E viruses. This is called non A–E hepatitis or hepatitis X. Scientists have identified several candidate viruses, but none have been proven to cause hepatitis. The search for the virus responsible for hepatitis X continues.

# Chapter 12

# *Assault and Homicide*

Dramatic increases in both homicide victimization and offending rates were experienced by young males, particularly young black males, in the late 1980s and early 1990s. During the past few years, homicide victimization rates have dropped for all groups. However, rates are not declining as rapidly as they did in the middle 1990s.

In addition, homicide victimization rates:

- For both black and white male teens and black female teens, showed similar patterns of an increase in the late 1980s and a more recent decline.

- For black male teens and young adults, declined more dramatically in recent years, but remain at relatively high levels.

- For white male teens, increased sharply several years later than those for black male teens.

- For white male teens and young adults, did not decline as rapidly as the rates for black male teens and young adults.

- For those over age 25 of all race and gender groups, generally declined over the past two decades.

- For male teens ages 14 to 17, which historically had been lower than those for older age groups, rose in the early 1990s to exceed

---

Reprinted from "Homicide Trends in the U.S.: Age, Gender, and Race Trends," Bureau of Justice Statistics, U.S. Department of Justice, updated January 2003, http://www.ojp.usdoj.gov/bjs/homicide/ageracesex.htm.

the rates for persons age 25 and older, but recently dropped back below the rates for persons age 25 and older.

- For black females in all age groups, were closer to those for white males than those for white females.

- For white females in all age groups, declined.

Homicide offending patterns are similar to victimization patterns. Homicide offending rates for:

- Adults (ages 25 and over) generally declined throughout the period from 1976 to 2000 for all racial and gender groups.

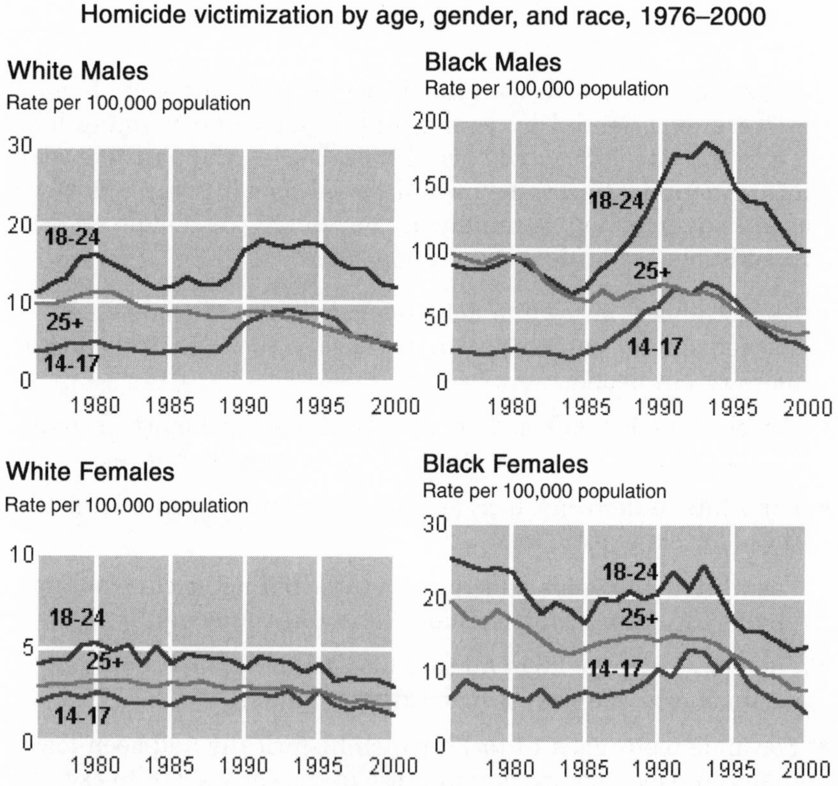

### Homicide victimization by age, gender, and race, 1976–2000

*Figure 12.1. Although homicide victimization rates for blacks and whites of both genders have declined in recent years, the rate of decrease has slowed.*

- Young adults (ages 18–24) are the highest among all groups.

- Black and white males under age 25 increased in the late 1980s.

- White males ages 18–24 did not decline as much as those for young black males and white males ages 14–17.

- Adult females declined over the past two decades for both races

- White female teens (ages 14–17) do not show a consistent pattern due to fairly modest shifts.

- Black female teens followed a pattern similar to that of male teens, both black and white, although without the dramatic increases.

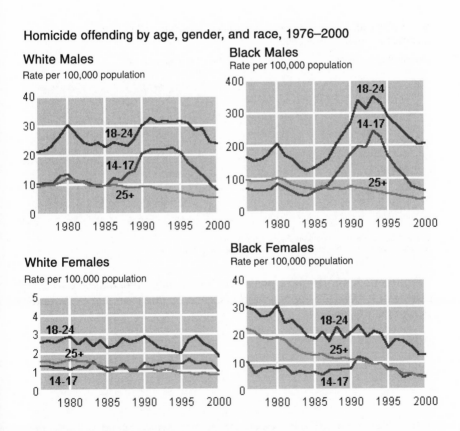

*Figure 12.2.* Like the rates for victimization, rates for homicide offense declined for blacks and whites of both genders.

Young males, particularly young black males, are disproportionately involved in homicide compared to their share of the population. The proportion of the population represented by:

• Young white males has declined, while the proportions of homicide victims and offenders who were young white males have been increasing.

• Young black males has remained at about 1 percent while the proportions of homicide victims and offenders who were young black males have increased dramatically from the mid 1980s to the early 1990s but have declined recently.

Young males as a proportion of the population, homicide victims, and homicide offenders, 1976–2000

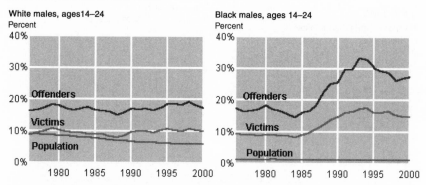

Source: FBI, Supplementary Homicide Reports, 1976–2000
Additional information about the data used in *Homicide trends in the U.S.*

*Figure 12.3.* Murder falls most heavily on young men. Males, particularly young black men, are represented disproportionately among both murderers and the murdered.

# Chapter 13

# Human Immunodeficiency Virus (HIV)

## Chapter Contents

197

## Section 13.1

# *HIV Infection and AIDS: An Overview*

Excerpted from "HIV Infection and AIDS: An Overview," National Institute of Allergy and Infectious Diseases, August 2002, http://www.niaid. nih.gov/factsheets/hivinf.htm,; and from "HIV Infection in Minority Populations," National Institute of Allergy and Infectious Diseases, June 2002, http://www.niaid.nih.gov/factsheets/Minor.htm.

AIDS—acquired immunodeficiency syndrome—was first reported in the United States in 1981 and has since become a major worldwide epidemic. AIDS is caused by the human immunodeficiency virus (HIV). By killing or damaging cells of the body's immune system, HIV progressively destroys the body's ability to fight infections and certain cancers. People diagnosed with AIDS may get life-threatening diseases called opportunistic infections, which are caused by microbes such as viruses or bacteria that usually do not make healthy people sick.

More than 790,000 cases of AIDS have been reported in the United States since 1981, and as many as 900,000 Americans may be infected with HIV. The epidemic is growing most rapidly among minority populations and is a leading killer of African American males ages 25 to 44. According to the U.S. Centers for Disease Control and Prevention (CDC), AIDS affects nearly seven times more African Americans and three times more Hispanics than whites.

### What Are the Early Symptoms of HIV Infection?

Many people do not have any symptoms when they first become infected with HIV. Some people, however, have a flu-like illness within a month or two after exposure to the virus. This illness may include:

- Fever
- Headache
- Tiredness
- Enlarged lymph nodes (glands of the immune system easily felt in the neck and groin)

These symptoms usually disappear within a week to a month and are often mistaken for those of another viral infection. During this period, people are very infectious, and HIV is present in large quantities in genital fluids.

More persistent or severe symptoms may not appear for 10 years or more after HIV first enters the body in adults, or within two years in children born with HIV infection. This period of "asymptomatic" infection is highly individual. Some people may begin to have symptoms within a few months, while others may be symptom-free for more than 10 years.

Even during the asymptomatic period, the virus is actively multiplying, infecting, and killing cells of the immune system. HIV's effect is seen most obviously in a decline in the blood levels of CD4+ T cells (also called T4 cells)—the immune system's key infection fighters. At the beginning of its life in the human body, the virus disables or destroys these cells without causing symptoms.

As the immune system worsens, a variety of complications start to take over. For many people, their first sign of infection is large lymph nodes, or "swollen glands," that may be enlarged for more than three months. Other symptoms often experienced months to years before the onset of AIDS include:

- Lack of energy
- Weight loss
- Frequent fevers and sweats
- Persistent or frequent yeast infections (oral or vaginal)
- Persistent skin rashes or flaky skin
- Pelvic inflammatory disease in women that does not respond to treatment
- Short-term memory loss

Some people develop frequent and severe herpes infections that cause mouth, genital, or anal sores or a painful nerve disease called shingles. Children may grow slowly or be sick a lot.

## What Is AIDS?

The term AIDS applies to the most advanced stages of HIV infection. CDC developed official criteria for the definition of AIDS and is responsible for tracking the spread of AIDS in the United States.

CDC's definition of AIDS includes all HIV-infected people who have fewer than 200 CD4+ T cells per cubic millimeter of blood. (Healthy adults usually have CD4+ T-cell counts of 1,000 or more.) In addition, the definition includes 26 clinical conditions that affect people with advanced HIV disease. Most of these conditions are opportunistic infections that generally do not affect healthy people. In people with AIDS, these infections are often severe and sometimes fatal because the immune system is so ravaged by HIV that the body cannot fight off certain bacteria, viruses, fungi, parasites, and other microbes.

Symptoms of opportunistic infections common in people with AIDS include:

- Coughing and shortness of breath
- Seizures and lack of coordination
- Difficult or painful swallowing
- Mental symptoms such as confusion and forgetfulness
- Severe and persistent diarrhea
- Fever
- Vision loss
- Nausea, abdominal cramps, and vomiting
- Weight loss and extreme fatigue
- Severe headaches
- Coma

People with AIDS are particularly prone to developing various cancers, especially those caused by viruses such as Kaposi's sarcoma and cervical cancer, or cancers of the immune system known as lymphomas. These cancers are usually more aggressive and difficult to treat in people with AIDS. Signs of Kaposi's sarcoma in light-skinned people are round brown, reddish, or purple spots that develop in the skin or in the mouth. In dark-skinned people, the spots are more pigmented.

During the course of HIV infection, most people experience a gradual decline in the number of CD4+ T cells, although some may have abrupt and dramatic drops in their CD4+ T-cell counts. A person with CD4+ T cells above 200 may experience some of the early symptoms of HIV disease. Others may have no symptoms even though their CD4+ T-cell count is below 200.

200

Many people are so debilitated by the symptoms of AIDS that they cannot hold steady employment or do household chores. Other people with AIDS may experience phases of intense, life-threatening illness followed by phases in which they function normally.

A small number of people first infected with HIV 10 or more years ago have not developed symptoms of AIDS. Scientists are trying to determine what factors may account for their lack of progression to AIDS, such as particular characteristics of their immune systems, whether they were infected with a less aggressive strain of the virus, or if their genes may protect them from the effects of HIV. Scientists hope that understanding the body's natural method of control may lead to ideas for protective HIV vaccines and use of vaccines to prevent the disease from progressing.

## How Is HIV Infection Diagnosed?

Because early HIV infection often causes no symptoms, a doctor or other health care provider usually can diagnose it by testing a person's blood for the presence of antibodies (disease-fighting proteins) to HIV. HIV antibodies generally do not reach detectable levels in the blood for one to three months following infection. It may take the antibodies as long as six months to be produced in quantities large enough to show up in standard blood tests.

People exposed to the virus should get an HIV test as soon as they are likely to develop antibodies to the virus—within six weeks to 12 months after possible exposure to the virus. By getting tested early, people with HIV infection can discuss with a health care provider when they should start treatment to help their immune systems combat HIV and help prevent the emergence of certain opportunistic infections (see section on treatment below). Early testing also alerts HIV-infected people to avoid high-risk behaviors that could spread the virus to others.

Most health care providers can do HIV testing and will usually offer counseling to the patient at the same time. Of course, individuals can be tested anonymously at many sites if they are concerned about confidentiality.

Health care providers diagnose HIV infection by using two different types of antibody tests: ELISA and Western Blot. If a person is highly likely to be infected with HIV yet both tests are negative, the health care provider may request additional tests. The person also may be told to repeat antibody testing at a later date, when antibodies to HIV are more likely to have developed.

## How Is HIV Infection Treated?

When AIDS first surfaced in the United States, there were no medicines to combat the underlying immune deficiency, and few treatments existed for the opportunistic diseases that resulted. During the past 10 years, however, researchers have developed drugs to fight both HIV infection and its associated infections and cancers.

The U.S. Food and Drug Administration (FDA) has approved a number of drugs for treating HIV infection. The first group of drugs used to treat HIV infection, called nucleoside reverse transcriptase (RT) inhibitors, interrupts an early stage of the virus making copies of itself. Included in this class of drugs (called nucleoside analogs) are AZT, ddC (zalcitabine), ddI (dideoxyinosine), d4T (stavudine), 3TC (lamivudine), abacavir (Ziagen®), and tenofovir (Viread®). These drugs may slow the spread of HIV in the body and delay the start of opportunistic infections.

Health care providers can prescribe non-nucleoside reverse transcriptase inhibitors (NNRTIs), such as delavirdine (Rescriptor®), nevirapine (Viramune®), and efavirenz (Sustiva®), in combination with other antiretroviral drugs.

More recently, FDA has approved a second class of drugs for treating HIV infection. These drugs, called protease inhibitors, interrupt virus replication at a later step in its life cycle. They include:

- Ritonavir (Norvir®)
- Amprenavir (Agenerase®)
- Saquinavir (Invirase®)
- Nelfinavir (Viracept®)
- Indinavir (Crixivan®)
- Lopinavir (Kaletra®)

Because HIV can become resistant to any of these drugs, health care providers must use a combination treatment to effectively suppress the virus. RT inhibitors and protease inhibitors are used in combination are referred to as highly active antiretroviral therapy, or HAART, which can be used by people who are newly infected with HIV as well as people with AIDS.

Researchers have credited HAART as being a major factor in significantly reducing the number of deaths from AIDS in this country. While HAART is not a cure for AIDS, it has greatly improved the health of many people with AIDS, and it reduces the amount of virus circulating in the blood to nearly undetectable levels. Researchers, however, have shown that HIV remains present in hiding places, such as the lymph nodes, brain, testes, and retina of the eye, even in patients who have been treated.

Despite the beneficial effects of HAART, side effects associated with the use of antiviral drugs can be severe. Some of the nucleoside RT inhibitors may cause a decrease of red or white blood cells, especially when taken in the later stages of the disease. Some may also cause inflammation of the pancreas and painful nerve damage.

There have been reports of complications and other severe reactions, including death, to some of the antiretroviral nucleoside analogs when used alone or in combination. Therefore, health care experts recommend that people on antiretroviral therapy be routinely seen and followed by their health care providers. The most common side effects associated with protease inhibitors include nausea, diarrhea, and other gastrointestinal symptoms. In addition, protease inhibitors can interact with other drugs resulting in serious side effects.

A number of drugs are available to help treat opportunistic infections to which people with HIV are especially prone. These drugs include:

- Foscarnet and ganciclovir to treat cytomegalovirus (CMV) eye infections

- Fluconazole to treat yeast and other fungal infections

- Trimethoprim/sulfamethoxazole (TMP/SMX) or pentamidine to treat *Pneumocystis carinii* pneumonia (PCP)

In addition to antiretroviral therapy, health care providers treat adults with HIV whose CD4+ T-cell counts drop below 200 to prevent the occurrence of PCP, which is one of the most common and deadly opportunistic infections associated with HIV. They give children PCP preventive therapy when their CD4+ T-cell counts drop to levels considered below normal for their age group. Regardless of their CD4+ T-cell counts, HIV-infected children and adults who have survived an episode of PCP take drugs for the rest of their lives to prevent a recurrence of the pneumonia.

HIV-infected individuals who develop Kaposi's sarcoma or other cancers are treated with radiation, chemotherapy, or injections of alpha interferon, a genetically engineered, naturally occurring protein.

## How Is HIV/AIDS Affecting American Minorities?

Minority populations in the United States, primarily African Americans and Hispanics, constitute 57 percent of the more than 700,000 cases of AIDS reported to the U.S. Centers for Disease Control and Prevention (CDC) since the epidemic began in 1981. African Americans make up almost 38 percent of all AIDS cases reported in the United States, yet according to the U.S. Census Bureau, they comprise only 12 percent of the U.S. population. Hispanics represent 19 percent of all AIDS cases; including residents of Puerto Rico, they represent 13 percent of the population in this country. According to CDC:

- As of June 2001, African Americans and Hispanics represented 51 percent of AIDS cases reported among males and 77 percent of those in females.

- As of June 2001, 58 percent of all women reported with AIDS are African American and 20 percent are Hispanic.

- African American children represent 58 percent of all pediatric AIDS cases.

- Of the 194 pediatric AIDS cases reported between July 2000 and June 2001, 163 (84 percent) were African Americans and Hispanics.

- In 1999, AIDS accounted for an estimated 50 percent of deaths among African Americans and 18 percent among Hispanics. It is the leading cause of death among African American men ages 25–44.

- Injection drug use is a major factor in the spread of HIV in minority communities. Through June 2001, injection drug users accounted for 20 percent of all AIDS cases among both African Americans and Hispanics.

## How Can HIV Infection Be Prevented?

Because no vaccine for HIV is available, the only way to prevent infection by the virus is to avoid behaviors that put a person at risk of infection, such as sharing needles and having unprotected sex.

Many people infected with HIV have no symptoms. Therefore, there is no way of knowing with certainty whether a sexual partner is infected unless he or she has repeatedly tested negative for the virus and has not engaged in any risky behavior.

People should either abstain from having sex or use male latex condoms or female polyurethane condoms, which may offer partial protection, during oral, anal, or vaginal sex. Only water-based lubricants should be used with male latex condoms.

Although some laboratory evidence shows that spermicides can kill HIV, researchers have not found that these products can prevent a person from getting HIV.

The risk of HIV transmission from a pregnant woman to her baby is significantly reduced if she takes AZT during pregnancy, labor, and delivery, and her baby takes it for the first six weeks of life.

## Section 13.2

# *HIV Transmission*

Reprinted from "HIV and Its Transmission," Divisions of HIV/AIDS Prevention, Centers for Disease Control, updated December 24, 2002, http://www.cdc.gov/hiv/pubs/facts/transmission.htm.

## *How HIV Is Transmitted*

HIV is spread by sexual contact with an infected person, by sharing needles and/or syringes (primarily for drug injection) with someone who is infected, or, less commonly (and now very rarely in countries where blood is screened for HIV antibodies), through transfusions of infected blood or blood-clotting factors. Babies born to HIV-infected women may become infected before or during birth or through breast-feeding after birth.

In the health care setting, workers have been infected with HIV after being stuck with needles containing HIV-infected blood or, less frequently, after infected blood gets into a worker's open cut or a mucous membrane (for example, the eyes or inside of the nose). There has been only one instance of patients being infected by a health care worker in the United States; this involved HIV transmission from one infected dentist to six patients. Investigations have been completed involving more than 22,000 patients of 63 HIV-infected physicians, surgeons, and dentists, and no other cases of this type of transmission have been identified in the United States.

Some people fear that HIV might be transmitted in other ways; however, no scientific evidence to support any of these fears has been found. If HIV were being transmitted through other routes (such as through air, water, or insects), the pattern of reported AIDS cases would be much different from what has been observed. For example, if mosquitoes could transmit HIV infection, many more young children and preadolescents would have been diagnosed with AIDS.

All reported cases suggesting new or potentially unknown routes of transmission are thoroughly investigated by state and local health departments with the assistance, guidance, and laboratory support from CDC. No additional routes of transmission have been recorded, despite a national sentinel system designed to detect just such an occurrence.

## Common Misperceptions about HIV Transmission

### HIV in the Environment

Scientists and medical authorities agree that HIV does not survive well in the environment, making the possibility of environmental transmission remote. HIV is found in varying concentrations or amounts in blood, semen, vaginal fluid, breast milk, saliva, and tears. To obtain data on the survival of HIV, laboratory studies have required the use of artificially high concentrations of laboratory-grown virus. Although these unnatural concentrations of HIV can be kept alive for days or even weeks under precisely controlled and limited laboratory conditions, CDC studies have shown that drying even these high concentrations of HIV reduces the amount of infectious virus by 90 to 99 percent within several hours. Since the HIV concentrations used in laboratory studies are much higher than those actually found in blood or other specimens, drying HIV-infected human blood or other body fluids reduces the theoretical risk of environmental transmission to that which has been observed—essentially zero. Incorrect interpretation of conclusions drawn from laboratory studies have unnecessarily alarmed some people.

Results from laboratory studies should not be used to assess specific personal risk of infection because (1) the amount of virus studied is not found in human specimens or elsewhere in nature, and (2) no one has been identified as infected with HIV due to contact with an environmental surface. Additionally, HIV is unable to reproduce outside its living host (unlike many bacteria or fungi, which may do so under suitable conditions), except under laboratory conditions; therefore, it does not spread or maintain infectiousness outside its host.

### Households

Although HIV has been transmitted between family members in a household setting, this type of transmission is very rare. These transmissions are believed to have resulted from contact between skin or mucous membranes and infected blood. To prevent even such rare occurrences, precautions should be taken in all settings, "including the home," to prevent exposures to the blood of persons who are HIV-infected or at risk for HIV infection or whose infection and risk status are unknown. For example:

- Gloves should be worn during contact with blood or other body fluids that could possibly contain visible blood, such as urine, feces, or vomit.

- Cuts, sores, or breaks on both the caregiver's and patient's exposed skin should be covered with bandages.

- Hands and other parts of the body should be washed immediately after contact with blood or other body fluids, and surfaces soiled with blood should be disinfected appropriately.

- Practices that increase the likelihood of blood contact, such as sharing of razors and toothbrushes, should be avoided.

- Needles and other sharp instruments should be used only when medically necessary and handled according to recommendations for health care settings. (Do not put caps back on needles by hand or remove needles from syringes. Dispose of needles in puncture-proof containers.)

### *Businesses and Other Settings*

There is no known risk of HIV transmission to co-workers, clients, or consumers from contact in industries such as food-service establishments. Food-service workers known to be infected with HIV need not be restricted from work unless they have other infections or illnesses (such as diarrhea or hepatitis A) for which any food-service worker, regardless of HIV infection status, should be restricted. CDC recommends that all food-service workers follow recommended standards and practices of good personal hygiene and food sanitation.

In 1985, CDC issued routine precautions that all personal-service workers (such as hairdressers, barbers, cosmetologists, and massage therapists) should follow, even though there is no evidence of transmission from a personal-service worker to a client or vice versa. Instruments that are intended to penetrate the skin (such as tattooing and acupuncture needles, ear-piercing devices) should be used once and disposed of or thoroughly cleaned and sterilized. Instruments not intended to penetrate the skin but which may become contaminated with blood (for example, razors) should be used for only one client and disposed of or thoroughly cleaned and disinfected after each use. Personal-service workers can use the same cleaning procedures that are recommended for health care institutions.

CDC knows of no instances of HIV transmission through tattooing or body piercing, although hepatitis B virus has been transmitted during some of these practices. One case of HIV transmission from acupuncture has been documented. Body piercing (other than ear piercing) is relatively new in the United States, and the medical complications for body piercing appear to be greater than for tattoos. Healing of piercings generally will take weeks, and sometimes even months, and the pierced tissue could conceivably be abraded (torn or cut) or inflamed even after healing. Therefore, a theoretical HIV transmission risk does exist if the unhealed or abraded tissues come into contact with an infected person's blood or other infectious body fluid. Additionally, HIV could be transmitted if instruments contaminated with blood are not sterilized or disinfected between clients.

## Kissing

Casual contact through closed-mouth, or "social," kissing is not a risk for transmission of HIV. Because of the potential for contact with blood during "French," or open-mouth, kissing, CDC recommends against engaging in this activity with a person known to be infected. However, the risk of acquiring HIV during open-mouth kissing is believed to be very low. CDC has investigated only one case of HIV infection that may be attributed to contact with blood during open-mouth kissing.

## Biting

In 1997, CDC published findings from a state health department investigation of an incident that suggested blood-to-blood transmission of HIV by a human bite. There have been other reports in the medical literature in which HIV appeared to have been transmitted by a bite. Severe trauma with extensive tissue tearing and damage and presence of blood was reported in each of these instances. Biting is not a common way of transmitting HIV. In fact, there are numerous reports of bites that did not result in HIV infection.

## Saliva, Tears, and Sweat

HIV has been found in saliva and tears in very low quantities from some AIDS patients. It is important to understand that finding a small amount of HIV in a body fluid does not necessarily mean that HIV can be transmitted by that body fluid. HIV has not been recovered from the sweat of HIV-infected persons. Contact with saliva, tears, or sweat has never been shown to result in transmission of HIV.

## *Insects*

From the onset of the HIV epidemic, there has been concern about transmission of the virus by biting and bloodsucking insects. However, studies conducted by researchers at CDC and elsewhere have shown no evidence of HIV transmission through insects—even in areas where there are many cases of AIDS and large populations of insects such as mosquitoes. Lack of such outbreaks, despite intense efforts to detect them, supports the conclusion that HIV is not transmitted by insects.

The results of experiments and observations of insect biting behavior indicate that when an insect bites a person, it does not inject its own or a previously bitten person's or animal's blood. Rather, it injects saliva, which acts as a lubricant or anticoagulant so the insect can feed efficiently. Such diseases as yellow fever and malaria are transmitted through the saliva of specific species of mosquitoes. However, HIV lives for only a short time inside an insect and, unlike organisms that are transmitted via insect bites, HIV does not reproduce (and does not survive) in insects. Thus, even if the virus enters a mosquito or another sucking or biting insect, the insect does not become infected and cannot transmit HIV to the next human it feeds on or bites. HIV is not found in insect feces.

There is also no reason to fear that a biting or bloodsucking insect, such as a mosquito, could transmit HIV from one person to another through HIV-infected blood left on its mouth parts. Two factors serve to explain why this is so—first, infected people do not have constant, high levels of HIV in their bloodstreams; and, second, insect mouth parts do not retain large amounts of blood on their surfaces. Further, scientists who study insects have determined that biting insects normally do not travel from one person to the next immediately after ingesting blood. Rather, they fly to a resting place to digest this blood meal.

Section 13.3

# HIV and Gay Men

Reprinted from "Need for Sustained HIV Prevention among Men Who Have Sex with Men," Divisions of HIV/AIDS Prevention, Centers for Disease Control, updated March 11, 2002, http://www.cdc.gov/hiv/pubs/facts/msm.htm.

In the United States, HIV-related illness and death historically have had a tremendous impact on men who have sex with men (MSM). Even though the toll of the epidemic among injection drug users (IDUs) and heterosexuals has increased during the last decade, MSM continue to account for the largest number of people reported with AIDS each year. In 2000 alone, 13,562 AIDS cases were reported among MSM, compared with 8,531 among IDUs and 6,530 among men and women who acquired HIV heterosexually.

Overall, the number of MSM of all races and ethnicities who are living with AIDS has increased steadily, partly as a result of the 1993 expanded AIDS case definition and, more recently, of improved survival (see Figure 13.1).

## Continuing Risk among Young MSM

Abundant evidence shows a need to sustain prevention efforts for each generation of young gay and bisexual men. We cannot assume that the positive attitudinal and behavioral change seen among older men also applies to younger men. Recent data on HIV prevalence and risk behaviors suggest that young gay and bisexual men continue to place themselves at considerable risk for HIV infection and other sexually transmitted diseases (STDs):

- Ongoing studies show that both HIV prevalence ratio (the proportion of people living with HIV in a population) and prevalence of risk behaviors remain high among some young MSM. In a sample of MSM 15–22 years old in seven urban areas, CDC researchers found that, overall, 7 percent already were infected with HIV. Higher percentages of African Americans (14 percent) and Hispanics (7 percent) were infected than were whites (3 percent).

- In the 34 areas with confidential HIV reporting, data show that substantial numbers of MSM still are being infected, especially young men. In 2000, 59 percent of reported HIV infections among adolescent males aged 13–19 and 53 percent of cases among men aged 20–24 were attributed to male-to-male sexual contact.

- Research among gay and bisexual men suggests that some individuals are now less concerned about becoming infected than in the past and may be inclined to take more risks. This is backed up by reported increases in gonorrhea among gay men in several large U.S. cities between 1993 and 1996. Despite medical advances, HIV infection remains a serious, usually fatal disease that requires complex, costly, and difficult treatment regimens that do not work for everyone. As better treatment options are developed, we must not lose sight of the fact that preventing HIV infection in the first place precludes the need for people to undergo these difficult and expensive therapies.

These data highlight the need to design more effective prevention efforts for gay and bisexual men of color. The involvement of community and opinion leaders in prevention efforts will be critical for overcoming cultural barriers to prevention, including homophobia. For example, there remains a tremendous stigma to acknowledging gay and bisexual activity in African American and Hispanic communities.

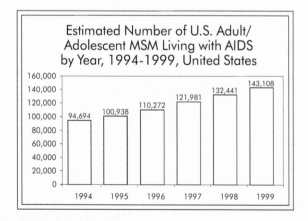

**Figure 13.1.** *As this graph shows, the number of American men who have sex with men and who also have AIDS has been growing each year.*

## *Need to Combat Other STDs*

Studies among MSM who are treated in STD clinics have shown consistently high percentages of HIV infection, ranging from nearly 4 percent in Seattle to a high of almost 36 percent in Atlanta. Some studies have shown that the likelihood of both acquiring and spreading HIV is two to five times greater in people with STDs, and that aggressively treating STDs in a community may help to reduce the rate of new HIV infections. Along with prompt attention to and treatment of STDs, efforts to reduce the behaviors that spread STDs are critical.

## *Prevention Services Must Reach Both Uninfected and Infected*

Research has shown that high-risk behavior is continuing in some populations of MSM, including those who are infected with HIV. Because HIV-infected gay and bisexual men are living longer and healthier lives, greater efforts must be made to reach them with behavioral interventions that can help them protect their own health and prevent transmission to others.

Overall, the number of MSM of all races and ethnicities who are living with AIDS has increased steadily, partly as a result of the 1993 expanded AIDS case definition and, more recently, of improved survival.

# Section 13.4

# *Preventing Sexual Transmission of HIV*

Updated June 4, 2003. © San Francisco AIDS Foundation.

## *Safe(er) Sex*

When thinking about "safe" sex, it is important to realize that risk from various sexual practices often falls along a continuum, rather than having a clear safe versus not safe boundary. Throughout this discussion, we will refer to "safer" sex, with the thought that by placing more or fewer "boundaries" around a particular sexual act, it can be made more safe or less safe.

Although in the early years of the epidemic we placed individual sexual practices in specific categories of risk, nowadays we stay away from the categories and emphasize the logic behind safer sex guidelines. In fact, the safety of an individual practice depends on how people are doing it.

Any sexual practice can be made safer or less safe. For instance, mutual masturbation can become unsafe if people touch their own genitals after getting a partner's infected semen, blood, or vaginal fluids on their hands. We hope to help you develop criteria to use to decide whether previous experiences you've had were safe or not, and how to stay safe in the future.

It is helpful to think about safer sex using a wide definition of sexuality. Many people think about sex fairly narrowly. For instance, thinking that sex only starts when penetration takes place may limit people's ability to protect themselves and to enhance their sexual lives through safer sex. We consider sexuality to include any practices that a person finds erotic and sexually exciting.

Remember, telephone hotline staffers are available to talk with you about any of these issues. Within California, call the San Francisco AIDS Foundation's California AIDS Hotline toll-free at (800) 367-AIDS. Outside California, call the CDC National AIDS Hotline toll-free at (800) 342-AIDS.

## Why Practice Safer Sex?

Most people are inclined to think that people who practice safer sex are only those who are concerned about getting HIV from their partners because they don't know their sexual partner(s)' HIV status or they know if their sexual partner(s) is (are) HIV-positive.

In fact, there are other reasons why some people decide to practice safer sex. Some examples:

- HIV-negative people who always practice safer sex so they don't lose the habit of protection. Also, if a person agrees, with ease, to practice safer sex, this is an indicator that the person has practiced safer sex with previous partners.

- HIV-negative people in a sexual relationship who want to avoid dealing with issues of trust between them. By practicing safer sex, there is no need to discuss whether they are being monogamous.

- HIV-negative people who agree to practice safer sex with each other for three months before they are tested again for antibodies, prior to conceiving a child.

- HIV-negative people who want to avoid getting sexually transmitted diseases other than HIV.

- HIV-positive people who want to avoid getting reinfected with HIV. Scientists believe that reinfection may accelerate the progression of the disease. Also, evidence presented at the 12th World AIDS Conference indicates that it is possible for someone with a drug-resistant strain of HIV to give it to another person, which could limit treatment options as well.

Of course, sexual partners who are HIV-negative, waited three months after their last risky activities to take the HIV-antibody test, and trust that neither one has current risks may practice sex without protection. Among these conditions, trust in their partners is sometimes the hardest one to achieve.

## Safer Sex and Pregnancy

One situation in which practicing safer sex is not an option is wanting to have a baby. Partners who are not sure of their antibody status can seek antibody testing to determine their status.

## Safer Sex Guidelines

The most general way in which we can define "safe" sex is the following:

Any sexual practice that does not let someone else's semen, blood, or vaginal fluids get into someone else's body. The parts of the body where HIV could enter the bloodstream are the anus and rectum, the vagina, the penis, the mouth, and the eyes. These body parts must be protected from contact with HIV-infected fluids. HIV cannot go through the skin unless there are open sores or bleeding cuts.

We hope to give you the tools with which you can make your own decisions about where you want to fit in on the continuum from safer sex to riskier sex. Each time you do a sexual activity, you choose (whether consciously or unconsciously) the level of risk you are comfortable with for that moment.

Safer sex often involves use of latex condoms, latex dental dams, plastic wrap, latex gloves, and finger cots as barriers between the infectious fluids and mucous membranes or open cuts (see Table 13.1.)

## Why Latex?

Latex has been proven effective in preventing the transmission of HIV. Latex is a very resilient and strong material that does not allow HIV to pass through it. When used properly, latex products offer the best possible barrier for HIV and other sexually transmitted diseases.

## Lubricant

There has been controversy over lubricant that contains nonoxynol-9 (N-9), a spermicide that is added to some products. Recent studies by the Centers for Disease Control, the World Health Organization, and the Population Council of New York have each demonstrated that hundreds of epithelial cells, which provide a protective membrane in the anus, were stripped away by products containing N-9.

Originally, N-9 was thought to help prevent HIV, because it killed the virus in a test tube, but now it's been documented that N-9 washes away the protective cells.

Due to public pressure, all lubricant manufacturers agreed to stop making lube with nonoxynol-9. There are however, still manufacturers that continue to make condoms laced with N-9 as it is legal and approved by the FDA. Time will tell if the FDA will change its position on this.

**Table 13.1.** Condoms and Other Safer Sex Devices

| | |
|---|---|
| **"Male" condoms** | A condom is a sleeve, closed at one end, which fits over the penis. There are three types of condoms: latex, polyurethane, and lambskin. The lambskin condoms may allow passage of HIV, and therefore are not recommended. Latex or polyurethane condoms are recommended because they do consistently prevent passage of HIV. |
| **"Female" condoms** | An approved alternative to the regular condom, the 'female' condom, is a disposable vaginal pouch made out of polyurethane. It is soft and thin and has a latex ring at each end. The ring at the closed end goes into the vagina and over the cervix (the opening of the uterus). The other end stays outside the vagina and covers the labia (vaginal lips). The polyurethane covers the cervix and the vaginal canal. The vaginal condom is currently marketed under the name Reality®. This condom is sometimes used by either men or women for anal sex, although it has not been designed for or tested for this usage. |
| **Latex dental dams** | Dental dams are squares made out of latex that dentists use to isolate the tooth on which they are working. AIDS educators have advocated their use for oral sex, either mouth-vagina or mouth-anus. Because they were not originally designed for sex, they tend to be thicker than condoms. |
| **"Dammit"** | This device consists of a couple of leather straps with snaps that can be adjusted around the legs to hold a dental dam in place, like a garter belt. This harness has several purposes: (1) one's hands are left free to hold or stimulate the partner, and (2) there is no risk of flipping the dental dam over and using the wrong (exposed to fluids) side for as long as the "dammit" is being used. |
| **Plastic wrap** | Plastic wrap is a common product in people's kitchens. It has been shown to prevent passage of HIV, and it is recommended as a barrier for oral sex, either mouth-vagina or mouth-anus. Although dental dams can also be used for these activities, plastic wrap has the advantage of being transparent, thinner, cheaper, and easier to get. |
| **Latex gloves** | Latex gloves are easy to find in drugstores and medical supply stores. They may be used to cover the hand when inserting the fingers or fist in the vagina or rectum. They may also be used by people who have open cuts in the hands or chronic skin problems such as eczema. Some people simply enjoy the feel of latex on their skin. |
| **Finger cots** | Finger cots are made out of latex and cover only one finger. They can be found in medical supply stores. |

## Types of Condoms

There are a wide variety of condoms on the market. They can be lubricated or nonlubricated. They come in different colors, shapes, sizes, textures, and thickness. There are condoms that are flavored, that glow in the dark, that play a short song when opened, etc. There is practically no limit to the selection.

Some men complain that condoms make them lose sensitivity in the penis during sex. We encourage these men to try out different brands and types of condoms and select the ones with which they are more comfortable (they can masturbate with them to get used to them and feel more comfortable during sex with their partners). Some people find that although they may lose their sensitivity at first, after using condoms for a while they can regain it. And, of course, they feel more relaxed about sex since they know they are protected.

There are no rules about what condom to use. Some men feel better with a thicker condom while others prefer a thinner one. Some people get excited about colors and flavors while others find these features boring or irrelevant. [See the subject of lubricants above and the concern over use of nonoxynol-9 (N-9).]

Some men claim that their penis is too big for a condom. We encourage them to try different brands (which fit different people in different ways; there are no "better" brands). There are also brands of condoms designed explicitly for men who have a large penis. Interestingly, few if any men say that their penises are too small for a condom.

## Using "Male" Condoms

- Pick up the condom by grabbing the "nose" (the reservoir tip) between your thumb and forefinger (to ensure that no air bubble gets trapped in the tip, which may cause breakage during intercourse).

- With both hands place the condom on the head of a fully erect penis (remember, you are holding the "nose" in one hand; you roll the condom down onto the penis with the other hand).

- Unroll the condom completely, all the way down to the base of the penis. Having used both hands and held onto the reservoir tip, you have just ensured that no air is trapped inside the condom. Not only does this prevent air bubbles popping the condom during the friction of intercourse, but it also creates a vacuum, which helps to keep the condom in place.

217

- Use plenty of water-based lubricant (some people use a single drop inside the tip to keep the air out).

- When pulling out, the man or his partner should hold the condom between the fingers so that it does not slip off and spill any semen inside the body.

## Preventing Condom Breakage

The main reason for condom breakage is user failure. Although condoms are very resilient, they may become weaker when affected by several factors:

- *Heat*. Condoms should never be left in places where they will be exposed to heat, such as glove compartments, under direct sunlight, or in pockets of tight jeans.

- *Old age*. Condoms should be fresh when used. We recommend not keeping condoms longer than a year. If there is any uncertainty about how old a condom is, it should be thrown out. Most condoms will have expiration dates on the package.

- *Insufficient lubrication*. It is important to use a lubricant (such as saliva or a commercial lubricant like KY jelly or another product) to reduce friction on the outside of the condom during sexual intercourse. When in doubt, more lubrication should be added.

- *Use of oil-based lubricant*. Oil-based lubricants affect the latex and make it break. Lubricants that should **never** be used include: Vaseline®, baby oil, Crisco®, hand lotion, massage oil, face cream, and so forth. Just look on the label for ingredients; water should be the first ingredient.

- *Air bubbles*. The main reason condoms break during sex is because air bubbles get trapped inside them, which make them break due to the motions of intercourse. The air must be pinched out of the condom's tip before putting it on.

## Using Condoms during Oral Sex

If you wish to perform safer oral sex on a man, you have the option of using nonlubricated condoms and also polyurethane condoms. Lubricated condoms do not taste good to most people, and if there is nonoxynol-9 on the condom, it may cause numbness of the lips lasting several hours. (See "Lubricant" above for more information on nonoxynol-9 and some concerns regarding it.) Some people don't like the white powder that covers nonlubricated condoms. That white powder is cornstarch and can be easily wiped off with a wet washcloth.

## Condom Availability

Condoms are, in general, very easy to find. Most drugstores carry them. However, in some places people have to ask the clerk for them, which can be embarrassing.

Condoms are usually inexpensive. Some stores have an arrangement of selling them at cost (that is, they charge only what the manufacturer charges them) to make them even more accessible. Some health departments, STD clinics, and nonprofit HIV/AIDS service organizations have condoms available for free.

We encourage you to keep a good supply of condoms available at home or at any place where you are likely to have sex. Having condoms readily available increases the probability of their being used.

## Using Dental Dams and Plastic Wrap for Oral Sex

The dam or plastic wrap can be placed between the mouth and the vagina or anus during oral sex to reduce risk of sexually transmitted diseases. It is very important that you use a different dam or piece of plastic wrap every time that you perform oral sex. It is not a good idea to set the barrier aside and use it again because it's too easy to flip it over and forget what side touched the vagina or anus.

Dental dams are not as readily available as plastic wrap. They can be bought from medical supply stores, and from some sex shops and drugstores. They can also be ordered by phone.

## Using Dildos and Other Sex Toys

Part of practicing safer sex is being creative. Sex toys can add to the pleasure and creativity of sex. However, some precautions are necessary when they are being used by more than one person.

It is best to have one's own personal sex toys and never share them. However, dildos and other toys may be washed with soap and water and then used by another person. Condoms may be placed on dildos and vibrators to avoid needing to wash them before a second person uses them. It is important to change the condom every time that the toy passes from one person to another.

## *Risk from Specific Sexual Practices*

**Anal Intercourse.** Anal intercourse without a condom is the riskiest activity for HIV transmission. The receptive partner is at risk because the anal area provides easy access to the bloodstream for HIV carried in semen. The insertive partner is also at risk because the membranes inside the urethra can provide an entry for HIV, possibly present in blood inside the anus, into the bloodstream.

Using a condom from start to finish greatly reduces the risk. However, the risk is not zero because the condom could break. It is important that you understand that condoms are only effective against HIV if they are used properly and do not break.

**Vaginal Intercourse.** In a heterosexual encounter, HIV passes more easily from male to female than vice versa. Therefore, the woman is at more risk. No matter what the gender of the partners, latex can reduce the risk of HIV transmission and other sexually transmitted diseases.

**Oral Sex.** This is the "grayest" area when discussing risk, and is very controversial.

In general, oral sex is much less risky for HIV transmission than anal or vaginal intercourse. But to properly assess risk, you must consider whether there is ejaculate, vaginal fluid, or blood present, because there are no absolute answers regarding oral sex and risk.

Risk assessments involve "what substance/fluid" and "where it goes." The mouth is a less likely path for transmission because the mucous membranes are more protective than those in the anus/rectum or vagina and because fluids can't remain in the mouth (they are swallowed or spit out). So the "where it goes" part of the risk equation means oral sex is inherently less risky than anal or vaginal sex.

However, you must consider the "what substance/fluid" as well. If there is infected ejaculate, vaginal fluid, or blood present, it increases the risk for infection. Blood contains the highest concentration of virus, followed by semen, vaginal fluid, and a distant last place, preseminal fluid.

How much does it increase the risk? We can't say for sure. Certainly, not to the level of risk from ejaculation inside anus or vagina. And we can definitely say that there are only a few documented cases of HIV in which the only possible source of infection was through oral sex, so the risk is still very low. But it is incorrect to equate the risk of oral sex with ejaculation to the risk of oral sex without.

A person receiving oral sex is generally not at risk, because that person is coming into contact only with saliva. (There is a *theoretical* risk of transmission if the person performing oral sex had blood in her/his mouth.) Many people find using a condom unacceptable and are practicing oral sex on men without ejaculation. They are coming into contact with pre-ejaculate fluid. There is no conclusive evidence that pre-ejaculate fluid transmits HIV, but some studies suggest that HIV is present in this fluid. Again, go back to the two questions: "Is HIV present?" and "How much HIV is present?" Although HIV may be present in pre-ejaculate fluid, it is in very small amounts, and the mouth is not an easy path for transmission. This means unprotected oral sex without ejaculation is a very low risk activity for HIV transmission.

Performing oral sex on a woman who is menstruating increases the risk because blood has more HIV than vaginal fluid. There is little data on how often HIV is transmitted via oral sex from an infected woman to an uninfected man.

**Urine in Sex or Sex Play.** Urine does not transmit HIV. Even if the urine contained small amounts of blood, the fragile virus would be battered by acid, heat, friction, enzymes, and dilution. And again, it's important to think about how this fluid is coming into contact with another person. To transmit HIV, there would have to be a source of bleeding, and then we're not talking about *urine* transmitting HIV, we're talking about blood.

**Oral-Anal Contact.** Feces may contain some blood, but it poses very minimal risk for HIV transmission. However, oral-anal contact is a risk for transmission of hepatitis, parasites, and many other sexually transmitted diseases. Safe oral-anal contact means using a dental dam or plastic wrap.

**Fisting**. Fisting refers to inserting the fingers or hand into the rectum or vagina. When people talk about fisting, they almost always mean anal fisting, but the precautions are the same for both. Fisting could be risky for the insertive partner if there is broken skin that would allow blood from the rectum or vagina into the bloodstream. Using a latex glove reduces the risk.

**Kissing.** This activity is not known to pose any risk for HIV infection. Saliva does not transmit HIV. One should be aware of cuts or sores in the mouth and, if concerned, not floss or brush right before

French kissing. "Dry" or "social" kissing (with the lips closed) poses no risk for transmitting HIV.

**Mutual Masturbation.** The skin is an effective barrier against all sorts of organisms, and will stop HIV. Any possibly infected fluid on the skin should be washed off. An intact scab is as effective as unbroken skin. Open cuts in the skin might allow passage of the virus, but the breaks need to be open and/or bleeding to pose a risk. If there is any question, latex gloves or finger cots should be used. It is not (if one wants to be perfectly safe) advisable to ejaculate on someone else's penis or labia, nor to touch the genitals with someone else's fresh semen or vaginal secretions on the hand.

**Solo Masturbation.** With solo masturbation there is no fear of self-infection as long as someone else's infectious fluids are not present.

**Body Massage, Hugging, Rubbing.** With only skin-to-skin contact, these activities are risk-free. This includes body-to-body rubbing ("frottage").

**Sadomasochistic (S&M) Activities.** Unless someone's blood, semen, or vaginal fluid enters the bloodstream of another person sadomasochistic activities pose little danger of transmission.

# Part Two

# Other Physical Concerns of Special Significance for Men

# Chapter 14

# *Hypertension*

## What Is High Blood Pressure?

Blood pressure is the force of blood against the walls of arteries. Blood pressure rises and falls throughout the day. But when the pressure stays elevated over time, then it's called high blood pressure.

The medical term for high blood pressure is hypertension. High blood pressure is dangerous because it makes the heart work too hard and contributes to atherosclerosis (hardening of the arteries). It increases the risk of heart disease and stroke, the first and third leading causes of death among Americans. High blood pressure also can result in other conditions, such as congestive heart failure, kidney disease, and blindness.

## Risk Factors for Heart Disease

Risk factors are conditions or behaviors that increase your likelihood of developing a disease. When you have more than one for heart disease, your risk greatly multiplies. So if you have high blood pressure, you need to take action. Fortunately, most of the heart disease risk factors are largely within your control.

Risk factors under your control are:

Adapted from "Facts about Lowering Blood Pressure," National Heart, Lung, and Blood Institute, National Institutes of Health (NIH), May 2000, http://www.nhlbi.nih.gov/health/public/heart/hbp/hbp_low/hbp_toc.htm. Available in hard copy as NIH Pub. No. 00-3281.

- High blood pressure
- High blood cholesterol
- Cigarette smoking

- Diabetes
- Overweight
- Physical inactivity

Risk factors beyond your control are:

- Age (45 or older for men)
- Family history of early heart disease (having a mother or sister who has been diagnosed with heart disease before age 65, or a father or brother diagnosed before age 55)

High blood pressure affects about 50 million—or one in four—American adults. Some people are more likely to develop it than others. It is especially common among African Americans, who tend to develop it earlier and more often than whites. Also, many Americans

**Table 14.1.** Blood Pressure Levels for Healthy Adults 18 and Older Not on Blood Pressure Medication

| Category | Systolic (in mm Hg) | Diastolic (in mm Hg) | Result |
|---|---|---|---|
| *Optimal* | less than 120 and | less than 80 | Good for you! |
| *Normal* | less than 130 and | less than 85 | Keep an eye on it. |
| *High Normal* | 130–139 or | 85–89 | Your blood pressure could be a problem. Make needed changes in what you eat and drink, get physical activity, and lose extra weight. If you also have diabetes, see the doctor. |

**Hypertension**

| | | | |
|---|---|---|---|
| *Stage 1* | 140–159 or | 90–99 | |
| *Stage 2* | 160–179 or | 100–109 | |
| *Stage 3* | 180 or higher or | 110 or higher | |

Source: The Sixth Report of the Joint National Committee on Prevention, Detection, Evaluation, and Treatment of High Blood Pressure, National High Blood Pressure Education Program, November 1997.

tend to develop high blood pressure as they get older, but hypertension is not a part of healthy aging. About 60 percent of all Americans age 60 and older have high blood pressure.

Others at high risk of developing hypertension are the overweight, those with a family history of high blood pressure, and those with a high-normal blood pressure (see Table 14.1). High blood pressure also is more common in the southeastern United States.

## How Is Blood Pressure Checked?

Blood pressure usually is measured in millimeters of mercury (mm Hg) and recorded as two numbers: systolic pressure (as the heart beats) "over" diastolic pressure (as the heart relaxes between beats)—for example, 130/80 mm Hg. Both numbers are important, although for some Americans systolic blood pressure is especially important.

The test to measure blood pressure is simple, quick, and painless. Typically, a blood pressure cuff called a sphygmomanometer (pronounced sfig'-mo-ma-nom-e-ter) is used. The cuff is placed around the upper arm and inflated with air until blood flow stops. Then, the cuff is slowly deflated, letting blood flow start again.

As the cuff is deflated, a stethoscope is used to listen to the blood flow in an artery at the inner elbow. The first thumping sound heard gives the blood pressure as the heart contracts—this is the systolic pressure. When the thumping sound is no longer heard, the blood pressure is between heartbeats—this is the diastolic pressure.

Because blood pressure changes and is affected by many factors, the test will be repeated on different days to confirm a reading of high blood pressure.

A systolic blood pressure of less than 120 and a diastolic blood pressure of less than 80 mm Hg are optimal. Systolic blood pressures of 140 or higher, or diastolic blood pressures of 90 or higher mm Hg are high. If systolic and diastolic pressures fall into different categories, go by the higher category. Even levels slightly above optimal can increase the risk of heart disease and other problems.

### *Watch That Systolic*

Both numbers in a blood pressure test are important but, for some, the systolic is especially meaningful. That's because, for those middle aged and older, the systolic pressure gives the most accurate diagnosis of high blood pressure.

Systolic blood pressure is the top number in a blood pressure reading. It is high if it is 140 mm Hg or above.

For American adults, the systolic pressure increases sharply with age, while the diastolic increases until about age 55 and then declines. Thus, many older Americans have only a high systolic pressure—a condition known as "isolated systolic hypertension," or ISH.

A high systolic pressure causes blood vessels to stiffen and can lead to cardiovascular disease and damage kidneys and other organs.

Clinical studies have proven that treating a high systolic pressure saves lives and greatly reduces illness. Yet, most Americans do not have their high systolic pressure under control.

Blood pressure must be controlled to under 140/90 mm Hg. The treatment is the same for ISH as for other forms of high blood pressure. So talk with your doctor. Ask about your blood pressure level—and especially your systolic blood pressure. If your blood pressure is too high, ask about adjusting your drug and making lifestyle changes to bring it to less than 140/90 mm Hg.

## How Can You Prevent or Control High Blood Pressure?

### Maintain a Healthy Weight

Carrying extra weight can promote high blood pressure and encourage other heart and lung diseases. Even the loss of 10 pounds can have a significant impact on your risk of blood-pressure problems. This section includes information about body mass index (BMI), an important measurement of obesity and overweight, and offers tips on how to lower or regulate your body weight.

Overweight increases your risk of developing high blood pressure. In fact, blood pressure rises as body weight increases. Losing even 10 pounds can lower blood pressure—and it has the biggest effect in those who are overweight and already have hypertension.

Overweight also is a risk factor for heart disease. And it increases your chance of developing high blood cholesterol and diabetes—two more risk factors for heart disease.

Two key measures are used to determine if someone is overweight. These are the body mass index, or BMI, and waist circumference.

BMI relates weight to height. It gives an approximation of total body fat—and that's what increases the risk of obesity-related diseases.

The formula for calculating BMI is: BMI = your weight in pounds (in underwear but no shoes) / (your height in inches) 2 x 703. Or, try this simple 3-step method:

1. Multiply your weight in pounds by 703

2. Divide the answer by your height (in inches)

3. Divide the answer again by your height (in inches) to get your BMI

For example: If you are 5'7" tall (or 67") and weigh 170 pounds, you would:

1. Multiply 170 x 703 = 119,510

2. Divide 119,510/67 = 1,785

3. Divide 1,785/67 = 26.6

4. BMI = 26.6

But BMI alone does not determine risk. For example, in someone who is very muscular or who has swelling from fluid retention (called edema), the BMI may overestimate body fat. BMI also may not accurately estimate total body fat in older persons or those losing muscle.

That's why waist measurement is often checked as well. Another reason is that too much body fat in the abdomen (or stomach area) also increases disease risk. A waist measurement of more than 35 inches in women and more than 40 inches in men is considered high.

Table 14.2 explains the meaning of BMI results. It tells if you are at increased risk for disease and if you need to lose weight. If you fall in the obese range, you should lose weight. You also should lose weight if you are overweight or have a high waist measurement and two or more heart disease risk factors. If you fall in the normal weight range or are overweight but do not need to lose pounds, you still should be careful not to gain weight.

If you have to lose weight, it's important to do so slowly. Lose no more than 1/2 to 2 pounds a week. Begin with a goal of losing 10 percent of your current weight. This is the healthiest way to lose weight and—importantly—it offers the best chance of long-term success.

There's no magic formula for weight loss. You have to eat fewer calories than you burn. Just how many calories you burn daily depends on factors such as your body size and how physically active you are.

One pound equals 3,500 calories. So, to lose one pound a week, you would need to eat 500 calories a day less or burn 500 calories a day more than you usually do. It's best to work out some combination of both eating less and being more physically active.

And remember to be careful of serving sizes. It's not only what you eat that adds calories, but also how much.

As you lose, be sure to eat a healthy diet, with a variety of foods.

### Be Physically Active

Being physically active is one of the most important steps you can take to prevent or control high blood pressure. It also helps to reduce your risk of heart disease.

It doesn't take a lot of effort to become physically active. All you need to do is 30 minutes of moderate-level activity on most, and preferably all, days of the week. Examples of moderate-level activity are brisk walking, bicycling, raking leaves, and gardening.

You can even divide the 30 minutes into shorter periods of at least 10 minutes each. For instance: Use stairs instead of an elevator; get off a bus one or two stops early; or park your car at the far end of the lot at work. If you already engage in 30 minutes a day, you can get added benefits by doing more. Do a moderate-level activity for a longer period each day or engage in a more vigorous activity.

Most people don't need to see a doctor before they start a moderate-level physical activity. You should check first with a doctor if you

**Table 14.2.** Body Mass Index (BMI) Categories

| | | |
|---|---|---|
| *Normal weight* | BMI = 18.5–24.9 | Good for you! Try not to gain weight. |
| *Overweight* | BMI = 25–29.9 | Do not gain any weight, especially if your waist measurement is high. You need to lose weight if you have two or more risk factors for heart disease and you are overweight or have a high waist measurement. |
| *Obese* | BMI = 30 or greater | You need to lose weight. Lose weight slowly—about 1/2–2 pounds a week. See your doctor or a nutritionist if you need help. |

*Source*: National Heart, Lung, and Blood Institute, in cooperation with the National Institute of Diabetes and Digestive and Kidney Diseases, National Institutes of Health, *Clinical Guidelines on the Identification, Evaluation, and Treatment of Overweight and Obesity in Adults*, June 1998.

have heart trouble or have had a heart attack, if you are over age 50 and are not used to doing a moderate-level activity, if you have a family history of heart disease at an early age, or if you have any other serious health problem.

## *Follow a Healthy Eating Plan*

Research has shown that what you eat affects the development of high blood pressure. A healthy eating plan can both reduce the risk of developing high blood pressure and lower an already-elevated blood pressure.

A key ingredient of healthy eating is choosing foods lower in salt (sodium chloride) and other forms of sodium. A recent study showed just how important lowering sodium is in keeping blood pressure at a healthy level. Here are some key results:

- The less sodium consumed, the lower the blood pressure.

- Blood pressure was lower in the Dietary Approaches to Stopping Hypertension (DASH) diet than in the control diet at all three sodium levels.

- The lowest blood pressures occurred with the DASH diet at the lower sodium level.

- Sodium level had a bigger effect in the control diet than in the DASH diet.

- The effects of sodium reduction were seen in all study participants—those with and without high blood pressure, men and women, and African Americans and others.

Most Americans eat more salt and sodium than they need. Some people, such as African Americans and the elderly, are especially sensitive to salt and sodium and may need to be particularly careful about how much they consume.

Most Americans should consume no more than 2.4 grams (2,400 milligrams) of sodium a day. That equals 6 grams (about one teaspoon) of table salt a day. For someone with high blood pressure, the doctor may advise less. The 6 grams includes all salt and sodium consumed, including that used in cooking and at the table.

Here are some tips for reducing salt and sodium:

- Buy fresh, plain frozen, or canned "with no salt added" vegetables.

231

- Use fresh poultry, fish, and lean meat rather than canned or processed types.

- Use herbs, spices, and salt-free seasoning blends in cooking and at the table.

- Cook rice, pasta, and hot cereals without salt. Cut back on instant or flavored rice, pasta, and cereal mixes, which usually have added salt.

- Choose "convenience" foods that are lower in sodium. Cut back on frozen dinners, mixed dishes such as pizza, packaged mixes, canned soups or broths, and salad dressings—these often have a lot of sodium.

- Rinse canned foods, such as tuna, to remove some sodium.

- When available, buy low- or reduced-sodium or no-salt-added versions of foods.

- Choose ready-to-eat breakfast cereals that are lower in sodium.

Sodium is found naturally in many foods. But processed foods account for most of the salt and sodium Americans consume. Processed foods with high amounts of salt include regular canned vegetables and soups, frozen dinners, lunch meats, instant and ready-to-eat cereals, and salty chips and other snacks. You should use food labels to choose products lower in sodium. Look for labels on cans, boxes, bottles, bags, and other products that say:

- Sodium free
- Very low sodium
- Low sodium
- Light in sodium
- Reduced or less sodium
- Unsalted or no salt added

Sodium also is found in many foods that may surprise you, such as baking soda, soy sauce, monosodium glutamate (MSG), seasoned salts, and some antacids—the range is wide.

Before trying salt substitutes, you should check with your doctor, especially if you have high blood pressure. These contain potassium chloride and may be harmful for those with certain medical conditions.

Table 14.3 provides a guide to the DASH eating plan based on 2,000 calories a day. The number of daily servings in a food group may vary from those listed depending on your caloric needs.

You should be aware that the DASH diet has more daily servings of fruits, vegetables, and grains than you may be used to eating. The servings make it high in fiber, which may temporarily cause bloating and diarrhea. To get used to the DASH diet, gradually increase your servings of fruits, vegetables, and grains. Here are some tips on making the switch:

**Table 14.3.** The DASH Eating Plan

| Food Group | Servings | Serving Size |
|---|---|---|
| Grains and grain products | 7–8 servings daily | 1 slice bread, 1 cup ready-to-eat cereal, 1/2 cup cooked rice, pasta, or cereal |
| Vegetables | 4–5 servings daily | 1 cup raw leafy vegetable, 1/2 cup cooked vegetable, 6 ounces vegetable juice |
| Fruits | 4–5 servings daily | 1 medium fruit; 1/4 cup dried fruit; 1/2 cup fresh, frozen, or canned fruit; 6 ounces fruit juice |
| Low-fat or fat-free dairy foods | 2–3 servings daily | 8 ounces milk, 1 cup yogurt, 1 1/2 ounces cheese |
| Lean meats, poultry, and fish | 2 or fewer servings daily | 3 ounces cooked lean meats, skinless poultry, or fish |
| Nuts, seeds, and dry beans | 4–5 servings weekly | 1/3 cup or 1 1/2 ounces nuts, 1 tablespoon or 1/2 ounce seeds, 1/2 cup cooked dry beans |
| Fats and oils | 2–3 servings daily | 1 teaspoon soft margarine, 1 tablespoon low-fat mayonnaise, 2 tablespoons light salad dressing, 1 teaspoon vegetable oil |
| Sweets | 5 servings weekly | 1 tablespoon sugar, 1 tablespoon jelly or jam, 1/2 ounce jelly beans, 8 ounces lemonade |

- Change gradually. Add a vegetable or fruit serving at lunch and dinner.

- Use only half the butter or margarine you do now.

- If you have trouble digesting dairy products, try lactase enzyme pills or drops—they're available at drugstores and groceries. Or buy lactose-free milk or milk with lactase enzyme added to it.

- Get added nutrients such as the B vitamins by choosing whole grain foods, including whole wheat bread or whole grain cereals.

- Spread out the servings. Have two servings of fruits and/or vegetables at each meal, or add fruits as snacks.

- Treat meat as one part of the meal, instead of the focus. Try casseroles, pasta, and stir-fry dishes. Have two or more meatless meals a week.

- Use fruits or low-fat foods as desserts and snacks.

A good way to change to the DASH diet is to keep a diary of your current eating habits. Write down what you eat, how much, when, and why. Note whether or not you snack on high-fat foods while watching television, or if you skip breakfast and eat a big lunch. Do this for several days. You'll be able to see where you can start making changes.

If you are trying to lose weight, you should choose an eating plan lower in calories. You can still use the DASH diet, but follow it at a lower calorie level. Again, a food diary can be helpful. It can tell you if there are certain times you eat but aren't really hungry, or when you can substitute lower-calorie foods for higher-calorie items.

### Consume Alcoholic Beverages in Moderation

Drinking too much alcohol can raise blood pressure. It also can harm the liver, brain, and heart. Furthermore, alcoholic drinks contain calories, which matter if you are trying to lose weight.

If you drink alcoholic beverages, have only a moderate amount—one drink a day for women, two drinks a day for men. Here are the amounts that count as one drink:

- 12 ounces of beer (regular or light, 150 calories)

- 5 ounces of wine (100 calories)

- 1 1/2 ounces of 80-proof whiskey (100 calories)

## *Take High Blood Pressure Medication As Directed*

If you have high blood pressure, the lifestyle habits noted above may not lower your blood pressure enough. If they don't, you will need to take medication.

However, even if you do need medication, you still must follow the lifestyle changes. Doing so will help your medication work better and may reduce how much of it you need.

There are many drugs available to lower high blood pressure. They work in various ways. Often, two or more drugs work better than one. Here's a rundown on the main types of drugs and how they work:

- *Diuretics.* These are sometimes called "water pills" because they work in the kidney and flush excess water and sodium from the body through urine. This reduces the amount of fluid in the blood. And, since sodium is flushed out of blood vessel walls, the vessels open wider. Pressure goes down. There are different types of diuretics. They are often used with other high blood pressure drugs.

- *Beta blockers.* These reduce nerve impulses to the heart and blood vessels. This makes the heart beat less often and with less force. Blood pressure drops and the heart works less hard.

- *Angiotensin converting enzyme (ACE) inhibitors.* These prevent the formation of a hormone called angiotensin II, which normally causes vessels to narrow. The blood vessels relax and pressure goes down.

- *Angiotensin antagonists.* These are a new type of high blood pressure drug. They shield blood vessels from angiotensin II. As a result, the vessels are wider and pressure lowers.

- *Calcium channel blockers (CCBs).* These keep calcium from entering the muscle cells of the heart and blood vessels. Blood vessels relax and pressure goes down. One short-acting type of CCB has been found to increase the chance of having another heart attack. Short-acting CCBs are taken several times a day. If you are on such a drug, you should talk with your doctor about other medication choices. The finding does not apply to the longer-acting types of CCB, which are taken once a day.

- *Alpha blockers.* These reduce nerve impulses to blood vessels, which allows blood to pass more easily. Results from a clinical study indicate that an alpha blocker may not be the best choice for an initial treatment for high blood pressure. If you now take an alpha blocker drug for high blood pressure, consult with your doctor about whether or not your treatment should be modified.

- *Alpha-beta blockers*. These work the same way as alpha blockers but also slow the heartbeat, as beta blockers do. As a result, less blood is pumped through the vessels.

- *Nervous system inhibitors*. These relax blood vessels by controlling nerve impulses.

- *Vasodilators*. These directly open blood vessels by relaxing the muscle in the vessel walls.

When you start on a medication, work with your doctor to get the right drug and dose level for you. If you have side effects, tell your doctor so the medication can be adjusted. If you're worried about cost, tell your doctor or pharmacist—there may be a less expensive drug or a generic form that can be used instead.

It's important that you take the medication as prescribed, including in the right amount. That can prevent a heart attack, stroke, and congestive heart failure, a serious condition in which the heart cannot pump enough blood for the body's needs.

But you can be taking medication and still not have your blood pressure under control. Everyone—and older Americans in particular—must be careful to control their blood pressure to below 140/90 mm Hg. If your blood pressure is higher than that, talk with your doctor about adjusting your medication or making any needed lifestyle changes to bring your blood pressure down.

### What Else Affects Blood Pressure?

Other factors have been reported to affect blood pressure. Here's a review of the latest findings.

**Potassium, Calcium, and Magnesium**. Potassium helps to prevent and control high blood pressure. Calcium and magnesium may help prevent high blood pressure, and are important nutrients for other reasons too.

The DASH eating plan is rich in various nutrients believed to benefit blood pressure and in other factors involved in good health. The amounts of the nutrients vary by how much you eat. If you eat about 2,000 calories a day on the plan, the nutrients you will get will include:

- 4,700 milligrams of potassium
- 500 milligrams of magnesium
- 1,240 milligrams of calcium
- 90 grams of protein
- 30 grams of fiber

The list below gives sources for each nutrient:

- **Potassium**
  - Catfish
  - Lean pork
  - Lean veal
  - Cod
  - Flounder
  - Trout
  - Milk
  - Yogurt
  - Pumpkin
  - Green beans
  - Apricots
  - Peaches
  - Bananas
  - Prunes and prune juice
  - Orange juice
  - Lima beans
  - Stewed tomatoes
  - Spinach
  - Plantain
  - Sweet potatoes
  - Dry peas and beans
  - Potatoes
  - Winter squash

- **Calcium**
  - Cheese
  - Milk
  - Yogurt
  - Broccoli
  - Spinach
  - Turnip greens
  - Tofu (made with calcium sulfate)
  - Mackerel
  - Perch
  - Salmon

- **Magnesium**
  - Whole wheat bread
  - Broccoli
  - Chard
  - Spinach
  - Okra
  - Plantain
  - Oysters
  - Scallops
  - Croaker
  - Mackerel
  - Sea bass
  - Beans
  - Soy milk
  - Tofu
  - Nuts and seeds
  - Whole grain, ready-to-eat and cooked cereals

**Fats**. Saturated fats and cholesterol in foods raise blood cholesterol, which increases the risk for heart disease. Foods high in fats also are high in calories, which must be reduced if you need to lose weight.

**Caffeine**. This may cause blood pressure to rise but only temporarily. Unless you are sensitive to caffeine, you do not have to limit how much you consume in order to prevent or control blood pressure.

**Garlic or Onions**. These have not been found to affect blood pressure. But they are tasty substitutes for salty seasonings and can be used often.

**Stress Management**. Stress too can make blood pressure go up for a while, and it has been thought to contribute to high blood pressure. But the long-term effects of stress are as yet unclear. Furthermore, stress management techniques do not seem to prevent high blood pressure. However, stress management techniques may help you control over eating.

## Here's a Recap

By preventing or controlling high blood pressure, you will reduce your risk for heart disease and stroke, as well as other conditions. The steps needed will help you feel healthier. Those steps are to:

- Maintain a healthy weight.

- Be physically active. It only takes 30 minutes of moderate-level physical activity on most, and preferably all, days of the week.

- Follow a healthy eating plan, which includes foods lower in salt and sodium. Have no more than 2,400 milligrams of sodium (6 grams of salt) a day. Also, try the DASH eating plan, which is low in saturated fat, total fat, and cholesterol and rich in fruits, vegetables, and low-fat dairy foods. The DASH eating plan offers plenty of potassium, as well as calcium, magnesium, fiber, and protein.

- If you drink alcoholic beverages, do so in moderation.

- If you have high blood pressure and are prescribed medication, take it as directed.

# Chapter 15

# Athlete's Foot and Jock Itch

## What is tinea?

Tinea is a fungus that can grow on your skin, hair, or nails. As it grows, it spreads out in a circle, leaving normal-looking skin in the middle. This makes it look like a ring. At the edge of the ring, the skin is lifted up by the irritation and looks red and scaly. To some people, the infection looks like a worm is under the skin. Because of the way it looks, tinea infection is often called "ringworm." However, there really isn't a worm under the skin.

## How did I get a fungal infection?

You can get a fungal infection by touching a person who has one. Some kinds of fungi live on damp surfaces, like the floors in public showers or locker rooms. You can easily pick up a fungus there. You can even catch a fungal infection from your pets. Dogs and cats, as well as farm animals, can be infected with a fungus. Often this infection looks like a patch of skin where fur is missing.

## What areas of the body are affected by tinea infections?

Fungal infections are named for the part of the body they infect.

Tinea corporis is a fungal infection of the skin on the body ("corporis" is the Latin word meaning "of the body"). If you have this infection, you may see small, red spots that grow into large rings almost anywhere on your arms, legs, or chest.

Tinea pedis is usually called athlete's foot ("pedis" is the Latin word for "of the foot"). The moist skin between your toes is a perfect place for a fungus to grow. The skin may become itchy and red, with a white, wet surface. The infection may spread to the toenails (tinea unguium; "unguium" comes from the Latin word for nail). Here it causes the toenails to become thick and crumbly. It can also spread to your hands and fingernails.

When a fungus grows in the moist, warm area of the groin, the rash is called tinea cruris ("cruris" is the Latin word meaning "of the leg"). The common name for this infection is "jock itch." Tinea cruris generally occurs in men, especially if they often wear athletic equipment.

Tinea capitis, which is called "ringworm," causes itchy, red areas, usually on the head ("capitis" is the Latin word meaning "of the head"). The hair is destroyed, leaving bald patches. This tinea infection is most common in children.

### *How do I know if I have a fungal infection?*

The best way to know for sure is to ask your doctor. Other skin problems can look just like a fungal infection but have very different treatments. To find out what is causing your rash, your doctor may scrape a small amount of the irritated skin onto a glass slide (or clip off a piece of nail or hair). Then he or she will look at the skin, nail, or hair under a microscope. After doing this, your doctor will usually be able to tell if your skin problem is caused by a fungus.

Sometimes a piece of your skin, hair, or nail will be sent to a lab to grow the fungus in a test tube. This is another way the lab can tell if your skin problem is caused by a fungus. They can also find out the exact type of fungus. This process takes a while because fungus grows slowly.

### *How do I get rid of a tinea infection?*

Once your doctor decides that you have a tinea infection, medicine can be used to get rid of it. You may only need to put a special cream on the rash for a few weeks. This is especially true for jock itch.

It can be harder to get rid of fungal infections on other parts of the body. Sometimes you have to take medicine by mouth. This medicine usually has to be taken for a long time, maybe even for months. Irritated skin takes time to heal. New hair or nails will have to grow back.

Some medicines can have unpleasant effects on the rest of your body, especially if you're also taking other medicines. There are some newer medicines that seem to work better with fewer side effects. You may need to have blood tests to make sure that your body is not having a bad reaction to the medicine.

### What can I do to prevent tinea infections?

Skin that is kept clean and dry is your best defense. However, you're also less likely to get a tinea infection if you do the following things:

- When you're at home, take your shoes off and expose your feet to the air.

- Change your socks and underwear every day, especially in warm weather.

- Dry your feet carefully (especially between the toes) after using a locker room or public shower.

- Avoid walking barefoot in public areas. Instead, wear "flip-flops," sandals, or water shoes.

- Don't wear thick clothing for long periods of time in warm weather. It will make you sweat more.

- Throw away worn-out exercise shoes. Never borrow other people's shoes.

- Check your pets for areas of hair loss. Ask your veterinarian to check them too. It's important to check pets carefully, because if you don't find out whether they're causing your fungal infection, you may get it again from them, even after treatment.

### Can tinea cause serious illness?

A fungus rarely spreads below the surface of the body to cause serious illness. Your body usually prevents this. However, people with weak immune systems, such as people with AIDS, may have a hard time getting well from a fungal infection.

Tinea infections usually don't leave scars after the fungus is gone. Sometimes, people don't even know they have a fungal infection and get better without any treatment.

Chapter 16

# *Duchenne-Becker*
# *Muscular Dystrophy*

### *What are muscular dystrophies?*

The muscular dystrophies are a group of muscle diseases which
have three features in common: They are hereditary; they are progressive; and each causes a characteristic, selective pattern of weakness.

This chapter deals only with the Duchenne-type muscular dystrophy (DMD) and Becker-type muscular dystrophy (BMD).

### *Why are DMD and BMD discussed together?*

DMD and BMD cause similar patterns of weakness and disability
and are inherited in the same way. Weakness and disability are more
severe in DMD than in BMD. Becker dystrophy is like a less severe
form of Duchenne dystrophy.

Recently it was shown that DMD and BMD are due to defects of
the same gene. The normal function of the gene is to enable muscle
fibers to make a particular chemical substance, a protein called dystrophin. Muscle fibers in people affected with DMD are extremely defi-
cient in dystrophin; in BMD the deficiency is less severe.

Reprinted with permission from "Muscular Dystrophies: Duchenne and
Becker," a fact sheet by the Muscular Dystrophy Association (MDA)–Australia,
http://www.mda.org.au. © 2003 MDA–Australia.

## Duchenne Muscular Dystrophy (DMD)

### What would make a doctor suspect Duchenne dystrophy (DMD)?

DMD affects only males, with rare exceptions. Unless a boy with DMD is known to be at risk because of his family history, he is unlikely to be diagnosed before the age of two or three years. Most boys with DMD walk alone at a later age than average. Then the parents are likely to be worried about something unusual in the way he walks, about frequent falling, or about difficulty rising from the ground or difficulty going up steps. Less often, concern arises because of intellectual handicap ("mental retardation"). Although intellectual handicap affects only a minority of boys with DMD, it is more frequent than in other children.

### How would the diagnosis of DMD be made?

Usually, by the time a doctor is consulted there is an effect on posture and gait — that is, in the way the affected boy stands, walks, runs, especially up hills or steps.

The doctor is likely to observe that the calf muscles and sometimes other muscles look very well developed or excessively large. Other muscles will be poorly developed.

There is usually a typical style of walking which can be recognized and which is something described as waddling.

Whether standing still or walking, the affected boy usually has an exaggeration of the forward curve of the lower part of the back. The medical term for this is lordosis; nonmedical people sometimes call it swayback.

A later development is a tendency to stand and walk on the forward part of the foot with the heels off the ground.

Testing individual muscles or muscle groups reveals a pattern of weakness which is typical of DMD.

### Can DMD be diagnosed before these features are obvious?

If parents have brought their son to a doctor at a very early stage of the disease, it may be difficult or impossible to detect anything definitely wrong on observing him. Doctors are therefore encouraged to test for DMD with a blood test, whether they strongly suspect the diagnosis or regard it as just a possibility.

## How does a blood test help?

The test is a measurement of the amount of a chemical, called creatine kinase, in the blood. It is a serum creatine kinase (SCK) measurement.

Creatine kinase is an important chemical in muscle fibers, and there is normally a small amount of it in the blood serum. (Serum is yellow fluid which is left when the blood cells have been allowed to clot and have been removed). In DMD and BMD, creatine kinase leaks out of the muscle fibers and is therefore found in greatly increased amounts in the serum. In young boys with DMD, the SCK level is nearly always at least five times as high as the maximum for unaffected people. It is sometimes 50 to 100 times as high.

The value of the test is:

- When there is reason to suspect DMD, a very high SCK level makes the diagnosis probable.

- A SCK level which is normal or only slightly raised means that the boy does not have DMD. The doctor may have to consider other muscle problems, but not DMD.

## Are any other tests necessary?

The diagnosis should be confirmed by muscle biopsy. Some doctors also recommended electromyography (EMG), which is an examination of the electrical activity generated by muscle when it contracts, recorded through a needle inserted in the muscle.

Muscle biopsy involves the removal of a small piece of muscle for examination. Since the discovery of the defect of dystrophin in DMD it has also been possible to arrange for muscle biopsy specimens to be examined for this specific defect.

## How does Duchenne dystrophy affect people as they get older?

At the time of writing there is no cure for DMD. The worsening of disability can be slowed by such measures as physiotherapy, but it cannot be stopped. On average, use of a wheelchair proceeds from occasional use at about age nine years to almost total dependence by the early teens, but there is a range of severity to either side of this.

As the ability to walk is lost, the function of the hands and arms becomes increasingly important in determining the affected person's abilities. Most affected people survive into their twenties. A small minority survive only to their late teens; another small number, to more than 30 years of age.

### Do affected people have other health problems?

Some people with DMD have additional problems. These include impaired intellectual development and problems with the joints, the spine, the heart, and the function of the lungs.

Intellectual handicap is more frequent in boys with DMD than in the general population but only affects a minority. Unlike the muscle weakness, it is not progressive. Whatever intelligence an affected boy has at birth, he retains unless it is affected by something else. This is so whether he is born with superior, average, or less than average intelligence.

Joints tend to become restricted in their range of movements. This is called contracture. The ankles are usually affected early, then the hips and knees, and lastly the joints of the upper limbs. Physiotherapy and occupational therapy are directed against this complication. The physiotherapist advises on exercises to stretch the joints, and the occupational therapist on good and bad sitting positions and activities.

Surgery is sometimes used to correct contractures. Medical opinions vary as to when surgery is advisable.

Curvature of the spine is a serious complication. It is called scoliosis. It is a curvature to the side, convex to one side and concave to the other. This is accompanied by rotation of the spine. Because the ribs are attached to the rotated spine, the chest wall becomes more prominent on one side.

Scoliosis, if severe, can be uncomfortable or painful and limits the function of the lungs and the upper limbs. It is also disfiguring.

Scoliosis worsens most rapidly when growth is most rapid, in the latter stages of puberty. If scoliosis is not severe by the time the peak rate of growth in height has been passed, it is unlikely to become severe.

Increasingly, scoliosis in people with DMD is treated surgically. This involves a major operation and the insertion of a metal rod to hold the spine straight.

The timing of surgical treatment is critical because the ability of a person with DMD to undergo such major surgery with safety is constantly diminishing with age. A decision about surgery is often taken before the scoliosis has become severe, in anticipation that it will do so if untreated.

Any suspicion that scoliosis is developing should be reported to the attending doctor or therapist.

The heart is a muscle and is affected in DMD, but usually without actually causing trouble. When the dystrophic process in the heart does cause symptoms, these usually respond to treatment.

The function of the lungs in people with DMD depends mostly on the strength of the muscles which move the chest in breathing and coughing. This usually determines the length of life for affected people, provided that the other complications do not occur.

When the muscles involved in breathing become very weak, lung function becomes inadequate so that there is not enough oxygen and too much carbon dioxide in the blood. This causes drowsiness, headaches, and a general lack of well-being. When this happens, assistance with breathing through a face mask, used during sleep, may return the blood oxygen and carbon dioxide levels to normal and relieve the symptoms.

A small number of affected people choose to have mechanically assisted breathing for 24 hours a day when their breathing muscles are so weak that they cannot otherwise support life.

## Becker Muscular Dystrophy (BMD)

### How is BMD different from DMD?

BMD is less severely disabling then DMD. An arbitrary means of distinguishing the two disorders depends on whether the affected person can still walk at age 16 years. Muscle biopsy tends to show more or less severe changes, related to the severity of disability.

Since the discovery that dystrophin is defective in DMD and BMD, but more severely defective in DMD, examination of dystrophin in muscle biopsy samples can be used to distinguish them.

### Are other muscular dystrophies difficult to distinguish from BMD?

Limb girdle muscular dystrophy (LGMD), which is most often of autosomal recessive inheritance, may be difficult or impossible to distinguish from BMD, which is X-linked recessive. The mode of inheritance and therefore the diagnosis may be revealed by the family tree or by blood tests (SCK) revealing carrier status in female relatives in the case of BMD.

However, the conclusive test to distinguish BMD and LGMD is the examination of dystrophin on the muscle biopsy specimen.

### Is BMD as predictable in its progress as DMD?

DMD is fairly predictable. There is a range of severity, and disability progresses more rapidly in some people than in others. Nevertheless, the range of severity is rather narrow.

BMD is much more variable. Some affected people are able to walk only until early adulthood, others to an advanced age. Survival in some is to middle age, but others have survived more than 80 years. Some develop heart trouble in early adulthood, others never do.

### Is the severity the same within families?

There are sometimes big differences in severity of BMD between affected individuals in the same family.

### How is BMD diagnosed?

The process is like that described for DMD, but the doctor's findings are in all respects generally less severe. The SCK level is increased, the EMG and muscle biopsy show changes consistent with the diagnosis. If a test for dystrophin in the muscle biopsy specimen can be arranged, the result will be diagnostic.

### Are the effects of BMD on the intelligence, joints, spine, heart, and lungs like those of DMD?

The intellect is not adversely affected in BMD. Like the muscle weakness, the effects of BMD on the joints and on the function of the lungs is mild in BMD compared with DMD. Scoliosis is seldom a problem because young people with BMD are usually still in relatively good condition at the time of the growth spurt at puberty.

Heart trouble is less frequent in BMD than in DMD but is occasionally serious in people who are otherwise very mildly affected.

## Genetic Counseling in DMD and BMD

DMD and BMD are due to defects in the same gene, which is now known to be the dystrophin gene, on the X chromosome. They are inherited as X-linked recessive diseases. This means:

- Only males are affected, with rare exceptions.

- Female relatives of affected males may be carriers.

- The mothers of affected males, in families with more than one affected male, are carriers.

- The mothers of affected males with no affected relatives are not always carriers, because their sons may have been affected by new mutations.

- The son of a carrier has a 50 percent probability of being affected.

- The daughter of a carrier has a 50 percent probability of being a carrier.

- The sons of an affected male are all unaffected; his daughters are all carriers.

### Will tests show whether an affected person's female relative is a carrier?

Sometimes tests will give a definite answer. Sometimes the best that can be achieved is a statement about the probability of carrier status.

### How useful are probabilities of carrier status for a prospective mother?

Certainty is better, but probabilities are still very useful. Often the probability that a woman is a carrier is so low that the risk of muscular dystrophy to her baby is much lower than the average risk of serious birth defect or genetic disease.

### How can it be certain that a woman is a carrier?

If a woman has an affected son and another affected relative, it is certain that she is a carrier. If she has two affected sons and no other affected relatives, it is very close to certain that she is a carrier.

If a woman is a possible carrier—for example, the sister or aunt or cousin of an affected male—a consistently abnormal SCK test on blood collected under proper conditions makes it almost certain that she is a carrier.

Finally, DNA tests sometimes demonstrate carrier status with certainly or high probability.

### What is DNA testing?

DNA is an abbreviation for the chemical which the genes are made of, deoxyribonucleic acid. It can be obtained from a blood specimen. DNA from a person with DMD or BMD can be tested to see if the genetic defect can be detected. If so, testing for that defect can be offered to other family members. This is called direct DNA testing.

### Is the DNA defect always the same in DMD or in BMD?

The defect is always in the dystrophin gene, but there are many ways in which the gene may be defective. The defect can be found by DNA testing on some but not all people with DMD or BMD.

### Is DNA testing useful in a family in which the gene defect cannot be found?

In such families the laboratory may be able to trace the defective gene and the normal gene by following markers called DNA polymorphisms. These are normal variants of DNA structure, close to the DMD/BMD region of the X chromosome.

If, in a family, one variant is found to be transmitted from mother to child with the normal gene, and another variant with the defective gene, the polymorphism is called "informative"; that is, diagnostically useful. This is called indirect DNA testing.

### Are direct and indirect DNA diagnostic tests equally good?

Direct testing is preferred so it is attempted first, if possible. The disadvantage of indirect testing are:

- Diagnosis is less than 100 percent reliable.
- It is usually more time-consuming for the laboratory staff.
- Any one marker is informative in only some families.

### What is DNA testing used for?

It is used to determine probabilities of carrier status and also for prenatal diagnosis.

### Has DNA testing replaced other tests like SCK measurement?

No. It is best to combine information from all available tests.

*—Dr. L. K. Shield, director of Neurology,*
*Royal Children's Hospital,*
*Melbourne, Australia*

# Chapter 17

# *Klinefelter Syndrome*

## *What Is Klinefelter Syndrome?*

In 1942, Dr. Harry Klinefelter and his co-workers at the Massachusetts General Hospital in Boston published a report about nine men who had enlarged breasts, sparse facial and body hair, small testes, and an inability to produce sperm.

By the late 1950s, researchers discovered that men with Klinefelter syndrome, as this group of symptoms came to be called, had an extra sex chromosome, XXY instead of the usual male arrangement, XY. (For a more complete explanation of the role this extra chromosome plays, see the following section, "Chromosomes and Klinefelter Syndrome.")

In the early 1970s, researchers around the world sought to identify males having the extra chromosome by screening large numbers of newborn babies. One of the largest of these studies, sponsored by the National Institute of Child Health and Human Development (NICHD), checked the chromosomes of more than 40,000 infants.

Based on these studies, the XXY chromosome arrangement appears to be one of the most common genetic abnormalities known, occurring as frequently as one in 500 to one in 1,000 male births. Although the syndrome's cause, an extra sex chromosome, is widespread, the syndrome

Reprinted from "Understanding Klinefelter Syndrome: A Guide for XXY Males and Their Families," National Institute of Child Health and Human Development, National Institutes of Health (NIH), August 1993, updated 1997, http://www.nichd.nih.gov/publications/pubs/klinefelter.htm. Also available as NIH Pub. No. 93-3202. Reviewed by David A. Cooke. M.D., June 14, 2003.

itself—the set of symptoms and characteristics that may result from having the extra chromosome—is uncommon. Many men live out their lives without ever even suspecting that they have an additional chromosome.

"I never refer to newborn babies as having Klinefelter's, because they don't have a syndrome," said Arthur Robinson, M.D., a pediatrician at the University of Colorado Medical School in Denver and the director of the NICHD-sponsored study of XXY males. "Presumably, some of them will grow up to develop the syndrome Dr. Klinefelter described, but a lot of them won't."

For this reason, the term "Klinefelter syndrome" has fallen out of favor with medical researchers. Most prefer to describe men and boys having the extra chromosome as XXY males.

In addition to occasional breast enlargement, lack of facial and body hair, and a rounded body type, XXY males are more likely than other males to be overweight, and tend to be taller than their fathers and brothers.

For the most part, these symptoms are treatable. Surgery, when necessary, can reduce breast size. Regular injections of the male hormone testosterone, beginning at puberty, can promote strength and facial hair growth, as well as bring about a more muscular body type.

A far more serious symptom, however, is one that is not always readily apparent. Although they are not mentally retarded, most XXY males have some degree of language impairment. As children, they often learn to speak much later than do other children and may have difficulty learning to read and write. And while they eventually do learn to speak and converse normally, the majority tend to have some degree of difficulty with language throughout their lives. If untreated, this language impairment can lead to school failure and its attendant loss of self esteem.

Fortunately, however, this language disability usually can be compensated for. Chances for success are greatest if begun in early childhood.

## Chromosomes and Klinefelter Syndrome

Chromosomes, the spaghetti-like strands of hereditary material found in each cell of the body, determine such characteristics as the color of our eyes and hair, our height, and whether we are male or female.

Women usually inherit two X chromosomes—one from each parent. Men tend to inherit an X chromosome from their mothers, and a

Y chromosome from their fathers. Most males with the syndrome Dr. Klinefelter described, however, have an additional X chromosomes for a total of two X chromosomes and one Y chromosome.

## Causes

No one knows what puts a couple at risk for conceiving an XXY child. Advanced maternal age increases the risk for the XXY chromosome count, but only slightly. Furthermore, recent studies conducted by NICHD grantee Terry Hassold, a geneticist at Case Western Reserve University in Cleveland, Ohio, show that half the time, the extra chromosome comes from the father.

Dr. Hassold explained that cells destined to become sperm or eggs undergo a process known as meiosis. In this process, the 46 chromosomes in the cell separate, ultimately producing two new cells having 23 chromosomes each. Before meiosis is completed, however, chromosomes pair with their corresponding chromosomes and exchange bits of genetic material. In women, X chromosomes pair; in men, the X and Y chromosome pair. After the exchange, the chromosomes separate, and meiosis continues.

In some cases, the Xs or the X chromosome and Y chromosome fail to pair and fail to exchange genetic material. Occasionally, this results in their moving independently to the same cell, producing either an egg with two Xs, or a sperm having both an X and a Y chromosome. When a sperm having both an X and a Y chromosome fertilizes an egg having a single X chromosome, or when a normal Y-bearing sperm fertilizes an egg having two X chromosomes, an XXY male is conceived.

## Diagnosis

Because they often don't appear any different from anyone else, many XXY males probably never learn of their extra chromosome. However, if they are to be diagnosed, chances are greatest at one of the following times in life: before or shortly after birth, early childhood, adolescence, and in adulthood (as a result of testing for infertility).

In recent years, many XXY males have been diagnosed before birth, through amniocentesis or chorionic villus sampling (CVS). In amniocentesis, a sample of the fluid surrounding the fetus is withdrawn. Fetal cells in the fluid are then examined for chromosomal abnormalities. CVS is similar to amniocentesis, except that the procedure is done in the first trimester, and the fetal cells needed for examination are taken from the placenta. Neither procedure is used routinely, except when there is a family history of genetic defects, the pregnant woman is older than 35, or other medical indications are present.

## Childhood

According to Dr. Robinson, the director of the NICHD-funded study, XXY babies differ little from other children their age. They tend to start life as what many parents call "good" babies—quiet, undemanding, and perhaps even a little passive. As toddlers, they may be somewhat shy and reserved. They usually learn to walk later than most other children, and may have similar delays in learning to speak.

In some, the language delays may be more severe, with the child not fully learning to talk until about age five. Others may learn to speak at a normal rate, and not meet with any problems until they begin school, where they may experience reading difficulties. A few may not have any problems at all in learning to speak or in learning to read.

XXY males usually have difficulty with expressive language—the ability to put thoughts, ideas, and emotions into words. In contrast, their faculty for receptive language—understanding what is said—is close to normal.

"It's one of the conflicts they have," said Melissa, the mother of an XXY boy. "My son can understand the conversations of other 10-year-olds. But his inability to use the language the way other 10-year-olds use it makes him stand out."

In addition to academic help, XXY boys, like other language-disabled children, may need help with social skills. Language is essential not only for learning the school curriculum, but also for building social relationships. By talking and listening, children make friends—in the process, sharing information, attitudes, and beliefs. Through language, they also learn how to behave, not just in the schoolroom, but also on the playground. If their sons' language disability seems to prevent them from fitting in socially, the parents of XXY boys may want to ask school officials about a social skills training program.

Throughout childhood—perhaps, even, for the rest of their lives—XXY boys retain the same temperament and disposition they first displayed as infants and toddlers. As a group, they tend to be shy, somewhat passive, and unlikely to take a leadership role. Although they do make friends with other children, they tend to have only a few friends at a time. Researchers also describe them as cooperative and eager to please.

## *Adolescence*

In general, XXY boys enter puberty normally, without any delay of physical maturity. But as puberty progresses, they fail to keep pace with other males. In chromosomally normal teenaged boys, the testes gradually increase in size, from an initial volume of about 2 milliliters, to about 15 milliliters. In XXY males, while the penis is usually of normal size, the testes remain at 2 milliliters, and cannot produce sufficient quantities of the male hormone testosterone. As a result, many XXY adolescents, although taller than average, may not be as strong as other teenaged boys, and may lack facial or body hair.

As they enter puberty, many boys will undergo slight breast enlargement. For most teenaged males, this condition, known as gynecomastia, tends to disappear in a short time. About one-third of XXY boys develop enlarged breasts in early adolescence slightly more than do chromosomally normal boys. Furthermore, in XXY boys, this condition may be permanent. However, only about 10 percent of XXY males have breast enlargement great enough to require surgery.

Most XXY adolescents benefit from receiving an injection of testosterone every two weeks, beginning at puberty. The hormone increases strength and brings on a more muscular, masculine appearance. More information about testosterone and XXY males can be found in the section titled "Testosterone Treatment."

Adolescence and the high school years can be difficult for XXY boys and their families, particularly in neighborhoods and schools where the emphasis is on athletic ability and physical prowess.

"They're usually tall, good-looking kids, but they tend to be awkward," Dr. Robinson said of the XXY teenagers he has met through his study. "They don't necessarily make good football players or good basketball players."

Lack of strength and agility, combined with a history of learning disabilities, may damage self-esteem. Unsympathetic peers, too, sometimes may make matters worse, through teasing or ridicule.

"Lots of kids have a tough time during adolescence," Dr. Robinson said. "But a higher proportion of XXY boys have a tough time. High school is very competitive, and these kids are not very good competitors, in general."

Dr. Robinson again stressed, however, that while XXY males share many characteristics, they cannot be pigeonholed into rigid categories. Several of his patients have played football, and one, in particular, is an excellent tennis player.

Damage to self-esteem may be more severe in XXY teenagers who are diagnosed in early or late adolescence. Teachers—and even parents—may have dismissed their scholastic difficulties as laziness. Lack of athletic prowess and the inability to use language properly in social settings may have helped to isolate them from their peers. Some may react by sliding quietly into depression and withdraw from contact with other people. Others may find acceptance in a dangerous crowd.

For these reasons, XXY males diagnosed as teenagers may need psychological counseling as well as help in overcoming their learning disabilities. Help with learning disabilities is available through public school systems for XXY males of high school age and under. Referrals to qualified mental health specialists may be obtained from family physicians.

## Testosterone Treatment

Ideally, XXY males should begin testosterone treatment as they enter puberty. XXY males diagnosed in adulthood are also likely to benefit from the hormone. A regular schedule of testosterone injections will increase strength and muscle size and promote the growth of facial and body hair.

In addition to these physical changes, testosterone injections often bring on psychological changes as well. As they begin to develop a more masculine appearance, the self-confidence of XXY males tends to increase. Many become more energetic and stop having sudden, angry changes in moods. What is not clear is whether these psychological changes are a direct result of testosterone treatment or are a side benefit of the increased self-confidence that the treatment may bring. As a group, XXY boys tend to suffer from depression, principally because of their scholastic difficulties and problems fitting in with other males their age. Sudden, angry changes in mood are typical of depressed people.

Other benefits of testosterone treatment may include decreased need for sleep, an enhanced ability to concentrate, and improved relations with others. But to obtain these benefits an XXY male must decide, on his own, that he is ready to stick to a regular schedule of injections.

Sometimes, younger adolescents, who may be somewhat immature, seem not quite ready to take the shots. It is an inconvenience, and many don't like needles.

Most physicians do not push the young men to take the injections. Instead, they usually recommend informing XXY adolescents and their parents about the benefits of testosterone injections and letting them take as much time as they need to make their decision.

Individuals may respond to testosterone treatment in different ways. Although the majority of XXY males ultimately will benefit from testosterone, a few will not.

To ensure that the injections will provide the maximum benefit, XXY males who are ready to begin testosterone injections should consult a qualified endocrinologist (a specialist in hormonal interactions) who has experience treating XXY males.

Side effects of the injections are few. Some individuals may develop a minor allergic reaction at the injection site, resulting in an itchy welt resembling a mosquito bite. Applying a nonprescription hydrocortisone cream to the area will reduce swelling and itching.

In addition, testosterone injections may result in a condition known as benign prostatic hyperplasia (BPH). This condition is common in chromosomally normal males as well, affecting more than 50 percent of men in their sixties, and as many as 90 percent in their seventies and eighties. In XXY males receiving testosterone injections, this condition may begin sometime after age 40.

The prostate is a small gland about the size of a walnut, which helps to manufacture semen. The gland is located just beneath the bladder and surrounds the urethra, the tube through which urine passes out of the body.

In BPH, the prostate increases in size, sometimes squeezing the bladder and urethra and causing difficulty urinating, "dribbling" after urination, and the need to urinate frequently.

XXY males receiving testosterone injections should consult their physicians about a regular schedule of prostate examinations. BPH can often be detected early by a rectal exam. If the prostate greatly interferes with the flow of urine, excess prostate tissue can be trimmed away by a surgical instrument that is inserted in the penis, through the urethra.

## Chromosomal Variations

Occasionally, variations of the XXY chromosome count may occur, the most common being the XY/XXY mosaic. In this variation, some of the cells in the male's body have an additional X chromosome, and the rest have the normal XY chromosome count. The percentage of cells containing the extra chromosome varies from case to case. In some instances, XY/XXY mosaics may have enough normally functioning cells in the testes to allow them to father children.

A few instances of males having two or even three additional X chromosomes have also been reported in the medical literature. In these individuals, the classic features of Klinefelter syndrome may be exaggerated, with low I.Q. or moderate to severe mental retardation also occurring.

In rare instances, an individual may possess both an additional X and an additional Y chromosome. The medical literature describes XXYY males as having slight to moderate mental retardation. They may sometimes be aggressive or even violent. Although they may have a rounded body type and decreased sex drive, experts disagree whether testosterone injections are appropriate for all of them.

One group of researchers reported that after receiving testosterone injections, an XXYY male stopped having violent sexual fantasies and ceased his assaults on teenage girls. In contrast, Dr. Robinson found that testosterone injections seemed to make an XXYY boy he had been treating more aggressive.

Scientists admit, however, that because these cases are so rare, not much is known about them. Most of the XXYY males who have been studied were referred to treatment because they were violent and got into trouble with the law. It is not known whether XXYY males are inherently aggressive by nature, or whether only a few extreme individuals come to the attention of researchers precisely because they are aggressive.

## Sexuality

The parents of XXY boys are sometimes concerned that their sons may grow up to be homosexual. This concern is unfounded, however, as there is no evidence that XXY males are any more inclined toward homosexuality than are other men.

In fact, the only significant sexual difference between XXY men and teenagers and other males their age is that the XXY males may have less interest in sex. However, regular injections of the male sex hormone testosterone can bring sex drive up to normal levels.

In some cases, testosterone injections lead to a false sense of security: After receiving the hormone for a time, XXY males may conclude they've derived as much benefit from it as possible and discontinue the injections. But when they do, their interest in sex almost invariably diminishes until they resume the injections.

## Infertility

The vast majority of XXY males do not produce enough sperm to allow them to become fathers. If these men and their wives wish to become parents, they should seek counseling from their family physician regarding adoption and infertility.

However, no XXY male should automatically assume he is infertile without further testing. In a very small number of cases, XXY males have been able to father children.

In addition, a few individuals who believe themselves to be XXY males may actually be XY/XXY mosaics. Along with having cells with the XXY chromosome count, these males may also have cells with the normal XY chromosome count. If the number of XY cells in the testes is great enough, the individual should be able to father children.

Karyotyping, the method traditionally used to identify an individual's chromosome count, may sometimes fail to identify XY/XXY mosaics. For this reason, a karyotype should never be used to predict whether an individual will be infertile or not.

## Health Considerations

Compared with other males, XXY males have a slightly increased risk of autoimmune disorders. In this group of diseases, the immune system, for unknown reasons, attacks the body's organs or tissues. The most well known of these diseases are type 1 (insulin dependent) diabetes, autoimmune thyroiditis, and lupus erythematosus. Most of these conditions can be treated with medication.

XXY males with enlarged breasts have the same risk of breast cancer as do women—roughly 50 times the risk XY males have. For this reason, these XXY adolescents and men need to practice regular breast self-examination. XXY males may also wish to consult their physicians about the need for more thorough breast examinations by medical professionals.

In addition, XXY males who do not receive testosterone injections may have an increased risk of developing osteoporosis in later life. In this condition, which usually afflicts women after the age of menopause, the bones lose calcium, becoming brittle and more likely to break.

## Adulthood

Unfortunately, comparatively little is known about XXY adults. Studies in the United States have focused largely on XXY males identified in infancy from large random samples. Only a few of these individuals have reached adulthood; most are still in adolescence. At this time, researchers simply do not know what kind of adults they will become.

259

"Some of them have really struggled through adolescence," said Dr. Bruce Bender, the psychologist for the NICHD-sponsored study of XXY males. "But we don't know whether they'll have serious problems in adulthood, or, like many troubled teenagers, overcome their problems and lead productive lives."

Comparatively few studies of XXY males diagnosed in adulthood have been conducted. By and large, the men who took part in these studies were not selected at random but identified by a particular characteristic, such as height. For this reason, it is not known whether these individuals are truly representative of XXY men as a whole or represent a particular extreme.

One study found a group of XXY males diagnosed between the ages of 27 and 37 to have suffered a number of setbacks, in comparison to a similar group of XY males. The XXY men were more likely to have had histories of scholastic failure, depression, and other psychological problems and to lack energy and enthusiasm.

But by the time the XXY men had reached their forties, most had surmounted their problems. The majority said that their energy and activity levels had increased, that they were more productive on the job, and that their relationships with other people had improved. In fact, the only difference between the XY males and the XXY males was that the latter were less likely to have been married.

That these men eventually overcame their troubled pasts is encouraging for all XXY males and particularly encouraging for those diagnosed in childhood. Had they received counseling, support, and testosterone treatments beginning in childhood, these men might have avoided the difficulties of their twenties and thirties.

Although a supportive environment through childhood and adolescence appears to offer the greatest chance for a well-adjusted adulthood, it is not too late for XXY men diagnosed as adults to seek help.

Research has shown that testosterone injections, begun in adulthood, can be beneficial. Psychological counseling also offers the best hope of overcoming depression and other psychological problems. For referrals to endocrinologists qualified to administer testosterone or to mental health specialists, XXY men should consult their physicians.

*—by Robert Bock, Office of Research Reporting, NICHD*

# Chapter 18

# *Hemophilia*

## *What Is It?*

Hemophilia is a bleeding disorder caused by a deficiency in one of the blood clotting factors. Hemophilia A (often called classic hemophilia) accounts for about 80 percent of all hemophilia cases. It is a deficiency in clotting factor VIII.

Hemophilia A is a hereditary disorder in which the clotting ability of the blood is impaired and excessive bleeding results. Small wounds and punctures are usually not a problem. But uncontrolled internal bleeding can result in pain and swelling and permanent damage, especially to joints and muscles.

Severity of symptoms can vary, and severe forms become apparent early on. Prolonged bleeding is the hallmark of hemophilia A and typically occurs when an infant is circumcised. Additional bleeding manifestations make their appearance when the infant becomes mobile. Mild cases may go unnoticed until later in life when there is excessive bleeding and clotting problems in response to surgery or trauma. Internal bleeding may happen anywhere, and bleeding into joints is common.

The incidence of hemophilia A is one out of 10,000 live male births. About 17,000 Americans have hemophilia. Women may have it, but

Reprinted with permission of the National Hemophilia Foundation from "Hemophilia A (Factor VIII Deficiency)," http://www.hemophilia.org/bdi/bdi_types1.htm. © 2003National Hemophilia Foundation; all rights reserved.

it's very rare. With treatment and management, the outcome is good. Most men with hemophilia are able to lead relatively normal lives.

## Inheritance Pattern

Hemophilia A is caused by an inherited sex-linked recessive trait with the defective gene located on the X chromosome. Females are carriers of this trait. Fifty percent of the male offspring of female carriers have the disease, and 50 percent of their female offspring are carriers. All female children of a male with hemophilia are carriers of the trait.

One-third of all cases of hemophilia A occur when there is no family history of the disorder. In these cases, hemophilia develops as the result of a new or spontaneous gene mutation.

Genetic counseling may be advised for carriers. Female carriers can be identified by testing.

A woman is definitely a hemophilia carrier if she is:

- The biological daughter of a man with hemophilia
- The biological mother of more than one son with hemophilia
- The biological mother of one hemophilic son and has at least one other blood relative with hemophilia

A woman may or may not be a hemophilia carrier if she is:

- The biological mother of one son with hemophilia
- The sister of a male with hemophilia
- An aunt, cousin, or niece of an affected male related through maternal ties
- The biological grandmother of one grandson with hemophilia

The only way a woman could ever have hemophilia is if her father has it and her mother carries the gene. Women who are carriers can also be symptomatic carriers, whereby they do experience factor deficiencies.

## Symptoms and Diagnosis

Hemophilia is caused by several different gene abnormalities. The severity of the symptoms of hemophilia A depends on how a particular gene abnormality affects the activity of factor VIII. When the activity is less than 1 percent of normal, episodes of severe bleeding occur and recur for no apparent reason.

Symptoms include:

- Bruising
- Spontaneous bleeding
- Bleeding into joints and associated pain and swelling
- Gastrointestinal tract and urinary tract hemorrhage
- Blood in the urine or stool
- Prolonged bleeding from cuts, tooth extraction, and surgery

People whose clotting activity is 5 percent of normal may have only mild hemophilia. They rarely have unprovoked bleeding episodes, but surgery or injury may cause uncontrolled bleeding, which can be fatal. Milder hemophilia may not be diagnosed at all, although some people whose clotting activity is 10 to 25 percent of normal may have prolonged bleeding after surgery, dental extractions, or a major injury.

Generally, the first bleeding episode occurs before 18 months of age, often after a minor injury. A child who has hemophilia bruises easily. Even an injection into a muscle can cause bleeding that results in a large bruise (hematoma). Recurring bleeding into the joints and muscles can ultimately lead to crippling deformities. Bleeding can swell the base of the tongue until it blocks the airway, making breathing difficult. A slight bump on the head can trigger substantial bleeding in the skull, causing brain damage and death.

A doctor may suspect hemophilia in a child whose bleeding is unusual. A laboratory analysis of blood samples can determine whether the child's clotting is abnormally slow. If it is, the doctor can confirm the diagnosis of hemophilia A and can determine the severity by testing the activity of factor VIII.

## Treatments

Hemophilia is treated by infusing the missing clotting factor. The amount infused depends upon the severity of bleeding, the site of the bleeding, and the size of the patient. In the past, mild hemophilia A was typically treated with infusion of cryoprecipitate or desmopressin acetate (DDAVP), which causes release of factor VIII that is stored within the body on the lining of blood vessels. Today, experts recommend desmopressin injection or Stimate™ nasal spray.

Clotting factors are found in plasma and, to a greater extent, in plasma concentrates. Some plasma concentrates are intended for home use and can be self-administered, either on a regular basis to prevent bleeding or at the first sign of bleeding. More often, they are administered three times a day, but both the dose and frequency depend on the severity of the bleeding problem. The dose is adjusted according to the results of periodic blood tests. During a bleeding episode, more clotting factors are needed.

To prevent a bleeding crisis, people with hemophilia and their families can be taught to administer factor VIII concentrates at home at the first signs of bleeding. People with severe forms of the disease may need regular prophylactic infusions, which bring factor levels higher than 1 percent to prevent bleeds.

Depending on the severity of the disease, DDAVP or factor VIII concentrate may be given prior to dental extractions and surgery to prevent bleeding. Immunization with hepatitis B vaccine is necessary because of the increased risk of exposure to hepatitis due to frequent infusions of blood products.

Gene therapy and fetal tissue implant techniques are under study as possible treatments.

People who have hemophilia should avoid situations that might cause bleeding. They should be conscientious about dental care so they won't need to have teeth extracted. People who have hemophilia should also avoid certain drugs that can aggravate bleeding problems:

- Aspirin
- Heparin
- Warfarin
- Certain analgesics such as nonsteroidal anti-inflammatory drugs

Treatment should be coordinated by a health care practitioner who is expert in the field, such as a hematologist or hemophilia treatment center nurse.

The National Hemophilia Foundation's Medical and Scientific Advisory Council (MASAC) made recommendations for treatment of hemophilia in November of 1999. They include:

- Factor VIII products for patients who are HIV seronegative, including recombinant factor VIII, especially for young and newly diagnosed patients who have not received any blood or plasma-derived products.

- Immunoaffinity purified factor VIII concentrates for patients who are HIV seropositive.

- Cryoprecipitate is not recommended because of the risk of HIV and hepatitis infection. Despite greatly improved screening and purification for viral inactivation in blood products, cryoprecipitate can still contain viruses.

- Mild hemophilia A should be treated with desmopressin, in a DDAVP injection or Stimate nasal spray.

## Complications

- Chronic joint deformities, caused by recurrent bleeding into the joint, may be managed by an orthopedic specialist.

- Intracerebral hemorrhage is another possible complication.

Some persons with hemophilia develop antibodies to transfused factor VIII. As a result, the transfusions are ineffective. If antibodies are detected in blood samples, the dosage of the plasma concentrates may be increased, or different types of clotting factors or drugs to reduce the antibody levels may be used.

In the past, the plasma concentrates carried the risk of transmitting blood-borne diseases such as hepatitis and AIDS. About 60 percent of persons with hemophilia who were treated with plasma concentrates in the early 1980s were infected with HIV. However, the risk of transmitting HIV infection through plasma concentrates has been virtually eliminated by today's use of screened and processed blood and a genetically engineered factor VIII (recombinant).

# Chapter 19

# *Sleep Apnea*

## *What is sleep apnea?*

Sleep apnea is a serious, potentially life-threatening condition that is far more common than generally understood. First described in 1965, sleep apnea is a breathing disorder characterized by brief interruptions of breathing during sleep. It owes its name to a Greek word, *apnea*, meaning "want of breath." There are two types of sleep apnea: central and obstructive. Central sleep apnea, which is less common, occurs when the brain fails to send the appropriate signals to the breathing muscles to initiate respirations. Obstructive sleep apnea is far more common and occurs when air cannot flow into or out of the person's nose or mouth although efforts to breathe continue.

In a given night, the number of involuntary breathing pauses or "apneic events" may be as high as 20 to 60 or more per hour. These breathing pauses are almost always accompanied by snoring between apnea episodes, although not everyone who snores has this condition. Sleep apnea can also be characterized by choking sensations. The frequent interruptions of deep, restorative sleep often leads to excessive daytime sleepiness and may be associated with an early morning headache.

Early recognition and treatment of sleep apnea is important because it may be associated with irregular heartbeat, high blood pressure, heart attack, and stroke.

---

Reprinted with permission from "Sleep Apnea," a brochure from the National Sleep Foundation, http://www.sleepfoundation.org. © 2002 National Sleep Foundation.

## Who gets sleep apnea?

Sleep apnea occurs in all age groups and both sexes but is more common in men (it may be underdiagnosed in women) and possibly young African Americans. It has been estimated that as many as 18 million Americans have sleep apnea. Four percent of middle-aged men and 2 percent of middle-aged women have sleep apnea along with excessive daytime sleepiness. People most likely to have or develop sleep apnea include those who snore loudly and also are overweight, or have high blood pressure, or have some physical abnormality in the nose, throat, or other parts of the upper airway. Sleep apnea seems to run in some families, suggesting a possible genetic basis.

## What causes sleep apnea?

Certain mechanical and structural problems in the airway cause the interruptions in breathing during sleep. In some people, apnea occurs when the throat muscles and tongue relax during sleep and partially block the opening of the airway. When the muscles of the soft palate at the base of the tongue and the uvula (the small fleshy tissue hanging from the center of the back of the throat) relax and sag, the airway becomes blocked, making breathing labored and noisy and even stopping it altogether. Sleep apnea also can occur in obese people when an excess amount of tissue in the airway causes it to be narrowed. With a narrowed airway, the person continues his or her efforts to breathe, but air cannot easily flow into or out of the nose or mouth. Unknown to the person, this results in heavy snoring, periods of no breathing, and frequent arousals (causing abrupt changes from deep sleep to light sleep). Ingestion of alcohol and sleeping pills increases the frequency and duration of breathing pauses in people with sleep apnea.

## How is normal breathing restored during sleep?

During the apneic event, the person is unable to breathe in oxygen and to exhale carbon dioxide, resulting in low levels of oxygen and increased levels of carbon dioxide in the blood. The reduction in oxygen and increase in carbon dioxide alert the brain to resume breathing and cause an arousal. With each arousal, a signal is sent from the brain to the upper airway muscles to open the airway; breathing is resumed, often with a loud snort or gasp. Frequent arousals, although necessary for breathing to restart, prevent the patient from getting enough restorative, deep sleep.

## *What are the effects of sleep apnea?*

Because of the serious disturbances in their normal sleep patterns, people with sleep apnea often feel very sleepy during the day and their concentration and daytime performance suffer. The consequences of sleep apnea range from annoying to life-threatening. They include symptoms suggesting depression, irritability, sexual dysfunction, learning and memory difficulties, and falling asleep while at work, on the phone, or driving. Untreated sleep apnea patients are three times (or more) likely to have automobile accidents; treatment reverses the increased risk. It has been estimated that up to 50 percent of sleep apnea patients have high blood pressure. It has recently been shown that sleep apnea contributes to high blood pressure. Risk for heart attack and stroke may also increase in those with sleep apnea.

## *When should sleep apnea be suspected?*

For many sleep apnea patients, their bed partners or family members are the first ones to suspect that something is wrong, usually from their heavy snoring and apparent struggle to breathe. Coworkers or friends of the sleep apnea victim may notice that the individual falls asleep during the day at inappropriate times (such as while driving a car, working, or talking). The patient often does not know he or she has a problem and may not believe it when told. It is important that the person see a doctor for evaluation of the sleep problem.

## *How is sleep apnea diagnosed?*

In addition to the primary care physician, pulmonologists, neurologists, or other physicians with specialty training in sleep disorders may be involved in making a definitive diagnosis and initiating treatment. Diagnosis of sleep apnea is not simple because there can be many different reasons for disturbed sleep. Several tests are available for evaluating a person for sleep apnea.

Polysomnography is a test that records a variety of body functions during sleep, such as the electrical activity of the brain, eye movement, muscle activity, heart rate, respiratory effort, air flow, and blood oxygen levels. These tests are used both to diagnose sleep apnea and to determine its severity.

The multiple sleep latency test (MSLT) measures the speed of falling asleep. In this test, patients are given several opportunities to fall asleep during the course of a day when they would normally be awake. For each opportunity, time to fall asleep is measured. Individuals who fall asleep in less than five minutes are likely to require some type of treatment for sleep disorders. The MSLT may be useful to measure the degree of excessive daytime sleepiness and to rule out other types of sleep disorders.

Diagnostic tests usually are performed in a sleep disorders center, but new technology may allow some sleep studies to be conducted in the patient's home.

### How is sleep apnea treated?

The specific therapy for sleep apnea is tailored to the individual patient based on medical history, physical examination, and the results of polysomnography. Medications are generally not effective in the treatment of sleep apnea. Oxygen is sometimes used in patients with central apnea caused by heart failure. It is not used to treat obstructive sleep apnea.

**Physical or mechanical therapy.** Nasal continuous positive airway pressure (CPAP) is the most common effective treatment for sleep apnea. In this procedure, the patient wears a mask over the nose during sleep, and pressure from an air blower forces air through the nasal passages. The air pressure is adjusted so that it is just enough to prevent the throat from collapsing during sleep. The pressure is constant and continuous. Nasal CPAP prevents airway closure while in use, but apnea episodes return when CPAP is stopped or it is used improperly.

Variations of the CPAP device attempt to minimize side effects that sometimes occur, such as nasal irritation and drying, facial skin irritation, abdominal bloating, mask leaks, sore eyes, and headaches. Some versions of CPAP vary the pressure to coincide with the person's breathing pattern, and other CPAPs start with low pressure, slowly increasing it to allow the person to fall asleep before the full prescribed pressure is applied.

Dental appliances that reposition the lower jaw and the tongue have been helpful to some patients with mild to moderate sleep apnea or who snore but do not have apnea. A dentist or orthodontist is often the one to fit the patient with such a device.

**Surgery.** Some patients with sleep apnea may need surgery. Although several surgical procedures are used to increase the size of the airway, none of them is completely successful or without risks. More than one procedure may need to be tried before the patient realizes any benefits.

Some of the more common procedures include removal of adenoids and tonsils (especially in children), nasal polyps or other growths, or other tissue in the airway and correction of structural deformities. Younger patients seem to benefit from these surgical procedures more than older patients.

Uvulopalatopharyngoplasty (UPPP) is a procedure used to remove excess tissue at the back of the throat (tonsils, uvula, and part of the soft palate). The success of this technique may range from 30 to 60 percent. The long-term side effects and benefits are not known, and it is difficult to predict which patients will do well with this procedure.

Laser-assisted uvulopalatoplasty (LAUP) is done to eliminate snoring but has not been shown to be effective in treating sleep apnea. This procedure involves using a laser device to eliminate tissue in the back of the throat. Like UPPP, LAUP may decrease or eliminate snoring but not eliminate sleep apnea itself. Elimination of snoring, the primary symptom of sleep apnea, without influencing the condition may carry the risk of delaying the diagnosis and possible treatment of sleep apnea in patients who elect to have LAUP. To identify possible underlying sleep apnea, sleep studies are usually required before LAUP is performed.

Somnoplasty is a procedure that uses radio waves to reduce the size of some airway structures such as the uvula and the back of the tongue. This technique is being investigated as a treatment for apnea.

Tracheostomy is used in persons with severe, life-threatening sleep apnea. In this procedure, a small hole is made in the windpipe and a tube is inserted into the opening. This tube stays closed during waking hours, and the person breathes and speaks normally. It is opened for sleep so that air flows directly into the lungs, bypassing any upper airway obstruction. Although this procedure is highly effective, it is an extreme measure that is rarely used.

Other procedures: Patients in whom sleep apnea is due to deformities of the lower jaw may benefit from surgical reconstruction. Finally, surgical procedures to treat obesity are sometimes recommended for sleep apnea patients who are morbidly obese.

**Nonspecific therapy.** Behavioral changes are an important part of the treatment program, and in mild cases behavioral therapy may be all that is needed. Overweight persons can benefit from losing weight. Even a 10 percent weight loss can reduce the number of apneic events for most patients. Individuals with apnea should avoid the use of alcohol and sleeping pills, which make the airway more likely to collapse during sleep and prolong the apneic periods. In some patients with mild sleep apnea, breathing pauses occur only when they sleep on their backs. In such cases, using pillows and other devices that help them sleep in a side position may be helpful.

### Should you seek medical help?

If you are experiencing sleepiness during the day, loud snoring or pauses in breathing during sleep or any other sleeping difficulties, make an appointment to discuss these problems with your doctor. Sleep disorders are treatable. Your doctor can evaluate your sleep problem and may refer you to a sleep specialist who has special training in sleep medicine. Many of these specialists work at sleep centers where overnight sleep studies can help determine whether you have a sleep disorder. For more information, contact the National Sleep Foundation or visit our website at www.sleepfoundation.org.

# Chapter 20

# 'Women's' Diseases: Men Get Them, Too

Seymour Kramer noticed a patch of what looked like blood on his pajama top three years ago and thought he had cut himself. But he wasn't scratched. His doctor tested the discharge and told the New Jersey man he had breast cancer.

Dan, 70, a retired Michigan engineer who asked that his last name not be used, was pulling weeds three years ago. For no apparent reason, he fractured two vertebrae. Doctors told him his bones were wasting away. He has osteoporosis.

As a teenager, Gary Grahl was obsessed with having a trim, "athletic" body. The Wisconsin resident shunned food and exercised excessively. Sometimes he'd do sit-ups and pushups for three hours before school. He ate little and shrank from 160 to an unhealthy 104 pounds. Over a six-year period, he was hospitalized four times. Now 26, Grahl says he is "completely recovered" from his eating disorder.

What do these men have in common? They all suffer from illnesses typically thought of as "women's diseases." Breast cancer, osteoporosis, and eating disorders all occur in men, too, though their prevalence is much greater in the female population. As a result, many men, unaware that the diseases affect both sexes, may fail to recognize symptoms. Likewise, doctors and families often don't suspect these illnesses. This can delay therapy and make disorders difficult to treat.

Reprinted from "Conditions Men Get, Too," U.S. Food and Drug Administration, published originally in *FDA Consumer* July–August 1995, http://www.fda.gov/fdac/features/695_men.html. Reviewed and revised by David A. Cooke, M.D., on July 2, 2003.

Medical experts say men may shy away from seeking medical treatment for disorders they feel are unmasculine. In support groups, men use terms like "very scared" and "ashamed" to describe initial feelings about their illnesses. Others express frustration at the difficulty in finding information and therapy.

## Osteoporosis

High on the list of such conditions is osteoporosis. Though women are four times more likely to acquire it, about 5 million men in this country have osteoporosis, according to the National Osteoporosis Foundation. A disorder in which bones become weakened, osteoporosis is sometimes called the "silent disease" because it has no symptoms. It often manifests itself in fractures of the hip, wrist, spine, and other bones. Among both sexes, it is responsible for 1.5 million fractures a year. Scientists are still piecing together just how osteoporosis develops, but it is well known that a key factor is deficiency of the mineral calcium. Leo Lutwak, M.D., Ph.D., a medical officer in FDA's Center for Drug Evaluation and Research, emphasizes that calcium intake over a person's lifetime is crucial to preventing bone loss. Ideally, he says, a diet adequate in calcium starting in childhood "can maximize peak bone mass," helping to ensure strong bones and make osteoporosis less likely. The revised food label that went into effect in 1994 can help consumers pinpoint calcium-rich foods.

About 99 percent of the body's calcium is stored in bones and teeth. Bone is continually being broken down and rebuilt. If the amount of calcium absorbed equals the amount lost, a state of balance occurs. When calcium absorption is greater than losses, the body accrues a "positive balance" that it can use for bone growth and repair. But when dietary intake of calcium can't meet the body's needs, the body draws the mineral from bones to allow a constant bloodstream supply. Ultimately, the breakdown process can exceed deposits, causing a possible reduction in bone mass and density.

Osteoporosis is seen less often in men than in women for several reasons. Men generally have greater bone mass than women, and in males, bone loss begins later and advances more slowly. But men do have a hormonal drop-off in testosterone similar to women's reduction of estrogen after menopause. Testosterone may diminish as a result of hypogonadism, a condition marked by decreased function of the testicles. Testosterone levels may naturally become lower as a man ages.

"Loss of sex hormone results in accelerated bone loss in whomever it occurs, whenever it occurs, for whatever reason," says Michael

Kleerekoper, M.D., deputy associate chairman of internal medicine at Wayne State University. "Whether that translates to osteoporosis depends on how much bone you have when the loss begins and how quickly you lose it." Women find relief from osteoporosis with estrogen therapy, and some men respond to testosterone injections. But successes with hormone therapy come most often from "seeing young men in the early stages" of the condition, Kleerekoper says.

While hormone replacement therapy is helpful for osteoporosis in women, it is less clear whether testosterone has similar benefits. Safety issues may limit the use of both drugs; estrogen-progesterone combinations were shown to have adverse effects that outweigh benefits in most women in a landmark 2002 study. No similar studies have been done for testosterone in men, and there is concern, albeit mostly theoretical, that testosterone therapy can increase a man's risk of prostate cancer.

Fortunately, effective nonhormonal treatments for osteoporosis have become available in the past several years. A class of drugs known as bisphosphonates have been shown to be quite effective in increasing bone density and reducing fracture risk. The most commonly used drugs of this type, alendronate (Fosamax™) and risedronate (Actonel™), have been approved for use in both men and women.

Another promising new therapy is teriparatide (Forteo™). A synthetic version of the parathyroid hormone normally produced by the body, it is a potent stimulator of bone growth. It has been approved for approved for use in both men and women. However, it must be taken by injection, and is very expensive.

Still another option to slow bone breakdown and reduce pain associated with fractures attributed to osteoporosis is the drug calcitonin, marketed as Miacalcin® or Calcimar®. FDA has not approved these drugs specifically for men, though some doctors prescribe them to males if they feel the patient will benefit.

Dan, the Michigan osteoporosis patient, receives biweekly testosterone injections and takes daily supplements of 1,500 milligrams of calcium with vitamin D. He also exercises in a swimming pool, where water provides a beneficial resistance to movement.

He says his two fractured vertebrae three years ago made him realize that osteoporosis gives no warnings.

Factors that raise the risk of osteoporosis include cigarette smoking, alcohol consumption in excess of two drinks a day, advanced age, and an inactive lifestyle.

Eric, 45, says years of inactivity helped bring on his osteoporosis. In his early twenties, the New York resident (who asked that his last name not be used) had several sports accidents that seriously impaired his mobility. An eating disorder in college also encouraged development of the condition, he suspects. Now, his bone loss is so severe that "anytime I have an x-ray, the doctors go into shock," he says. He risks injury by simply taking a walk and cannot stand barefoot on a hard floor without excruciating pain. He is taking calcitonin, which he hopes will stabilize his bone loss and allow him to do more walking.

Though osteoporosis cannot be cured, it can be slowed down and steps can be taken to prevent it. The National Osteoporosis Foundation suggests these preventive measures:

- Eat a balanced diet rich in calcium.

- Exercise regularly, especially in weight-bearing activities.

- Don't smoke.

- If you drink alcohol, do so in moderation.

## Breast Cancer

Primarily associated with women, breast cancer also occurs in men, although rarely. According to the American Cancer Society (ACS), men will make up 1,400 of the 183,400 new cases of breast cancer expected in 1995.

Men typically do not perform breast self-examinations to detect tumors, and doctors do not ordinarily examine men for breast cancer during physicals. Unlike women, men do not get routine mammograms. Consequently, a tumor may be present and go undiscovered.

As with breast cancer in women, symptoms include the presence of a breast lump that is usually firm and painless. The nipple can have an abnormality such as retraction, crusting, or a discharge. Patients frequently are over 60.

Seymour Kramer was 70 when a gooey, bloodlike discharge from his nipple prompted him to seek medical attention. After analyzing the secretion, doctors told him he had breast cancer and recommended a lumpectomy, in which the nipple and a small amount of breast tissue are taken out. He also had several lymph nodes removed, and he underwent five weeks of radiation therapy to help ensure that residual cancer cells were killed. Though his prognosis appears very good, Kramer won't say he's been cured. But he expresses optimism: "Just because I had cancer doesn't mean my life is over."

The ACS says risk factors for male breast cancer include:

- Hyperestrogenism, or abnormal secretion of the hormone estrogen

- Klinefelter syndrome, a male disorder characterized by reduced or absent sperm production, small testicles, and enlarged breasts

- Gynecomastia, or enlargement of the male breast

Though medical professionals typically don't recommend detection exams for the general male population, doctors may advise men with gynecomastia to perform periodic breast self-examinations.

Breast cancer in men does not appear to be more aggressive than the same disease in women. However, because it is so rarely suspected in male patients, it tends to be found in a more advanced stage. Often, the tumor has already spread by the time of diagnosis, so radical mastectomy—removal of breast tissue and pectoral muscle—is often the initial treatment. But if the cancer is found before it spreads to surrounding tissue or to the lymph nodes, a lumpectomy can be performed. Radiation sometimes is used without surgery, but the verdict is still out on its effectiveness. As in Kramer's case, radiation also can be employed after surgery to reduce the chance of local recurrence and to relieve symptoms in advanced cases. If cancer has spread into the lymph nodes, some physicians use chemotherapy. A therapeutic "tumor vaccine" for men and women to treat breast cancer that has already spread is in clinical trials now.

Possible complications after surgery or radiation include decreased shoulder function, fluid retention in the arm, and pain or stiffness in the operated or radiated area. The ACS emphasizes that besides tending to the physical consequences of breast cancer therapy, "attention should be paid to the psychological aftereffects."

Patients also need follow-up monitoring—including regular exams, blood chemistry, imaging (such as magnetic resonance imaging), and bone scans—to discover any recurring tumors quickly.

Kramer says his experience of being blindsided by the disease put him on "a crusade" to inform men and medical professionals about breast cancer in males. "During a routine physical exam, I think doctors should run their hands across a man's breast to see if there's anything irregular," he says. "I'm not saying men have to go out and get wholesale mammograms. But [as a rule] doctors don't do this [touch test] and men don't inspect themselves. Those men who are not aware need to be shocked into the fact that, 'Hey, guys, this could happen to you.'"

## Eating Disorders

Though many people associate eating disorders with women, these illnesses also occur in males. In one disorder, anorexia nervosa, the person limits food intake to the point of starvation. In another, bulimia nervosa, sufferers alternate between eating large amounts of food and ridding the body of it through vomiting or laxative use. About half of those with anorexia also have bulimia symptoms.

According to the National Association of Anorexia Nervosa and Associated Disorders (ANAD), men make up about one million of the 8 million Americans with eating disorders.

"It's a myth that these are illnesses of rich, white, perfectionist women," says Chris Athas, ANAD vice president. "Just as a man or woman may become an alcoholic, either may fall victim to an eating disorder."

Medical professionals say the disorders most often surface during the teen years, but in rare cases, men as old as 60 and boys as young as eight can be afflicted. In both sexes, the illnesses can lead to life-long medical and psychological complications. An estimated 6 percent of cases result in death. Most people find it difficult to halt the behavior without professional assistance. Though some men ultimately seek help, many continue untreated with the disorders, often for years and sometimes for a decade or more.

Diagnosis is complicated by a reluctance some men have to seek medical help for disorders that are "still primarily women's," Athas says. "We live in a 'macho' society. Many men simply are ashamed to have an illness of this type." Thus, they suffer in silence.

Another problem, says ANAD, is that a great number of doctors and health-care professionals are not trained to identify or treat male eating disorders, especially anorexia. Families, too, often fail to see the diseases' symptoms. The illnesses then can progress to a more advanced stage where they are harder to treat.

During recovery, men sometimes are unwilling to participate in support-group sessions because the groups are mostly female. "Men as a whole are not comfortable in eating disorder support groups," says Athas. "But we encourage them to go anyway."

Unlike many women, who acquire eating disorders because they "feel" fat, men often are medically obese at some point in the illness and feel pressure to be thin. Sometimes athletic activities induce this struggle to be lean, prompting not only the eating disorder but also compulsive exercising. Men also may adopt disease behaviors when teased or criticized about being fat at critical development stages, such as puberty.

Treatment can be very effective, according to Arnold Andersen, M.D., an expert on eating disorders in men who has written a book on the subject. He describes a regimen of inpatient or outpatient hospital treatment, depending on the illness severity. Conditions such as anemia or depression are treated, and patients gradually relearn proper eating habits. Treatment also usually includes psychotherapy, which helps patients understand why they have the illness.

One antidepressant drug, Prozac® (fluoxetine hydrochloride), has been approved by FDA as a treatment for bulimia. Other antidepressants may also be effective, and are being studied. One, Wellbutrin® (bupropion), was shown to induce seizures in both anorexia and bulimia patients, and therefore should not be prescribed for these diagnoses. Doctors sometimes prescribe tricyclic drugs—a class that includes Elavil® (amitriptyline), Tofranil® (imipramine), and Norpramin® (desipramine). FDA has approved tricyclics for other uses but not specifically for eating disorders. However, doctors may prescribe approved drugs for "off-label" uses if, in their judgment, the patient will benefit.

Patients also undergo what Andersen calls "nutritional rehabilitation," which allows them to regain a desirable body weight. Treatment is followed by weeks, months, even years of follow-up to ensure complete recovery.

Men in support groups for eating disorders, as well as those for breast cancer and osteoporosis, say the public gradually is becoming more aware that these disorders can occur in men. They also say there's a long way to go. Some think doctors need to be enlightened. Others bemoan the lack of research. But most seem to agree that men should be educated about the disorders and how to detect them.

As breast cancer patient Seymour Kramer says: "Men need to get the word that, yes, this is a woman's disease. But you're not immune. It can happen to you."

—by John Henkel

# Part Three

# Reproductive and Sexual Concerns

# Chapter 21

# *The Male Reproductive System*

All living things, including humans, reproduce; it's one of the things that set us apart from nonliving matter. And because all living things eventually die, new creatures of the same kind must constantly be born to perpetuate a particular species. Interestingly, although the reproductive system is essential to keeping a species alive, unlike other body systems, it is not essential to keeping an individual being alive.

In the reproductive process, two kinds of sex cells, or gametes, are involved. The male gamete, or sperm, and the female gamete, the egg or ovum, meet in the female's reproductive system to create a new individual.

## *How Is the Male Reproductive System Important for Living?*

The male reproductive system is essential to the perpetuation of life: The female is dependent on the male for fertilization of her egg, even though it is she who carries the offspring through pregnancy and childbirth.

---

This information was provided by KidsHealth, one of the largest resources online for medically reviewed health information written for parents, kids, and teens. For more articles like this one, visit www.KidsHealth.org or www. TeensHealth.org. © 2001 The Nemours Center for Children's Health Media, a division of The Nemours Foundation.

Testosterone, the hormone that allows boys to become mature men, is produced by the male reproductive system. Without it, men wouldn't be able to make sperm, and reproduction would be impossible.

## Basic Anatomy

Most species have male and female organisms. Each sex has its own unique reproductive system. They are different in shape and structure, but both produce, nourish, and transport either the egg or sperm.

Unlike its female counterpart, whose sex organs are inside the body, the male reproductive system includes sex organs, or genitals, that are situated both inside and outside the body (see Figure 21.1). These are the testicles; duct system, including the epididymis and vas deferens; accessory glands; and penis. The two testicles, or testes, produce and store the tiny sperm cells. The counterpart of the ovaries in the female, the testicles are oval shaped and grow to be about one inch long. The testicles also produce hormones, including testosterone, which stimulates the production of sperm and facilitates male maturation.

The duct system includes the epididymis and the vas deferens, a muscular tube that passes upward alongside the testes and transports the sperm-containing fluid called semen. Each epididymis is a set of coiled tubes that lies against the testes, connecting them with the vas deferens. With the testes, they hang in a pouch-like structure behind the penis called the scrotum.

The accessory glands, including the seminal vesicles and the prostate gland, provide fluids that lubricate the duct system and nourish the sperm. The seminal vesicles are sac-like structures attached to the vas deferens to the side of the bladder. The prostate gland, which produces some of the components of semen, surrounds the ejaculatory ducts at the base of the urethra, just below the bladder. The urethra carries the semen through the penis, a cylindrical structure located between the legs, to the outside. The urethra also discharges urine, which is filtered in the kidneys and stored in the bladder.

## Normal Physiology

The male sex organs work together to produce semen and to release the sperm into the reproductive system of the female during sexual intercourse. They also produce and secrete sex hormones.

During puberty, sex hormones help a male to develop into a sexually mature man. At this time, usually between the ages of nine and

14, the pituitary gland secretes hormones that stimulate the testicles to produce testosterone, which is responsible for bringing about a series of sexual changes. These changes may occur at different rates but generally follow a set sequence.

The first stage of sexual maturation involves the growth of the scrotum and testes. Next, the penis becomes longer, and the seminal vesicles and prostate gland grow. Hair begins to appear in the pubic area, and about two years later, it grows on the face and underarms. The voice deepens, and males may experience their first ejaculation. Most males will also undergo a growth spurt during adolescence,

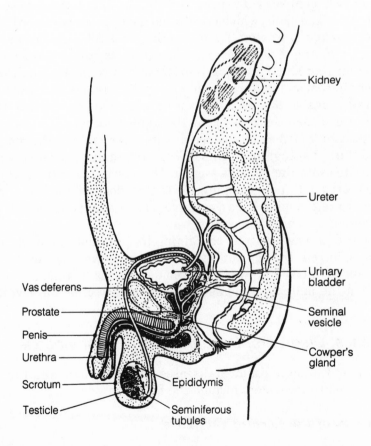

*Figure 21.1.* A cross-section of the male reproductive system. Source: *National Cancer Institute Visuals Online, 2001.*

reaching their adult height and weight. The onset of sexual maturation may be delayed or brought on earlier by certain genetic abnormalities or illnesses.

An adult male produces several million sperm cells every day. Sperm develop in the testicles within a system of tubes called seminiferous tubules. When a male baby is born, his tubules contain simple round cells, but during puberty testosterone and other hormones cause these cells to divide and change until they are thin, with a head and short tail, like tadpoles. The head contains genetic material (genes). The sperm use their tails to propel themselves into the epididymis, where they complete their development.

The sperm then move to the vas deferens, or sperm duct. The seminal vesicles and prostate gland produce a whitish fluid called seminal fluid, which mixes with sperm to form semen as a result of sexual stimulation. The penis, which usually hangs limp, becomes hard when a male is sexually excited. Tissues in the penis fill with blood and it becomes stiff and erect. When the erect penis is stimulated, muscles around the reproductive organs contract and force the semen through the duct system and urethra. Semen is expelled from the body through the urethra inside the penis. This process is called ejaculation. Each milliliter of semen contains about 100 million sperm.

The rigidity of the erect penis aids its insertion into the female's vagina during sexual intercourse. When the male ejaculates, semen is deposited into the female's vagina. The sperm make their way up to the uterus with help from uterine contractions. If a mature egg is in one of the fallopian tubes, a single sperm may penetrate it, and fertilization or conception occurs.

The cell is now a zygote, containing its full quota of 46 chromosomes, half from the egg, and half from the sperm. The cell divides again and again as it grows in the female's uterus. The genetic material from the male and female has combined to create a new individual.

## Diseases, Disorders, Conditions, and Dysfunctions

Some of the more common diseases and conditions affecting the male reproductive system include the following.

### Disorders of the Scrotal Contents

Conditions affecting the scrotal contents may involve the testicles, epididymis, or the scrotum itself.

## Testicular Disorders

- *Testicular trauma.* Even the slightest injury to the testicles can cause severe pain, bruising, or swelling. Most testicular injuries occur when the testicles are struck, hit, kicked, or crushed, usually during sports. To protect their testicles from trauma, boys and men should always wear athletic cups during contact sports.

- *Testicular torsion.* This testicular problem occurs most frequently in males between the ages of 12 and 18. Within the scrotum, the testicles are secured by a structure called the spermatic cord. When the testicle twists on this cord, the blood supply to the testicle is cut off. Torsion might occur as the result of trauma to the testicles, strenuous activity, or for no apparent reason at all. In the United States, testicular torsion occurs in one out of 4,000 males younger than 25.

- *Undescended testicles.* A male baby may be born with his testicles not having descended into the scrotum. The testes form in the abdominal cavity in the early stages of fetal development, and then descend in the month before birth. If the testicles do not drop by themselves, surgery can bring them down.

- *Testicular cancer.* Although rare, this is one of the most common cancers in men younger than 40. It occurs when cells in the testicle divide and form a tumor. If detected early, the cure rate is excellent. Lance Armstrong, champion U.S. cyclist, survived testicular cancer that was not detected early and had spread to his abdomen, lungs, and brain. Teens should be encouraged to perform self-examinations, because early detection of testicular cancer can be life-saving.

- *Epididymitis* is inflammation of the epididymis, the coiled tubes that connect the testes with the vas deferens. It is usually caused by infection or by the sexually transmitted disease chlamydia, and results in pain and swelling at the back of one testicle.

- *Hydrocele.* A hydrocele—fluid in the membranes surrounding the testes—may be present at birth or may develop later in life. Hydroceles may cause swelling of the testicle but are generally painless. If a large amount of fluid is present, a doctor may need to draw it out with a needle.

- *Inguinal hernias.* When a portion of the intestines pushes through the abdominal wall and into the groin or scrotum, it is known as an inguinal hernia. The hernia is apparent as a bulge or swelling in the groin area. It can be corrected with surgery.

## Penile Disorders

Disorders affecting the penis include the following:

- *Hypospadias*, a birth defect in which the opening of the urethra is in the wrong place, such as the underside of the penis. Surgery can correct it.

- *Phimosis*, a tightening of the foreskin of the penis, which is common in newborns and young children and usually resolves without treatment. If it interferes with urination, circumcision may be recommended.

- *Ambiguous genitalia*, a very rare condition in which a child is born with genitals that aren't clearly male or female. In most boys born with this disorder, the penis may be very small or nonexistent but testicular tissue is present. In a small number of cases, the child may have both testicular and ovarian tissue.

- *Micropenis*, another rare disorder where the penis, although normally formed, falls well below the average size, as determined by standard measurements.

## Circumcision

Although circumcision is not a penile disorder or dysfunction, it is something that parents of newborn boys may find themselves thinking a lot about. Usually performed during the first few days of life, circumcision is a procedure in which the foreskin is surgically removed, exposing the end of the penis. Parents who choose circumcision often do so based on religious beliefs, concerns about hygiene, or cultural or social reasons.

## Sterility/Infertility

If a male is sterile, either his body doesn't produce sperm at all or it doesn't produce enough sperm. This may occur as a result of abnormalities of the reproductive organs, inflammation in the genitals, alcoholism, or sexually transmitted diseases. Some men may also have trouble ejaculating. In vitro fertilization and artificial insemination can aid infertility.

# Chapter 22

# Sexual Orientation: Straight or Gay

## What is sexual orientation?

Sexual orientation is an enduring emotional, romantic, sexual, or affectional attraction to another person. It is easily distinguished from other components of sexuality including biological sex, gender identity (the psychological sense of being male or female), and the social gender role (adherence to cultural norms for feminine and masculine behavior).

Sexual orientation exists along a continuum that ranges from exclusive homosexuality to exclusive heterosexuality and includes various forms of bisexuality. Bisexual persons can experience sexual, emotional, and affectional attraction to both their own sex and the opposite sex. Persons with a homosexual orientation are sometimes referred to as gay (both men and women) or as lesbian (women only).

Sexual orientation is different from sexual behavior because it refers to feelings and self-concept. Persons may or may not express their sexual orientation in their behaviors.

## What causes a person to have a particular sexual orientation?

There are numerous theories about the origins of a person's sexual orientation; most scientists today agree that sexual orientation is most

Reprinted from "Answers to Your Questions about Sexual Orientation and Homosexuality," APA Online, American Psychological Association, http://www. apa.org/pubinfo/answers.html. Copyright © 2003 by the American Psychological Association. Reprinted with permission.

likely the result of a complex interaction of environmental, cognitive, and biological factors. In most people, sexual orientation is shaped at an early age. There is also considerable recent evidence to suggest that biology, including genetic or inborn hormonal factors, plays a significant role in a person's sexuality. In summary, it is important to recognize that there are probably many reasons for a person's sexual orientation and the reasons may be different for different people.

### Is sexual orientation a choice?

No, human beings cannot choose to be either gay or straight. Sexual orientation emerges for most people in early adolescence without any prior sexual experience. Although we can choose whether to act on our feelings, psychologists do not consider sexual orientation to be a conscious choice that can be voluntarily changed.

### Can therapy change sexual orientation?

No. Even though most homosexuals live successful, happy lives, some homosexual or bisexual people may seek to change their sexual orientation through therapy, sometimes pressured by the influence of family members or religious groups to try and do so. The reality is that homosexuality is not an illness. It does not require treatment and is not changeable.

However, not all gay, lesbian, and bisexual people who seek assistance from a mental health professional want to change their sexual orientation. Gay, lesbian, and bisexual people may seek psychological help with the coming-out process or for strategies to deal with prejudice, but most go into therapy for the same reasons and life issues that bring straight people to mental health professionals.

### What about so-called "conversion therapies"?

Some therapists who undertake so-called conversion therapy report that they have been able to change their clients' sexual orientation from homosexual to heterosexual. Close scrutiny of these reports, however, show several factors that cast doubt on their claims. For example, many of the claims come from organizations with an ideological perspective which condemns homosexuality. Furthermore, their claims are poorly documented. For example, treatment outcome is not followed and reported over time as would be the standard to test the validity of any mental health intervention.

The American Psychological Association is concerned about such therapies and their potential harm to patients. In 1997, the Association's Council of Representatives passed a resolution reaffirming psychology's opposition to homophobia in treatment and spelling out a client's right to unbiased treatment and self-determination. Any person who enters into therapy to deal with issues of sexual orientation has a right to expect that such therapy would take place in a professionally neutral environment absent of any social bias.

### *Is homosexuality a mental illness or emotional problem?*

No. Psychologists, psychiatrists, and other mental health professionals agree that homosexuality is not an illness, mental disorder, or emotional problem. Over 35 years of objective, well-designed scientific research has shown that homosexuality, in and of itself, is not associated with mental disorders or emotional or social problems. Homosexuality was once thought to be a mental illness because mental health professionals and society had biased information. In the past, the studies of gay, lesbian, and bisexual people involved only those in therapy, thus biasing the resulting conclusions. When researchers examined data about these people who were not in therapy, the idea that homosexuality was a mental illness was quickly found to be untrue.

In 1973 the American Psychiatric Association confirmed the importance of the new, better designed research and removed homosexuality from the official manual that lists mental and emotional disorders. Two years later, the American Psychological Association passed a resolution supporting the removal. For more than 25 years, both associations have urged all mental health professionals to help dispel the stigma of mental illness that some people still associate with homosexual orientation.

### *Can lesbians, gay men, and bisexuals be good parents?*

Yes. Studies comparing groups of children raised by homosexual and by heterosexual parents find no developmental differences between the two groups of children in four critical areas: their intelligence, psychological adjustment, social adjustment, and popularity with friends. It is also important to realize that a parent's sexual orientation does not dictate his or her children's.

Another myth about homosexuality is the mistaken belief that gay men have more of a tendency than heterosexual men to sexually molest children. There is no evidence to suggest that homosexuals are more likely than heterosexuals to molest children.

## Why do some gay men, lesbians, and bisexuals tell people about their sexual orientation?

Because sharing that aspect of themselves with others is important to their mental health. In fact, the process of identity development for lesbians, gay men, and bisexuals called "coming out," has been found to be strongly related to psychological adjustment—the more positive the gay, lesbian, or bisexual identity, the better one's mental health and the higher one's self-esteem.

## Why is the "coming-out" process difficult for some gay, lesbian, and bisexual people?

For some gay and bisexual people the coming-out process is difficult; for others it is not. Often lesbian, gay, and bisexual people feel afraid, different, and alone when they first realize that their sexual orientation is different from the community norm. This is particularly true for people becoming aware of their gay, lesbian, or bisexual orientation as children or adolescents, which is not uncommon. And, depending on their families and where they live, they may have to struggle against prejudice and misinformation about homosexuality. Children and adolescents may be particularly vulnerable to the deleterious effects of bias and stereotypes. They may also fear being rejected by family, friends, co-workers, and religious institutions. Some gay people have to worry about losing their jobs or being harassed at school if their sexual orientation became well known. Unfortunately, gay, lesbian, and bisexual people are at a higher risk for physical assault and violence than are heterosexuals. Studies done in California in the mid-1990s showed that nearly one-fifth of all lesbians who took part in the study and more than one-fourth of all gay men who participated had been the victims of a hate crime based on their sexual orientation. In another California study of approximately 500 young adults, half of the young men participating in the study admitted to some form of antigay aggression from name-calling to physical violence.

## What can be done to overcome the prejudice and discrimination that gay men, lesbians, and bisexuals experience?

Research has found that the people who have the most positive attitudes toward gay men, lesbians, and bisexuals are those who say they know one or more gay, lesbian, or bisexual person well—often as a friend or co-worker. For this reason, psychologists believe negative attitudes toward gay people as a group are prejudices that are not grounded in actual experiences but are based on stereotypes and prejudice.

Furthermore, protection against violence and discrimination is very important, just as it is for other minority groups. Some states include violence against an individual on the basis of his or her sexual orientation as a "hate crime," and 10 U.S. states have laws against discrimination on the basis of sexual orientation.

### Why is it important for society to be better educated about homosexuality?

Educating all people about sexual orientation and homosexuality is likely to diminish antigay prejudice. Accurate information about homosexuality is especially important to young people who are first discovering and seeking to understand their sexuality—whether homosexual, bisexual, or heterosexual. Fears that access to such information will make more people gay have no validity—information about homosexuality does not make someone gay or straight.

### Are all gay and bisexual men HIV-infected?

No. This is a commonly held myth. In reality, the risk of exposure to HIV is related to a person's behavior, not his or her sexual orientation. What's important to remember about HIV/AIDS is it is a preventable disease through the use of safe sex practices and by not using drugs.

Chapter 23

# *Circumcision*

## *How do I decide about circumcision?*

Deciding whether to have your newborn son circumcised may be difficult. You will need to consider both the benefits and the risks of circumcision. Other factors, such as your culture, religion, and personal preference, will also affect your decision.

The information about circumcision in this chapter may help you make your decision. After you have read the information, talk with your doctor about any concerns you have. The decision about whether to have your son circumcised should be made before your baby is born.

## *What is circumcision?*

During a circumcision, the prepuce of the foreskin, which is the skin that covers the tip of the penis, is removed. Circumcision is usually performed on the first or second day after birth. It becomes more complicated and riskier in infants older than two months and in boys and men. The procedure takes only about five to 10 minutes. A local anesthetic (numbing medicine) can be given to your baby so he does not feel pain from the procedure.

---

## Are there any benefits from circumcision?

Studies about the benefits of circumcision have provided conflicting results. Some studies show certain benefits, while other studies do not. The American Academy of Pediatrics (AAP) says the benefits of circumcision are not significant enough to recommend circumcision as a routine procedure and that circumcision is not medically necessary. The American Academy of Family Physicians believes parents should discuss with their son's doctor the potential benefits and the risks involved when making their decision.

A recent AAP report stated that circumcision does offer some benefit in preventing urinary tract infections in infants. Circumcision also offers some benefit in preventing penile cancer in adult men. However, this disease is very rare in all men, whether or not they have been circumcised. Circumcision may reduce the risk of sexually transmitted diseases. A man's sexual practices (e.g., if he uses condoms, if he has more than one partner, etc.) have more to do with STD prevention than whether or not he is circumcised.

Study results are mixed about whether circumcision may help reduce the risk of cervical cancer in female sex partners, and whether it helps prevent certain problems with the penis, such as infections and unwanted swelling. Some studies show that keeping the penis clean can help prevent these problems just as well as circumcision. Infections and unwanted swelling are not serious and can usually be easily treated if they do occur.

## What are the risks of circumcision?

Like any surgical procedure, circumcision has some risks. However, the rate of problems after circumcision is low. Bleeding and infection in the circumcised area are the most common problems. Sometimes the skin of the newly exposed glans becomes irritated by the pressure of diapers and ammonia in the urine. The irritation is usually treated with petroleum ointment (Vaseline®) put directly on the area. This problem will usually lessen after a few days.

## How do I care for my baby's penis after a circumcision?

Gently clean the area with water every day and whenever the diaper area becomes soiled. Some swelling of the penis is normal after a circumcision. A clear crust will probably form over the area. It normally takes seven to 10 days for the penis to heal after a circumcision.

After the circumcision, you may notice a small amount of blood on the baby's diaper. If the bloodstain is larger than the size of a quarter, call your doctor right away. In addition, you should call your doctor if a Plastibell™ device was used during the circumcision and the device doesn't fall off within 10 to 12 days. If there is a bandage on the penis instead of a Plastibell, the bandage should be changed each time you change your son's diaper. This will help prevent infection. Signs of infection also signal the need to call your doctor. These signs include a temperature of 100.4°F or higher, redness, swelling, and/or a yellowish discharge.

When to call your doctor:

- If the wound does not stop bleeding

- If your son does not have a wet diaper within six to eight hours after the circumcision

- If the redness and swelling around the tip of the penis do not go away or get worse after three to five days

- If there is a yellow discharge or coating around the tip of the penis after seven days

- If the Plastibell device does not fall off within 10 to 12 days

### How do I care for my baby's penis if I choose not to have him circumcised?

Simply keeping the penis clean with soap and water helps reduce the risk of problems or infections.

In older boys and adult men, the foreskin slides back and forth over the penis, allowing the area underneath to be cleaned. The foreskin doesn't retract in boys for a few years. Don't try to force the foreskin to retract, because this can damage the penis and cause problems. When the foreskin is ready to retract, you can teach your son how to retract it himself and clean the skin underneath. He should wash his foreskin every day while bathing.

# Chapter 24

# *Benign Prostatic Hyperplasia*

## *The Prostate Gland*

The prostate is a walnut-sized gland that forms part of the male reproductive system. The gland is made of two lobes, or regions, enclosed by an outer layer of tissue. The prostate is located in front of the rectum and just below the bladder, where urine is stored. The prostate also surrounds the urethra, the canal through which urine passes out of the body.

Scientists do not know all the prostate's functions. One of its main roles, though, is to squeeze fluid into the urethra as sperm move through during sexual climax. This fluid, which helps make up semen, energizes the sperm and makes the vaginal canal less acidic.

## *BPH: A Common Part of Aging*

It is common for the prostate gland to become enlarged as a man ages. Doctors call the condition benign prostatic hyperplasia (BPH), or benign prostatic hypertrophy.

As a man matures, the prostate goes through two main periods of growth. The first occurs early in puberty, when the prostate doubles in size. At around age 25, the gland begins to grow again. This second growth phase often results, years later, in BPH.

Reprinted from "Prostate Enlargement: Benign Prostatic Hyperplasia," National Kidney and Urologic Diseases Information Clearinghouse, June 2002, http://www.niddk.nih.gov/health/urolog/pubs/prostate/, NIH Pub. No. 02-3012.

Though the prostate continues to grow during most of a man's life, the enlargement doesn't usually cause problems until late in life. BPH rarely causes symptoms before age 40, but more than half of men in their sixties and as many as 90 percent in their seventies and eighties have some symptoms of BPH.

As the prostate enlarges, the layer of tissue surrounding it stops it from expanding, causing the gland to press against the urethra like a clamp on a garden hose. The bladder wall becomes thicker and irritable. The bladder begins to contract even when it contains small amounts of urine, causing more frequent urination. Eventually, the bladder weakens and loses the ability to empty itself. Urine remains in the bladder. The narrowing of the urethra and partial emptying of the bladder cause many of the problems associated with BPH.

Many people feel uncomfortable talking about the prostate, since the gland plays a role in both sex and urination. Still, prostate enlargement is as common a part of aging as gray hair. As life expectancy rises, so does the occurrence of BPH. In the United States alone, 375,000 hospital stays each year involve a diagnosis of BPH.

It is not clear whether certain groups face a greater risk of getting BPH. Studies done over the years suggest that BPH occurs more often among married men than single men and is more common in the United States and Europe than in other parts of the world. However, these findings have been debated, and no definite information on risk factors exists.

## Why BPH Occurs

The cause of BPH is not well understood. For centuries, it has been known that BPH occurs mainly in older men and that it doesn't develop in men whose testes were removed before puberty. For this reason, some researchers believe that factors related to aging and the testes may spur the development of BPH.

Throughout their lives, men produce both testosterone, an important male hormone, and small amounts of estrogen, a female hormone. As men age, the amount of active testosterone in the blood decreases, leaving a higher proportion of estrogen. Studies done with animals have suggested that BPH may occur because the higher amount of estrogen within the gland increases the activity of substances that promote cell growth.

Another theory focuses on dihydrotestosterone (DHT), a substance derived from testosterone in the prostate, which may help control its growth. Most animals lose their ability to produce DHT as they age.

However, some research has indicated that even with a drop in the blood's testosterone level, older men continue to produce and accumulate high levels of DHT in the prostate. This accumulation of DHT may encourage the growth of cells. Scientists have also noted that men who do not produce DHT do not develop BPH.

Some researchers suggest that BPH may develop as a result of "instructions" given to cells early in life. According to this theory, BPH occurs because cells in one section of the gland follow these instructions and "reawaken" later in life. These "reawakened" cells then deliver signals to other cells in the gland, instructing them to grow or making them more sensitive to hormones that influence growth.

## Symptoms

Many symptoms of BPH stem from obstruction of the urethra and gradual loss of bladder function, which results in incomplete emptying of the bladder. The symptoms of BPH vary, but the most common ones involve changes or problems with urination, such as:

- A hesitant, interrupted, weak stream
- Urgency and leaking or dribbling
- More frequent urination, especially at night

The size of the prostate does not always determine how severe the obstruction or the symptoms will be. Some men with greatly enlarged glands have little obstruction and few symptoms while others, whose glands are less enlarged, have more blockage and greater problems.

Sometimes a man may not know he has any obstruction until he suddenly finds himself unable to urinate at all. This condition, called acute urinary retention, may be triggered by taking over-the-counter cold or allergy medicines. Such medicines contain a decongestant drug, known as a sympathomimetic. A potential side effect of this drug may be to prevent the bladder opening from relaxing and allowing urine to empty. When partial obstruction is present, urinary retention also can be brought on by alcohol, cold temperatures, or a long period of immobility.

It is important to tell your doctor about urinary problems such as those described above. In eight out of 10 cases, these symptoms suggest BPH, but they also can signal other, more serious conditions that require prompt treatment. These conditions, including prostate cancer, can be ruled out only by a doctor's exam.

301

Severe BPH can cause serious problems over time. Urine retention and strain on the bladder can lead to urinary tract infections, bladder or kidney damage, bladder stones, and incontinence. If the bladder is permanently damaged, treatment for BPH may be ineffective. When BPH is found in its earlier stages, there is a lower risk of developing such complications.

## Diagnosis

You may first notice symptoms of BPH yourself, or your doctor may find that your prostate is enlarged during a routine checkup. When BPH is suspected, you may be referred to a urologist, a doctor who specializes in problems of the urinary tract and the male reproductive system. Several tests help the doctor identify the problem and decide whether surgery is needed. The tests vary from patient to patient, but the following are the most common.

### Digital Rectal Exam (DRE)

This exam is usually the first test done. The doctor inserts a gloved finger into the rectum and feels the part of the prostate next to the rectum. This exam gives the doctor a general idea of the size and condition of the gland.

### Prostate Specific Antigen (PSA) Blood Test

In order to rule out cancer as a cause of urinary symptoms, your doctor may recommend a PSA blood test. PSA, a protein produced by prostate cells, is frequently present at elevated levels in the blood of men who have prostate cancer. The U.S. Food and Drug Administration has approved a PSA test for use in conjunction with a digital rectal exam to help detect prostate cancer in men age 50 or older and for monitoring prostate cancer patients after treatment. However, much remains unknown about the interpretation of PSA levels, the test's ability to discriminate cancer from benign prostate conditions, and the best course of action following a finding of elevated PSA.

Because many unanswered questions surround the issue of PSA screening, the relative magnitude of its potential risks and benefits is unknown. Both PSA and ultrasound tests enhance detection when added to DRE screening. But they are known to have relatively high false-positive rates, and they may identify a greater number of medically insignificant tumors. Thus, PSA screening might lead to treatment of unproven benefit that could result in morbidity (including impotence and incontinence) and mortality. It cannot be determined from earlier studies whether PSA screening will reduce prostate cancer mortality. Ongoing studies are addressing this issue.

### *Rectal Ultrasound*

If there is a suspicion of prostate cancer, your doctor may recommend a test with rectal ultrasound. In this procedure, a probe inserted in the rectum directs sound waves at the prostate. The echo patterns of the sound waves form an image of the prostate gland on a display screen.

### *Urine Flow Study*

Sometimes the doctor will ask a patient to urinate into a special device that measures how quickly the urine is flowing. A reduced flow often suggests BPH.

### *Intravenous Pyelogram (IVP)*

IVP is an x-ray of the urinary tract. In this test, a dye is injected into a vein, and the x-ray is taken. The dye makes the urine visible on the x-ray and shows any obstruction or blockage in the urinary tract.

### *Cystoscopy*

In this exam, the doctor inserts a small tube through the opening of the urethra in the penis. This procedure is done after a solution numbs the inside of the penis so all sensation is lost. The tube, called a cystoscope, contains a lens and a light system, which help the doctor see the inside of the urethra and the bladder. This test allows the doctor to determine the size of the gland and identify the location and degree of the obstruction.

## Treatment

Men who have BPH with symptoms usually need some kind of treatment at some time. However, a number of recent studies have questioned the need for early treatment when the gland is just mildly enlarged. These studies report that early treatment may not be needed because the symptoms of BPH clear up without treatment in as many as one-third of all mild cases. Instead of immediate treatment, they suggest regular checkups to watch for early problems. If the condition begins to pose a danger to the patient's health or causes a major inconvenience to him, treatment is usually recommended.

Since BPH may cause urinary tract infections, a doctor will usually clear up any infection with antibiotics before treating the BPH itself. Although the need for treatment is not usually urgent, doctors generally advise going ahead with treatment once the problems become bothersome or present a health risk.

## *Drug Treatment*

Over the years, researchers have tried to find a way to shrink or at least stop the growth of the prostate without using surgery. The Food and Drug Administration (FDA) has approved four drugs to relieve common symptoms associated with an enlarged prostate.

Finasteride (marketed under the name Proscar®), FDA-approved in 1992, inhibits production of the hormone DHT, which is involved with prostate enlargement. Its use can actually shrink the prostate in some men.

FDA also approved the drugs terazosin (marketed as Hytrin®) in 1993, doxazosin (marketed as Cardura®) in 1995, and tamsulosin (marketed as Flomax®) in 1997 for the treatment of BPH. All three drugs act by relaxing the smooth muscle of the prostate and bladder neck to improve urine flow and to reduce bladder outlet obstruction. Terazosin, doxazosin, and tamsulosin belong to the class of drugs known as alpha blockers. Terazosin and doxazosin were developed first to treat high blood pressure. Tamsulosin is the first alpha blocker developed specifically to treat BPH.

The Medical Therapy of Prostatic Symptoms (MTOPS) Trial of the National Institute of Diabetes and Digestive and Kidney Diseases (NIDDK) recently found that using finasteride and doxazosin together is more effective than either drug alone to relieve symptoms and prevent BPH progression. The two-drug regimen reduced the risk of BPH progression by 67 percent, compared to 39 percent for doxazosin alone and 34 percent for finasteride alone.

## *Nonsurgical Treatment*

Because drug treatment is not effective in all cases, researchers in recent years have developed a number of procedures that relieve BPH symptoms but are less invasive than surgery.

*Transurethral Microwave Procedures*

In May 1996, FDA approved the Prostatron®, a device that uses microwaves to heat and destroy excess prostate tissue. In the procedure called transurethral microwave thermotherapy (TUMT), the Prostatron sends computer-regulated microwaves through a catheter to heat selected portions of the prostate to at least 111° Fahrenheit. A cooling system protects the urinary tract during the procedure.

A similar microwave device, the Targis™ System, received FDA approval in September 1997. Like the Prostatron, the Targis System delivers microwaves to destroy selected portions of the prostate and uses a cooling system to protect the urethra. A heat-sensing device inserted in the rectum helps monitor the therapy.

Both procedures take about one hour and can be performed on an outpatient basis without general anesthesia. Neither procedure has been reported to lead to impotence or incontinence.

While microwave therapy does not cure BPH, it reduces urinary frequency, urgency, straining, and intermittent flow. It does not correct the problem of incomplete emptying of the bladder. Ongoing research will determine any long-term effects of microwave therapy and who might benefit most from this therapy.

*Transurethral Needle Ablation*

In October 1996, FDA approved VidaMed's minimally invasive Transurethral Needle Ablation (TUNA®) System for the treatment of BPH.

The TUNA System delivers low-level radiofrequency energy through twin needles to burn away a well-defined region of the enlarged prostate. Shields protect the urethra from heat damage. The TUNA System improves urine flow and relieves symptoms with fewer side effects when compared with transurethral resection of the prostate (TURP). No incontinence or impotence has been observed.

## Surgical Treatment

Most doctors recommend removal of the enlarged part of the prostate as the best long-term solution for patients with BPH. With surgery for BPH, only the enlarged tissue that is pressing against the urethra is removed; the rest of the inside tissue and the outside capsule are left intact. Surgery usually relieves the obstruction and incomplete emptying caused by BPH.

*Transurethral Surgery*

In this type of surgery, no external incision is needed. After giving anesthesia, the surgeon reaches the prostate by inserting an instrument through the urethra.

A procedure called TURP (transurethral resection of the prostate) is used for 90 percent of all prostate surgeries done for BPH. With TURP, an instrument called a resectoscope is inserted through the penis. The resectoscope, which is about 12 inches long and one-half inch in diameter, contains a light, valves for controlling irrigating fluid, and an electrical loop that cuts tissue and seals blood vessels.

During the 90-minute operation, the surgeon uses the resectoscope's wire loop to remove the obstructing tissue one piece at a time. The pieces of tissue are carried by the fluid into the bladder and then flushed out at the end of the operation.

Most doctors suggest using TURP whenever possible. Transurethral procedures are less traumatic than open forms of surgery and require a shorter recovery period.

Another surgical procedure is called transurethral incision of the prostate (TUIP). Instead of removing tissue, as with TURP, this procedure widens the urethra by making a few small cuts in the bladder neck, where the urethra joins the bladder, and in the prostate gland itself. Although some people believe that TUIP gives the same relief as TURP with less risk of side effects such as retrograde ejaculation, its advantages and long-term side effects have not been clearly established.

*Open Surgery*

In the few cases when a transurethral procedure cannot be used, open surgery, which requires an external incision, may be used. Open surgery is often done when the gland is greatly enlarged, when there are complicating factors, or when the bladder has been damaged and needs to be repaired. The location of the enlargement within the gland and the patient's general health help the surgeon decide which of the three open procedures to use.

With all the open procedures, anesthesia is given and an incision is made. Once the surgeon reaches the prostate capsule, he scoops out the enlarged tissue from inside the gland.

*Laser Surgery*

In March 1996, FDA approved a surgical procedure that employs side-firing laser fibers and Nd:YAG lasers to vaporize obstructing prostate tissue. The doctor passes the laser fiber through the urethra into the prostate using a cystoscope and then delivers several bursts of energy lasting 30 to 60 seconds. The laser energy destroys prostate tissue and causes shrinkage. Like TURP, laser surgery requires anesthesia and a hospital stay. One advantage of laser surgery over TURP is that laser surgery causes little blood loss. Laser surgery also allows for a quicker recovery time. But laser surgery may not be effective on larger prostates. The long-term effectiveness of laser surgery is not known.

## Your Recovery after Surgery in the Hospital

If you have surgery, you'll probably stay in the hospital from three to 10 days depending on the type of surgery you had and how quickly you recover.

At the end of surgery, a special catheter is inserted through the opening of the penis to drain urine from the bladder into a collection bag. Called a Foley catheter, this device has a water-filled balloon on the end that is placed in the bladder, which keeps it in place.

This catheter is usually left in place for several days. Sometimes, the catheter causes recurring painful bladder spasms the day after surgery. These may be difficult to control, but they will eventually disappear.

You may also be given antibiotics while you are in the hospital. Many doctors start giving this medicine before or soon after surgery to prevent infection. However, some recent studies suggest that antibiotics may not be needed in every case, and your doctor may prefer to wait until an infection is present to give them.

After surgery, you will probably notice some blood or clots in your urine as the wound starts to heal. If your bladder is being irrigated (flushed with water), you may notice that your urine becomes red once the irrigation is stopped. Some bleeding is normal, and it should clear up by the time you leave the hospital. During your recovery, it is important to drink a lot of water (up to eight cups a day) to help flush out the bladder and speed healing.

## Do's and Don'ts

Take it easy the first few weeks after you get home. You may not have any pain, but you still have an incision that is healing—even with transurethral surgery, where the incision can't be seen. Since many people try to do too much at the beginning and then have a setback, it is a good idea to talk to your doctor before resuming your normal routine. During this initial period of recovery at home, avoid any straining or sudden movements that could tear the incision. Here are some guidelines:

- Continue drinking a lot of water to flush the bladder.
- Avoid straining when moving your bowel.
- Eat a balanced diet to prevent constipation. If constipation occurs, ask your doctor if you can take a laxative.
- Don't do any heavy lifting.
- Don't drive or operate machinery.

## Getting Back to Normal

Even though you should feel much better by the time you leave the hospital, it will probably take a couple of months for you to heal completely. During the recovery period, the following are some common problems that can occur.

### Problems Urinating

You may notice that your urinary stream is stronger right after surgery, but it may take awhile before you can urinate completely normally again. After the catheter is removed, urine will pass over the surgical wound on the prostate, and you may initially have some discomfort or feel a sense of urgency when you urinate. This problem will gradually lessen, though, and after a couple of months you should be able to urinate less frequently and more easily.

### Inability to Control Urination (Incontinence)

As the bladder returns to normal, you may have some temporary problems controlling urination, but long-term incontinence rarely occurs. Doctors find that the longer problems existed before surgery, the longer it will take for the bladder to regain its full function after the operation.

### Bleeding

In the first few weeks after transurethral surgery, the scab inside the bladder may loosen, and blood may suddenly appear in the urine. Although this can be alarming, the bleeding usually stops with a short period of resting in bed and drinking fluids. However, if your urine is so red that it is difficult to see through or if it contains clots or if you feel any discomfort, be sure to contact your doctor.

## Sexual Function after Surgery

Many men worry about whether surgery for BPH will affect their ability to enjoy sex. Some sources state that sexual function is rarely affected, while others claim that it can cause problems in up to 30 percent of all cases. However, most doctors say that even though it takes a while for sexual function to return fully, with time, most men are able to enjoy sex again.

Complete recovery of sexual function may take up to one year, lagging behind a person's general recovery. The exact length of time depends on how long after symptoms appeared that BPH surgery was done and on the type of surgery. Following is a summary of how surgery is likely to affect various aspects of sexual function.

### Erections

Most doctors agree that if you were potent (able to maintain an erection) shortly before surgery, you will probably be able to have erections afterward. Surgery rarely causes a loss of potency. However, surgery cannot usually restore potency that was lost before the operation.

### Ejaculation

Although most men are able to continue having erections after surgery, a prostatectomy frequently makes them sterile (unable to father children) by causing a condition called "retrograde ejaculation" or "dry climax."

During sexual activity, sperm from the testes enter the urethra near the opening of the bladder. Normally, a muscle blocks off the entrance to the bladder, and the semen is expelled through the penis. However, the coring action of prostate surgery cuts this muscle as it widens the neck of the bladder. Following surgery, the semen takes the path of least resistance and enters the wider opening to the bladder rather than being expelled through the penis. Later it is harmlessly flushed out with urine.

### Orgasm

Most men find little or no difference in the sensation of orgasm, or sexual climax, before and after surgery. Although it may take some time to get used to retrograde ejaculation, you should eventually find sex as pleasurable after surgery as before.

Many people have found that concerns about sexual function can interfere with sex as much as the operation itself. Understanding the surgical procedure and talking over any worries with the doctor before surgery often help men regain sexual function earlier. Many men also find it helpful to talk to a counselor during the adjustment period after surgery.

## Is Further Treatment Needed?

In the years after your surgery, it is important to continue having a rectal exam once a year and to have any symptoms checked by your doctor.

Since surgery for BPH leaves behind a good part of the gland, it is still possible for prostate problems, including BPH, to develop again. However, surgery usually offers relief from BPH for at least 15 years. Only 10 percent of the men who have surgery for BPH eventually need a second operation for enlargement. Usually these are men who had the first surgery at an early age.

Sometimes, scar tissue resulting from surgery requires treatment in the year after surgery. Rarely, the opening of the bladder becomes scarred and shrinks, causing obstruction. This problem may require a surgical procedure similar to transurethral incision. More often, scar tissue may form in the urethra and cause narrowing. This problem can usually be solved during an office visit when the doctor stretches the urethra.

### Prostatic Stents

Stents are small devices inserted through the urethra to the narrowed area and allowed to expand, like a spring. The stent pushes back the prostatic tissue, widening the urethra. FDA approved the UroLume® Endoprosthesis in 1996 to relieve urinary obstruction in men and improve ability to urinate. The device is approved for use in men for whom other standard surgical procedures to correct urinary obstruction have failed.

### BPH and Prostate Cancer: No Apparent Relation

Although some of the signs of BPH and prostate cancer are the same, having BPH does not seem to increase the chances of getting

prostate cancer. Nevertheless, a man who has BPH may have undetected prostate cancer at the same time or may develop prostate cancer in the future. For this reason, the National Cancer Institute and
the American Cancer Society recommend that all men over 40 have
a rectal exam once a year to screen for prostate cancer.

After BPH surgery, the tissue removed is routinely checked for
hidden cancer cells. In about one out of 10 cases, some cancer tissue
is found, but often it is limited to a few cells of a nonaggressive type
of cancer, and no treatment is needed.

# Chapter 25

# *Prostatitis*

You or someone you know may have been diagnosed as having a type of prostatitis, a common and painful disease of the prostate gland and its surrounding structures. The following has been designed to answer your questions about prostatitis.

### *What is the prostate?*

The prostate is a part of the male reproductive system; it is about the same size and shape of a walnut and weighs about an ounce. It is located below the bladder and in front of the rectum and surrounds the urethra, the tube-like structure that carries urine from the bladder out through the penis. The main function of the prostate is to produce ejaculatory fluid.

### *What are the different types of prostatitis and their causes?*

Acute bacterial prostatitis is the least common type of prostatitis and is always caused by bacterial infection. It is usually easy to identify because of the sudden onset of symptoms severe enough that a visit to a doctor or even the hospital may be required. Acute bacterial prostatitis can affect any age group but commonly occurs in young and middle-aged men.

Another type that is caused by bacterial infection is chronic bacterial prostatitis, which may exist for several years without producing any symptoms. When symptoms do appear, they are generally less severe than acute bacterial prostatitis but often recur. This condition can also affect any age group but is most common in young and middle-aged men.

Nonbacterial prostatitis is the most common type of prostatitis. The exact cause of nonbacterial prostatitis is not known, but it is due to an inflammation rather than an infection. Other types include prostatodynia and asymptomatic prostatic inflammation.

### What causes prostatitis?

The bacteria that cause acute and chronic bacterial prostatitis get into the prostate from the urethra by backward flow of infected urine into the prostate ducts. Bacterial prostatitis is not contagious and is not considered to be a sexually transmitted disease. A sexual partner cannot catch this infection.

Certain conditions or medical procedures increase the risk of contracting bacterial prostatitis. There is a higher risk if the man has recently had a catheter or other instrument inserted into his urethra, an abnormality of his urinary tract, or a recent bladder infection.

Chronic nonbacterial prostatitis results in similar inflammation of the prostate gland, but it may not be due to the typical bacteria that cause urine infections. It may be caused by organisms called chlamydia or mycoplasma. Some of these organisms may be transmitted by sexual contact. It may also be due to a chemical or immunologic reaction, perhaps even to urine itself flowing backwards into the prostate ducts.

There is no known cause for prostatodynia. It does not appear to be related to bacteria or inflammation of the prostate gland but may be related to a disorder of the nerves and muscles surrounding the prostate gland.

### What are the symptoms of prostatitis?

The symptoms of the various prostatitis syndromes are extremely variable, and although they depend on the type of disease you have, there is much overlap.

In acute bacterial prostatitis, the symptoms are severe and sudden and may cause the patient to seek emergency medical care. Chills, fever, severe burning during urination, and the inability to completely empty the bladder are common.

In chronic bacterial prostatitis, the symptoms are similar but much less severe. They include: burning during urination; urinary frequency, especially at night; perineal, testicular, bladder, and low back pain; and painful ejaculation. The physician may note, in bacterial prostatitis, that the prostate is swollen and tender upon examination.

The symptoms of chronic nonbacterial prostatitis include difficult and sometimes painful urination, discomfort or pain in the perineum, bladder, testicles and penis as well as difficult and painful ejaculation. In some cases, these symptoms can be indistinguishable from those described above for chronic bacterial prostatitis.

The symptoms of prostatodynia include difficult and sometimes painful urination, discomfort or even pain in the perineum and penis, as well as difficult and painful ejaculation. These symptoms can be indistinguishable from those described above for chronic nonbacterial prostatitis.

## *How is prostatitis diagnosed?*

The correct diagnosis is very important because the treatment is different for the different types of prostatitis syndromes. In addition, it is extremely important to make sure that the symptoms are not caused by urethritis, cystitis, an enlarged prostate, or cancer. To help make an accurate diagnosis, several types of examinations are useful.

To examine the prostate gland, the physician will perform a digital rectal examination (DRE). This is a simple examination in which the doctor will pass a lubricated, gloved finger into the rectum. Because the prostate is located just in front of the rectum, it can be easily pressed. The physician will be able to determine whether the prostate is enlarged or tender. Lumps or firm areas can suggest the presence of prostate cancer. The physician will also assess the degree of pain or discomfort the patient experiences as he presses the muscles and ligaments of the pelvic floor and perineum. If a man has prostatitis, this examination may produce momentary pain or discomfort, but it causes neither damage nor significant prolonged pain.

If the physician requires a closer look at the prostate gland or decides that a biopsy is necessary, he may order a transrectal ultrasound, which allows him to visualize the prostate gland. If you are at risk for cancer, your physician will consider ordering a PSA test.

If your physician suspects that you have prostatitis or one of the other prostate problems, he may refer you to a urologist, a doctor who specializes in diseases of the urinary tract and male reproductive system, to confirm the diagnosis.

The urologist will repeat some of the examinations already performed by the first physician. The urologist will also assess the degree of pain or discomfort the patient experiences as he presses the prostate as well as the muscles and ligaments of the pelvic floor and perineum. The urologist may analyze various urine specimens as well as a specimen of prostatic fluid obtained by massaging the prostate gland during DRE. The various urine specimens and prostatic fluid will be analyzed for signs of inflammation and infection. These samples will help the urologist determine whether your problem is inflammation or infection and whether the problem is in the urethra, bladder, or prostate.

Other tests the urologist may consider employing include cystoscopy in which a small telescope is passed through the urethra into the bladder permitting examination of the urethra, prostate, and bladder. The urologist may also order urine flow studies, which help measure the strength of your urine flow and any obstruction caused by the prostate, urethra, or pelvic muscles.

### *How should prostatitis be treated?*

Your treatment depends on the type of prostatitis you have.

If acute bacterial prostatitis is diagnosed, the patient will need to take antibiotics for a minimum of 14 days. Sometimes, this means being admitted to the hospital and being given intravenous antibiotics. A catheter is sometimes required if the patient has difficulty urinating. Almost all acute infections can be cured with this treatment. Frequently, the antibiotics will be continued for as long as four weeks.

If chronic bacterial prostatitis is diagnosed, the patient will require antibiotics for a longer period of time, usually four to 12 weeks. About 60 percent of all cases of chronic bacterial prostatitis clear up with this treatment. Sometimes the symptoms recur and antibiotic therapy is again required. For cases that do not respond to this treatment, long-term antibiotic therapy may be recommended to relieve the symptoms. Other medications (such as those used for nonbacterial prostatitis) or other treatments (e.g., prostate massage therapy) may also be used in difficult cases. In some rare cases, surgery on either the urethra or prostate may be recommended. Surgery for chronic bacterial prostatitis should not be taken lightly, and a second opinion is advisable.

The patient may not need antibiotics, if he is diagnosed with chronic nonbacterial prostatitis. Frequently, physicians have difficulty trying to decide whether a patient has bacterial or nonbacterial prostatitis.

316

This is because of the difficulties in obtaining a specimen; sometimes previous antibiotic therapy obscures the diagnosis. An organism that responds to antibiotics but is difficult to diagnose may also cause non-bacterial prostatitis. For these reasons, antibiotics are usually prescribed, at least initially, even when a definitive diagnosis of bacterial prostatitis has not been made with the appropriate tests. Your response to the antibiotic therapy will decide whether or not it should be continued. Depending on your symptoms you may receive one of a variety of other treatments. These may consist of alpha blockers, anti-inflammatory drugs, plant extracts (or vitamins), repetitive prostatic massage (to drain the prostate ducts), and various heat therapies.

The treatment for prostatodynia is difficult since physicians do not really understand what causes this type of disease. Muscle relaxants, alpha blockers, biofeedback, and relaxation exercises may alleviate some of the symptoms. Once a correct diagnosis has been made, one of the best therapies may be that of reassurance that the patient does not have a serious condition.

Treatment for asymptomatic prostatitic inflammation is usually not required.

### *Why do physicians have trouble diagnosing prostatitis?*

The diagnosis of the various types of prostatitis can be very difficult and sometimes quite frustrating for the patient and his physician. The symptoms are variable, and there is much overlap in symptoms between the various types of prostatitis. Once the patient has been treated with antibiotics, it can be difficult to differentiate a bacterial prostatitis from a nonbacterial prostatitis.

### *How will prostatitis affect a patient?*

Prostatitis is an extremely frustrating disease for both the patient and his physician. It can seriously affect a patient's quality of life. The correct diagnosis of the prostatitis problem is difficult, and it cannot always be cured. However, prostatitis is a treatable disease and one can usually get relief from major symptoms by following the recommended treatment.

### *Why are some patients not cured after they have been diagnosed with prostatitis?*

Most cases of acute bacterial prostatitis respond completely to therapy. Unfortunately, the treatment for the chronic prostatitis syndrome is far from perfect. Patients with chronic bacterial prostatitis can have persistence of their infectious problem despite antibiotic use. This is because of the difficulty antibiotics have in penetrating the prostate gland to completely kill all the bacteria deep within the prostatic ducts. Repetitive or frequent prostate massages may be helpful in these cases. The patients who have had chronic bacterial prostatitis and have been cured are susceptible to recurrences, and each recurrence may be more difficult to treat than the last. Many patients with nonbacterial prostatitis and prostatodynia fail therapy. Patients may find that they have to learn to live with their symptoms while the inflammation hopefully "burns itself out."

### What are some of the most important facts about prostatitis?

- Correct diagnosis is the key to the management of prostatitis.

- Prostatitis cannot always be cured but can be managed.

- Treatment should be followed even if symptoms have improved.

- Patients with prostatitis are not at higher risk for developing prostate cancer.

- There is no reason to discontinue normal sexual relations unless they are uncomfortable, usually during an acute phase.

- One can live a reasonably normal life with prostatitis.

# Chapter 26

# *Peyronie Disease*

As the channel for semen and urine, the penis serves two important functions in men. But a disease described as early as the mid-eighteenth century by a French physician, Francois Gigot de la Peyronie, which causes hardened patches on the penile shaft, can severely impact a man's sexual performance. If you have pain and penile curvature characteristic of Peyronie disease, the following information should help you understand your condition.

## *What happens under normal conditions?*

The penis is a cylindrical organ consisting of three chambers: paired corpora cavernosa that are surrounded by a protective tunica albuginea; a dense, elastic membrane or sheath under the skin; and the corpus spongiosum, a singular channel, located centrally beneath and surrounded by a thinner connective tissue sheath. It contains the urethra, the narrow tube that carries urine and semen out of the body.

These three chambers are made up of highly specialized, sponge-like erectile tissue filled with thousands of venous cavities, spaces that remain relatively empty of blood when the penis is soft. But during erection, blood fills the cavities, causing the corpora cavernosa to balloon and push against the tunica albuginea. While the penis hardens and stretches, the skin remains loose and elastic to accommodate the changes.

## What is Peyronie disease?

Peyronie disease (also known as fibrous cavernositis) is an acquired inflammatory condition of the penis. It is the formation of a plaque or hardened scar tissue beneath the skin of the penis. This scarring is noncancerous, but often leads to painful erection and curvature of the erect penis (a "crooked penis").

## What are the symptoms of Peyronie disease?

This scarring, or plaque, typically develops on the upper side of the penis (dorsum). It reduces the elasticity of the tunica albuginea in that area and, as a result, causes the penis to bend upward during an erection. Although Peyronie plaque is most commonly located on the top of the penis, it may occur on the underside or on the lateral side of the penis, causing a downward or lateral bend. Some patients may even develop a plaque that goes all the way around the penis, causing a "waisting" or "bottleneck" deformity of the penile shaft. The majority of patients complain of generalized shrinkage or shortening of their penis.

Painful erections and difficulty with intercourse usually lead men with Peyronie disease to seek medical help. Since there is great variability in this condition, sufferers may complain of any combination of symptoms: penile curvature, obvious penile plaques, painful erection, and diminished ability to achieve an erection.

Any of those physical deformities make Peyronie disease a quality-of-life issue. Not surprising, it is linked to erectile dysfunction in 20 to 40 percent of sufferers. While studies have shown that 77 percent of men demonstrate significant psychological effects, the numbers, medical researchers believe, are underreported. Instead, many men affected with this truly devastating condition suffer in silence.

## How frequently does Peyronie disease occur?

Peyronie disease affects a reported 1 to 3.7 percent (about one to four in 100) of males between ages 40 and 70, even though severe cases have been reported in younger men. Medical researchers believe the actual prevalence may be higher due to patient embarrassment and limited reporting by physicians. Since the introduction of sildenafil citrate, an oral therapy for impotence, doctors have reported increased incidence of Peyronie cases. With more men being treated successfully for erectile dysfunction in the future, an increasing number of cases presenting to urologists is anticipated.

## What causes Peyronie disease?

Ever since Francois Gigot de la Peyronie, personal physician to King Louis XV, first reported penile curvature in 1743, scientists have been mystified by the causes of this well-recognized disorder. Yet medical researchers have speculated on a variety of factors that might be at work.

Most experts believe that acute or short-term cases of Peyronie disease are likely the consequence of a minor penile trauma, sometimes caused by sports injuries, but more often by vigorous sexual activity (e.g., the penis accidentally being jammed into a mattress). In injuring the tunica albuginea, that trauma triggers a cascade of inflammatory and cellular events resulting in the abnormal fibrosis (excess fibrous tissue), plaque, and calcifications characteristic of this disease.

Such trauma, however, may not account for those Peyronie cases that begin slowly and become so severe that they require surgery. Researchers believe genetics or relationship with other connective tissue disorders may play a role. Studies already suggest that if you have a relative with Peyronie disease you have a greater risk of developing it yourself.

## How is Peyronie disease diagnosed?

A physical examination is sufficient to diagnose curvature of the penis. The hard plaques can be felt with or without erection. It may be necessary to use injectable medications to induce an erection for proper evaluation of the penile curvature. The patient may also provide pictures of the erect penis for evaluation by the physician. Ultrasound of the penis may demonstrate the lesions in the penis but is not always necessary.

## How is Peyronie disease treated?

Because Peyronie disease is a wound-healing disorder, changes are constantly occurring in the early stages. In fact, this disease can be classified into two stages: 1) an acute inflammatory phase persisting for six to 18 months during which men experience pain, slight penile curvature, and nodule formations; and 2) a chronic phase during which men develop a stable plaque, significant penile curvature, and erectile dysfunction.

Occasionally the condition regresses spontaneously with symptoms resolving themselves. In fact, some studies show that approximately 13 percent of patients have complete resolution of their plaques within a year. There is no change in 40 percent of cases, with progression or worsening of symptoms in 40 to 45 percent. For these reasons, most physicians recommend a nonsurgical approach for the first 12 months.

**Conservative approaches.** Instead of requiring invasive diagnostic procedures or treatments, men who experience only small plaques, minimal penile curvature, and no pain or sexual limitations need only be reassured that the condition will not lead to malignancy or another chronic disease. Pharmaceutical agents have shown promise for early-stage disease, but there are drawbacks. Because of a lack of controlled studies, scientists have yet to establish their true effectiveness. For instance:

- *Oral vitamin E*: It remains a popular treatment for early-stage disease because of its mild side effects and low cost. While uncontrolled studies as far back as 1948 demonstrated decreases in penile curvature and plaque size, investigation continues concerning its effectiveness.

- *Potassium aminobenzoate*: Recent controlled studies have shown that this B-complex substance popular in Central Europe yields some benefits. But it is somewhat expensive, requiring 24 pills each day for three to six months. It is also often associated with gastrointestinal issues, making compliance low.

- *Tamoxifen*: This nonsteroidal, anti-estrogen medication has been used in the treatment of desmoid tumors, a condition with properties similar to Peyronie disease. Researchers claim that inflammation and the production of scar tissue are inhibited. But early-stage disease studies in England have found only marginal improvement with tamoxifen. Like other research in this area, however, these studies include few patients, and no controls, objective improvement measures, or long-term follow up.

- *Colchicine*: Another anti-inflammatory agent that decreases collagen development, colchicine has been shown to be slightly beneficial in a few small, uncontrolled studies. Unfortunately, up to 50 percent of patients develop gastrointestinal upset and must discontinue the drug early in treatment.

**Injections.** Injecting a drug directly into the penile plaque is an attractive alternative to oral medications, which do not specifically target the lesion, or invasive surgical procedures, which carry the inherent risks of general anesthesia, bleeding, and infection. Intralesional injection therapies introduce drugs directly into the plaque with a small needle after appropriate anesthesia. Because they offer a minimally invasive approach, these options are popular among men who have early-phase disease or who are reluctant to have surgery. Yet their effectiveness is also under investigation. For instance:

- *Verapamil*: Early uncontrolled studies demonstrated that this substance interferes with calcium, a factor shown by in vitro cattle connective tissue cell studies to support collagen transport. As such, intralesional verapamil reduced penile pain and curvature while improving sexual function. Other studies have concluded that it is a reasonable treatment in men with non-calcified plaques and penile angles of less than 30 degrees.

- *Interferon*: The use of these naturally occurring antiviral, antiproliferative, and antitumorigenic glycoproteins to treat Peyronie disease was born out of experiments demonstrating the antifibrotic effect on skin cells of two different disorders— keloids, overgrowth of collagenous scar tissue and scleroderma, a rare autoimmune disease affecting the body's connective tissue. In addition to inhibiting proliferation of fibroblast cells, interferons, such as alpha-2b, also stimulate collagenase, which breaks down collagen and scar tissue. Several uncontrolled studies have demonstrated intralesional interferon's effectiveness in reducing penile pain, curvature, and plaque size while improving some sexual function. A current multi-institutional, placebo-controlled trial will hopefully answer many of the questions about intralesional therapy in the near future.

**Other Investigative Therapies.** The medical literature is replete with reports on less invasive methods for treating Peyronie disease. But the effectiveness of treatments such as high-intensity focused ultrasound and radiation therapy, topical verapamil, and iontophoresis (introducing soluble salt ions into the tissue via electric current) must still be investigated before these alternative therapies are considered clinically useful. Likewise, controlled studies using larger patient groups with longer follow-ups are necessary to prove that the same high-energy shock waves used to break up kidney stones will have positive effects on Peyronie disease.

**Surgery.** Surgery is reserved for men with severe disabling penile deformities that prevent satisfactory sexual intercourse. But, in most cases, it is not recommended for the first six to 12 months, until the plaque has stabilized. Since a spin-off of this disease is an abnormal blood supply to the penis, a vascular evaluation with vasoactive agents (drugs that cause erections by opening the vessels) is done prior to any surgery. A penile ultrasound can also illustrate the anatomy of the deformity. The images allow the urologist to determine which patients are most likely to benefit from reconstructive procedures versus a penile prosthesis. The three surgical approaches include:

- *Nesbit procedure*: First described to correct congenital penile curvature by cutting a portion of tissue from the tunica albuginea and shortening the unaffected side of the penis, this procedure is used by many surgeons today for Peyronie disease. Variations on the approach include the plication technique, where sutured tucks are placed into the side of maximum curvature to shorten and straighten the penis, and the corporoplasty technique, where a longitudinal or lengthwise incision is closed transversely to correct the curvature. Nesbit and its variations are simple to perform and involve limited risk. They are most beneficial in men with ample penile length and lesser degrees of curvatures. But they are not recommended in individuals with short penises or severe curvatures as this procedure is recognized to shorten the penis somewhat.

- *Grafting procedures*: When plaques are large and curvatures severe, the surgeon may choose to incise or cut out the hardened area and replace the tunica defect with a graft material of some type. While the choice of materials depends on the doctor's experience, preferences, and what is available, some are more attractive than others. For instance:

  - *Autograft tissue grafts*: Taken from the patient's body during surgery and thus less likely to cause an immunologic reaction, these materials usually require a second incision. They are also known to undergo postoperative contracture or tightening and scarring.

  - *Synthetic inert substances*: Materials such as Dacron® mesh or Gore-Tex® can cause significant fibrosis, a spreading of connective tissue cells. Occasionally palpated or felt by the patient, these grafts may cause more scarring.

- *Allografts or xenografts*: Harvested human or animal tissues are the focus of most grafting material today. These substances are uniformly strong, easy to work with, and readily available because they are "off-the-shelf" in the operating room, so to speak. They act as scaffolds for the tunica albuginea tissue to grow over as the graft is naturally dissolved by the patient's body.

- *Penile prostheses*: A penile prosthesis may be the only good option for Peyronie disease patients with significant erectile dysfunction and insufficient blood vessels verified by ultrasound. In most cases, implanting such a device alone will straighten the penis, correcting its rigidity. But when that does not work, the surgeon may manually "model" the organ, bending it against the plaque to break the deformity, or the surgeon may need to remove the plaque over the prosthesis and apply a graft to completely straighten the penis.

### What can be expected after treatment for Peyronie disease?

Routinely, a light pressure dressing is applied for 24 to 48 hours after the surgery to prevent any accumulation of blood. The Foley catheter is removed after the patient recovers from anesthesia, and most patients are discharged later the same day or the following morning. During the healing process, medications to counteract erections are usually prescribed. The patient is also asked to take antibiotics for seven to 10 days postoperatively to ward off infection, and analgesics for any discomfort. If patients have no penile pain or other complications, they can resume sexual intercourse in six to eight weeks.

### What happens to the cells following penile trauma?

In theory, following any penile trauma, there is a release of growth factors and cytokines or daughter cells that activate fibroblasts, cells that produce connective tissue. They, in turn, cause abnormal collagen deposition or scarring, which damages the internal elastic framework of the penis. Similar wound-healing disorders are commonly seen in the practice of dermatology, with conditions such as keloids and hypertrophic scarring, both involving tissue overgrowth in wound healing.

## *Are Peyronie disease sufferers prone to other related conditions?*

About 30 percent of Peyronie disease sufferers also develop other systemic fibrosis in other connective tissue in the body. Common sites are the hands and feet. In Dupuytren contracture, scarring or thickening of the fibrosis tissue in the palm leads progressively to a permanent bending of the pinkie and ring fingers into the hand. While the fibrosis occurring in both diseases is similar, it is not clear yet what causes either plaque type or why men with Peyronie disease are more likely to develop Dupuytren's contracture.

## *Will Peyronie disease evolve into cancer?*

No. There are no documented cases of progression of Peyronie disease to malignancy. However, if your doctor observes other findings that are not typical with this disease—such as external bleeding, obstructed urination, prolonged severe penile pain—he or she may elect to perform a biopsy on the tissue for pathological examination.

## *What should men remember about Peyronie disease?*

Peyronie disease is a well-recognized but poorly understood urological condition. Interventions need to be individualized to each patient, based on the timing and severity of the disease. The objective of any treatment should be on reducing pain, normalizing penile anatomy so that intercourse is comfortable, and restoring erectile function in patients who suffer erectile dysfunction. Although surgical correction is ultimately successful in the majority of cases, the early acute phase of this disease is customarily treated by either oral and/or intralesional approaches. As medical researchers continue to develop basic and clinical research for a better understanding of this disease, more therapies and targets for intervention will become available.

# Chapter 27

# *Sex and Aging*

Sexual feelings and desires exist throughout the life cycle. In recent years, there has been an increase in research on sexuality in middle and later life. This chapter presents some of the research that brings important insight into the sexual behavior, health, attitudes, values, and beliefs of individuals from their forties through their eighties and older.

Many of the researchers cited in this chapter did not define "sex" or "sexual activity" when they asked individuals about their sexual behaviors and beliefs. Each of the researchers also phrased their questions differently and surveyed varied age groups. Therefore, direct comparison of these studies is not possible. Percentages cited do not always total 100 percent because some participants chose not to respond to specific questions. Although most of the research was weighted in order to generalize the results to the overall population in these age groups, some of the research (particularly among the oldest participants) is based on small samples.

## *The Importance of Sexual Relationships*

- The Harris Interactive study reported that 80 percent of post-menopausal women under the age of 55 who are married, living with a partner, or currently involved in a sexual relationship considered sex to be either "very important" or "somewhat important." In contrast, 20 percent consider sex to be either "not very important" or "not important at all." (*Harris Interactive Sexual Communications Survey*, p. 5)

- The Harris Interactive study reported that 82 percent of male partners of menopausal women believe that sex is either "very important" or "somewhat important" to their relationship. In contrast, 18 percent believe it is "not very important" or "not important at all." (*Harris Interactive Sexual Communications Survey*, p. 10)

- The American Association of Retired Persons (AARP) study reported that 74 percent of men 45–59 years of age, 61 percent 60–74 years of age, and 50 percent 75 years of age and older believe that "a satisfying sexual relationship" is important to their quality of life. (*AARP/Modern Maturity Sexuality Study*, p. 24)

- The AARP study found that 66 percent of women 45–59 years of age, 48 percent 60–74 years of age, and 44 percent 75 years of age and older believe that "a satisfying sexual relationship" is important to their quality of life. (*AARP/Modern Maturity Sexuality Study*, p. 24)

- The AARP study reported that 50 percent of men and 53 percent of women 45 years of age and older agree that "sexual activity is a pleasurable, but not necessary, part of a good relationship." (*AARP/Modern Maturity Sexuality Study*, p. 10)

## Sexual Partners

- The AARP study reported that 84 percent of men 45–59 years of age, 79 percent 60–74 years of age, and 58 percent 75 years of age and older currently have a sexual partner. (*AARP/Modern Maturity Sexuality Study*, p. 31)

- The AARP study reported that 78 percent of women 45–59 years of age, 53 percent 60–74 years of age, and 21 percent 75 years of age and older currently have a sexual partner. (*AARP/Modern Maturity Sexuality Study*, p. 31)

## Sexual Activity

- The Association of Reproductive Health Professionals (ARHP) study reported that 62 percent of men 50–59 years of age, 52 percent 60–69 years of age, and 36 percent 70 years of age and older considered themselves sexually active. (*ARHP Sexual Activity Survey*, Chart Q1)

- The ARHP study reported that 50 percent of women 50–59 years of age, 9 percent 60–69 years of age, and 18 percent 70 years of age and older considered themselves sexually active. (*ARHP Sexual Activity Survey*, Chart Q1)

## Frequency of Sexual Activity

- The Harris Interactive study reported that 59 percent of post-menopausal women under the age of 55 have sex at least once a week. In contrast, 35 percent reported having sex less than once a week. (*Harris Interactive Sexual Communications Survey*, p. 5)

- The Harris Interactive study reported that 47 percent of post-menopausal women under the age of 55 experienced a decrease in sexual activity since they entered menopause, 36 percent reported no change at all, and 10 percent reported an increase in sexual activity. (*Harris Interactive Sexual Communications Survey*, p. 6)

- The Harris Interactive study reported that 48 percent of male partners of menopausal women reported having sex at least once a week, the same number (48 percent), reported having sex less often than once a week. (*Harris Interactive Sexual Communications Survey*, p. 10)

- The Harris Interactive study reported that 66 percent of male partners of menopausal women have noticed a decrease in sexual activity since their partner entered menopause. (*Harris Interactive Sexual Communications Survey*, p. 10)

- The ARHP study reported that 52 percent of men 50–59 years of age, 26 percent 60–69 years of age, and 27 percent 70 years of age and older engaged in any form of sexual activity more than once a week. (*ARHP Sexual Activity Survey*, Chart Q4)

- The ARHP study reported that 41 percent of women 50–59 years of age, 10 percent 60–69 years of age, and 20 percent 70 years of age and older engaged in any form of sexual activity more than once a week. (*ARHP Sexual Activity Survey*, Chart Q4)

- The National Council on Aging (NCOA) study reported that 71 percent of men in their sixties, 57 percent in their seventies, and

27 percent in their eighties or older engaged in sexual activity once a month or more during the past year. (The National Council on Aging Study, *Healthy Sexuality and Vital Aging*, p. 5)

- The NCOA study reported that 51 percent of women in their sixties, 30 percent in their seventies, and 18 percent in their eighties or older engaged in sexual activity once a month or more during the past year. (National Council on Aging, *Healthy Sexuality and Vital Aging*, p. 5)

- The NCOA study reported that men 60 and older (56 percent) were more likely than women 60 and older (25 percent) to say that they would like to have sex more often than they do now. (National Council on Aging, *Healthy Sexuality and Vital Aging*, p. 6)

- The National Health and Social Life Survey (NHSLS) study reported that 44 percent of men 40–44 years of age, 33 percent 45–49 years of age, 45 percent 50–54 years of age, and 42 percent 55–59 years of age have had sex a few times per month in the past year. (*National Health and Social Life Survey*, p. 88)

- The NHSLS study reported that 46 percent of women 40–44 years of age, 41 percent 45–49 years of age, 40 percent 50–54 years of age, and 30 percent 55–59 years of age have had sex a few times per month in the past year. (*National Health and Social Life Survey*, p. 88)

## Sexual Behaviors

- The AARP study reported that during the past six months, men with partners have engaged in the following sexual activities about once a week or more often: kissing and hugging (85 percent), sexual touching or caressing (76 percent), sexual intercourse (52 percent), self stimulation (22 percent), and oral sex (17 percent). (*AARP/Modern Maturity Sexuality Study*, p. 43)

- The AARP study reported that during the past six months, women with partners have engaged in the following sexual activities about once a week or more often: kissing and hugging (86 percent), sexual touching or caressing (73 percent), sexual intercourse (55 percent), oral sex (18 percent), and self-stimulation (3 percent). (*AARP/Modern Maturity Sexuality Study*, p. 43)

- The NHSLS study reported that 29 percent of men 40–44 years of age, 27 percent 45–49 years of age, 14 percent 50–54 years of age, and 10 percent 55–59 years of age masturbate at least once a week. (*National Health and Social Life Survey*, p. 82)

- The NHSLS study reported that 9 percent of women 40–44 years of age, 9 percent 45–49 years of age, 2 percent 50–54 years of age, and 2 percent 55–59 years of age masturbate at least once a week. (*National Health and Social Life Survey*, p. 82)

- The NHSLS study reported that on average, men 40–59 years of age find the following "very appealing": vaginal intercourse (86 percent), watching their partner undress (43 percent), receiving oral sex (35 percent), and giving oral sex (26 percent). (*National Health and Social Life Survey*, p. 152)

- The NHSLS study reported that on average, women 40–59 years of age find the following "very appealing": vaginal intercourse (75 percent), watching their partner undress (19 percent), receiving oral sex (17 percent), and giving oral sex (11 percent). (*National Health and Social Life Survey*, p. 152)

- The NHSLS study reported that 11 percent of men 40–49 years of age and 9 percent 50–59 years of age have engaged in any form of same-gendered sexual activity at some time in their life since puberty. (*National Health and Social Life Survey*, p. 305)

- The NHSLS study reported that 5 percent of women 40–49 years of age and 2 percent 50–59 years of age have engaged in any form of same-gendered sexual activity at some time in their life since puberty. (*National Health and Social Life Survey*, p. 305)

## Sexual Satisfaction

- The Harris Interactive study reported that 72 percent of post-menopausal women under the age of 55 were either "very satisfied" or "somewhat satisfied" with their sex life. In contrast, 27 percent responded that they were "not very satisfied" or "not satisfied at all." (*Harris Interactive Sexual Communications Survey*, p. 5)

- The Harris Interactive study reported that 63 percent of male partners of menopausal women were either "very satisfied" or "somewhat satisfied" with their sex life. In contrast, 25 percent were "not very satisfied" and 11 percent were "not satisfied at all." (*Harris Interactive Sexual Communications Survey*, p. 10)

- The AARP study reported that 63 percent of men 45–59 years of age, 50 percent 60–74 years of age, and 35 percent 75 years of age and older were "extremely" or "somewhat" satisfied with their sex life. (*AARP/Modern Maturity Sexuality Study*, p. 32)

- The AARP study reported that 61 percent of women 45–59 years of age, 49 percent 60–74 years of age, and 37 percent 75 years of age and older were "extremely" or "somewhat" satisfied with their sex life. (*AARP/Modern Maturity Sexuality Study*, p. 32)

- The ARHP study reported that 70 percent of men 50–59 years of age, 62 percent 60–69 years of age, and 50 percent 70 years of age and older were either "very" or "somewhat" satisfied with their sex lives. In contrast, 14 percent of men 50–59 years of age, 18 percent 60–69 years of age, and 36 percent 70 years of age and older were "very" or "somewhat" dissatisfied with their sex life. (*ARHP Sexual Activity Survey*, Chart Q2)

- The ARHP study reported that 60 percent of women 50–59 years of age, 49 percent 60–69 years of age, and 65 percent 70 years of age and older were "very" or "somewhat" satisfied with their sex lives. In contrast, 16 percent of women 50–59 years of age, 9 percent 60–69 years of age, and no women 70 years of age and older were "very" or "somewhat" dissatisfied with their sex life. (*ARHP Sexual Activity Survey*, Chart Q2)

- The NCOA study reported that 35 percent of men in their sixties, 34 percent in their seventies, and 38 percent in their eighties or older are satisfied with how often they have sex. (National Council on Aging, *Healthy Sexuality and Vital Aging*, p. 6)

- The NCOA study reported that 53 percent of women in their sixties, 38 percent in their seventies, and 26 percent 80 years of age and older are satisfied with how often they have sex. (National Council on Aging, *Healthy Sexuality and Vital Aging*, p. 6)

- The Harris Interactive study reported that 35 percent of post-menopausal women under the age of 55 have experienced a decrease in sexual satisfaction since entering menopause, 46 percent have experienced no change at all, and 7 percent have experienced an increase in sexual satisfaction. (*Harris Interactive Sexual Communications Survey*, p. 6)

- The ARHP study reported that 56 percent of men 50–59 years of age, 47 percent 60–69 years of age, and 44 percent 70 years of age and older were "more" or "equally" satisfied with their sex life compared to when they were younger. In contrast, 25 percent of men 50–59 years of age, 33 percent 60–69 years of age, and 38 percent 70 years of age and older were "less" satisfied with their sex life compared to when they were younger. (*ARHP Sexual Activity Survey*, Chart Q5)

- The ARHP study reported that 52 percent of women 50–59 years of age, 42 percent 60–69 years of age, and 49 percent 70 years of age and older were "more" or "equally" satisfied with their sex life compared to when they were younger. In contrast, 22 percent of women 50–59 years of age, 8 percent 60–69 years of age, and 10 percent 70 years of age and older were "less" satisfied with their sex life compared to when they were younger. (*ARHP Sexual Activity Survey*, Chart Q5)

- The NCOA study reported that 24 percent of men and 14 percent of women 60 years of age or older considered their sex life physically "more satisfying," 25 percent of men and 25 percent of women considered their sex life physically "unchanged," and 46 percent of men and 41 percent of women considered their sex life physically "less satisfying" compared to their sex life in their forties. (National Council on Aging, *Healthy Sexuality and Vital Aging*, p. 8)

- The NCOA study reported that 31 percent of men and 17 percent of women 60 years of age or older considered their sex life emotionally "more satisfying," 29 percent of men and 26 percent of women considered their sex life emotionally "unchanged," and 36 percent of men and 37 percent of women considered their sex life emotionally "less satisfying" compared to their sex life in their forties. (National Council on Aging, *Healthy Sexuality and Vital Aging*, p. 9)

- The AARP study reported that men 45 years of age and older believe the following factors would improve their sexual satisfaction: better health for themselves (30 percent), better health for their partners (22 percent), less stress (20 percent), more free time (18 percent), better financial situation (15 percent), better relationship with their partners (13 percent), and finding a partner (12 percent). In contrast, 22 percent of men 45 and older believed no change was needed. (*AARP/Modern Maturity Sexuality Study*, p. 17)

- The AARP study reported that women 45 years of age and older believe the following factors would improve their sexual satisfaction: less stress (20 percent), better health for their partners (19 percent), better health for themselves (16 percent), finding a partner (15 percent), more free time (14 percent), and better relationship with their partners (11 percent). In contrast, 28 percent of women 45 and older believed no change was needed. (*AARP/Modern Maturity Sexuality Study*, p. 17)

## Orgasm

- The AARP study reported that during the last six months, 70 percent of men and 29 percent of women 45 years of age and older always had an orgasm during sexual activity, 22 percent of men and 33 percent of women usually had an orgasm, 40 percent of men and 19 percent of women sometimes had an orgasm, 2 percent of men and 8 percent of women rarely had an orgasm, and 3 percent of men and 10 percent of women never had an orgasm. (*AARP/Modern Maturity Sexuality Study*, p. 14)

- The National Health and Social Life Survey (NHSLS) reported that 78 percent of men 40–44 years of age, 81 percent 45–49 years of age, 69 percent 50–54 years of age, and 75 percent 55–59 years of age always had an orgasm with their partner. (*National Health and Social Life Survey*, p. 116)

- NHSLS reported that 33 percent of women 40–44 years of age, 34 percent 45–49 years of age, 26 percent 50–54 years of age, and 25 percent 55–59 years of age always had an orgasm with their partner. (*National Health and Social Life Survey*, p. 116)

## Sexual Desire

- The Harris Interactive study reported that 41 percent of postmenopausal women under the age of 55 have experienced "lack of sexual desire." (*Harris Interactive Sexual Communications Survey*, p. 1)

- The Harris Interactive study reported that 45 percent of postmenopausal women under the age of 55 have experienced a decrease in sexual desire since the onset of menopause, that 37 percent reported no change at all, and that 10 percent reported an increase in sexual desire. (*Harris Interactive Sexual Communications Survey*, p. 6)

- The Harris Interactive study reported that 62 percent of male partners of menopausal women have noticed a decrease in their partner's sexual desire since entering menopause. (*Harris Interactive Sexual Communications Survey*, p. 10)

- The AARP study reported that 57 percent of men 45 years of age and older reported that they feel sexual desire at least two or three times a week compared to 22 percent of women 45 and older. (*AARP/Modern Maturity Sexuality Study*, p. 12)

- The Harris Interactive study reported that on average, 46 percent of obstetricians/gynecologists and 45 percent of primary care physicians estimate that nearly 50 percent of their menopausal patients suffer from a loss of sexual desire or a decrease in sexual satisfaction as a consequence of menopause. (*Harris Interactive Sexual Communications Survey*, p. 13)

## Sexual Attitudes, Values, and Beliefs

- The AARP study reported that 30 percent of men and 25 percent of women 45–59 years of age, 45 percent of men and 47 percent of women 60–74 years of age, and 57 percent of men and 52 percent of women 75 years of age and older agree that "sex become less important to people as they age." (*AARP/Modern Maturity Sexuality Study*, p. 25)

- The AARP study reported that 32 percent of men and 24 percent of women 45–59 years of age, 32 percent of men and 26 percent of women 60–74 years of age, and 38 percent of men and 38 percent of women 75 years of age and older agree that "sexual activity is a duty to one's spouse/partner." (*AARP/Modern Maturity Sexuality Study*, p. 25)

- The AARP study reported that one percent of men and 9 percent of women 45–59 years of age, 5 percent of men and 28 percent of women 60–74 years of age, and 5 percent of men and 36 percent of women 75 years of age and older agree that "I would be quite happy never having sex again." (*AARP/Modern Maturity Sexuality Study*, p. 25)

- The AARP study reported that 28 percent of men and 36 percent of women 45–59 years of age, 38 percent of men and 53 percent of women 60–74 years of age, and 50 percent of men and 66 percent of women 75 years of age and older agree that "people

should not have a sexual relationship if they are not married."
(*AARP/Modern Maturity Sexuality Study*, p. 25)

- The NCOA study reported that 53 percent of men and women 60 years of age and older agree that new prescription medicines will have a positive impact on the way older men view sexuality in later life; 50 percent of men and women 60 years of age and older agree these medicines will have a positive impact on the way society in general views sexuality in later life; and 45 percent of men and women 60 years of age and older agree that they will have a positive impact on the way older women view sexuality in later life. (National Council on Aging, *Healthy Sexuality and Vital Aging*, p. 12)

- The NCOA study reported that 81 percent of respondents correctly agreed with the statement that older people are just as susceptible to sexually transmitted diseases—such as AIDS—as younger people. (National Council on Aging, *Healthy Sexuality and Vital Aging*, p. 4)

- The NHSLS study reported that 49 percent of men 40–44 years of age, 48 percent 45–49 years of age, 57 percent 50–54 years of age, and 49 percent 55–59 years of age felt guilty after masturbation. (*National Health and Social Life Survey*, p. 82)

- The NHSLS study reported that 46 percent of women 40–44 years of age, 35 percent 45–49 years of age, 53 percent 50–54 years of age, and 50 percent 55–59 years of age felt guilty after masturbation. (*National Health and Social Life Survey*, p. 82)

- The ARHP study reported that 54 percent of men 50–59 years of age, 38 percent 60–69 years of age, and 34 percent 70 years of age and older considered themselves to be better lovers than in the past. (*ARHP Sexual Activity Survey*, Chart Q7)

- The ARHP study reported that 38 percent of women 50–59 years of age, 28 percent 60–69 years of age, and 24 percent 70 years of age and older considered themselves to be better lovers than in the past. (*ARHP Sexual Activity Survey*, Chart Q7)

## Sexual Health and Functioning

- The NCOA study reported that 63 percent of men 60 years of age and older, who have had one or more sex partners in the past 12 months, have been able to consistently get and maintain an erection sufficient for sex in the past six months, compared to 37 percent who were not able to maintain an erection. (National Council on Aging, *Healthy Sexuality and Vital Aging,* p. 10)

- The NCOA study reported that 63 percent of women 60 years of age and older, who have had one or more sex partners in the past 12 months, have been able to consistently become and stay lubricated sufficient for sex in the last six months, compared to 33 percent that were not able to become and stay lubricated. (National Council on Aging, *Healthy Sexuality and Vital Aging,* p. 11)

- The NHSLS study reported that on average men 40–59 years of age reported the following: climax too early (28 percent), lacked interest in sex (19 percent), unable to keep an erection (16 percent), anxiety about performance (16 percent), inability to orgasm (10 percent), sex is not pleasurable (8 percent), and pain during sex (3 percent). (*National Health and Social Life Survey*, p. 370)

- The NHSLS study reported that on average women 40–59 years of age reported the following: lacked interest in sex (34 percent), had trouble lubricating (21 percent), unable to orgasm (20 percent), sex not pleasurable (16 percent), pain during sex (10 percent), anxiety about performance (8 percent), and climax too early (8 percent). (*National Health and Social Life Survey*, p. 371)

- The AARP study reported that 26 percent of men 45 years of age and older describe themselves as being either "completely" or "moderately" impotent. (*AARP/Modern Maturity Sexuality Study*, p. 15)

- The Harris Interactive study reported that 56 percent of post-menopausal women under the age of 55 say that they would be most likely to discuss sexual problems such as lack of desire or a decrease in sexual satisfaction with their physician, 16 percent would seek help from their sexual partner, 10 percent from their friend, and 2 percent from a family member. (*Harris Interactive Sexual Communications Survey*, p. 3)

- The AARP study reported that 28 percent of men 45 years of age and older and 14 percent of women 45 years of age and older have ever sought treatment from personal physicians, specialists, mental health professionals, or sex therapists for any problems related to sexual functioning. (*AARP/Modern Maturity Sexuality Study*, p. 60)

- The AARP study reported that 11 percent of men 45 years of age and older and 7 percent of women 45 years of age and older are currently using, or have ever used, medications, hormones, or other treatments to improve sexual function and activity. (*AARP/Modern Maturity Sexuality Study*, p. 61)

## Research

The information in this chapter is based on the research of the following organizations.

### Harris Interactive/PRIME PLUS/Red Hot Mamas (HI/PP)

These separate surveys of physicians (301), menopausal women (580), and partners of menopausal women (1,352) were conducted by mail and online in January 2000, supported by an unrestricted grant from Solvay Pharmaceuticals. Survey recipients were drawn from the Harris Poll Online database of approximately 5.3 million registered participants. Complete interviews were weighted to figures obtained from the Current Population Survey as well as key questions administered in Harris Poll monthly phone surveys of national cross-sectional samples of 1,000 adults 18 years of age and older. Demographic variables such as gender, age, education, race, and ethnicity, as well as a variable representing the propensity of an individual respondent to be online, were used to generalize survey results to the national population. (*Harris Interactive Sexual Communications Survey*, Harris Interactive/PRIME PLUS/Red Hot Mamas, Ridgefield, Connecticut, 2000)

### American Association of Retired Persons (AARP)

The *AARP/Modern Maturity Sexuality Study* of 1,384 Americans 45 years of age and older was conducted by National Family Opinion Research, Inc. (NFO) in 1999. It surveyed the NFO national consumer panel by mail. The final data were weighted to reflect U.S. Census estimates for age and gender in the over-45 population. (*AARP/Modern Maturity Sexuality Study*, Washington, D.C., 1999)

### Association of Reproductive Health Professionals (ARHP)

The ARHP *Sexual Activity Survey* of 1,000 Americans 18 years of age and older—reporting results for ages 50–59, 60–69, and 70 and older—was conducted by OmniTel, a weekly national phone omnibus service of Bruskin/Goldring Research in 1999. All completed interviews were weighted to ensure accurate and reliable representation of the total population 18 years and older. Weighting variables included age, gender, education, race, and geographic region. The weighted total of those 50 years of age and older was 355. The unweighted number of those 70 years of age or older was 90 (34 men and 56 women). Each interviewee was asked seven multiple-choice questions related to sexual behavior and attitudes. (*ARHP Sexual Activity Survey*, Association of Reproductive Health Professionals, Washington, D.C., 1999)

### National Council on Aging (NCOA)

The NCOA study of 1,292 Americans 60 years of age or older, *Healthy Sexuality and Vital Aging*, was conducted by Roper Starch Worldwide in 1998. The study relied on National Panel Data, a market research firm, for the nationally representative, randomly selected sample receiving the mailed questionnaire. Analyses of data from the respondents were weighted for gender, age, marital status, race, and household income to reflect true proportions among the general U.S. population in the older age groups, and balanced to match the 1997 Current Population Survey findings. (*Healthy Sexuality and Vital Aging*, National Council on Aging, Washington, D.C., 1998)

### National Health and Social Life Survey (NHSLS)

The University of Chicago's *National Health and Social Life Survey* (NHSLS) of 3,432 Americans 18 to 59 years of age was conducted by the National Opinion Research Center (NORC) in 1992. The study is based on personal interviews. Results reported from the study are included in the book *The Social Organization of Sexuality: Sexual Practices in the United States*. (*National Health and Social Life Survey*, Chicago, Illinois, 1992)

# Chapter 28

# *Erectile Dysfunction*

Erectile dysfunction, sometimes called impotence, is the repeated inability to get or keep an erection firm enough for sexual intercourse. The word "impotence" may also be used to describe other problems that interfere with sexual intercourse and reproduction, such as lack of sexual desire and problems with ejaculation or orgasm. Using the term "erectile dysfunction" makes it clear that those other problems are not involved.

Erectile dysfunction, or ED, can be a total inability to achieve erection, an inconsistent ability to do so, or a tendency to sustain only brief erections. These variations make defining ED and estimating its incidence difficult. Estimates range from 15 million to 30 million, depending on the definition used. According to the National Ambulatory Medical Care Survey (NAMCS), for every 1,000 men in the United States, 7.7 physician office visits were made for ED in 1985. By 1999, that rate had nearly tripled to 22.3. The increase happened gradually, presumably as treatments such as vacuum devices and injectable drugs became more widely available and discussing erectile function became accepted. Perhaps the most publicized advance was the introduction of the oral drug sildenafil citrate (Viagra®) in March 1998. NAMCS data on new drugs show an estimated 2.6 million mentions of Viagra at physician office visits in 1999, and one-third of those mentions occurred during visits for a diagnosis other than ED.

---

Reprinted from "Erectile Dysfunction," National Kidney and Urologic Diseases Information Clearinghouse, September 2002, http://www.niddk.nih.gov/health/urolog/pubs/impotnce/impotnce.htm, NIH Pub. No. 03-3823.

In older men, ED usually has a physical cause, such as disease, injury, or side effects of drugs. Any disorder that causes injury to the nerves or impairs blood flow in the penis has the potential to cause ED. Incidence increases with age: About 5 percent of 40-year-old men and between 15 and 25 percent of 65-year-old men experience ED. But it is not an inevitable part of aging.

ED is treatable at any age, and awareness of this fact has been growing. More men have been seeking help and returning to normal sexual activity because of improved, successful treatments for ED. Urologists, who specialize in problems of the urinary tract, have traditionally treated ED; however, urologists accounted for only 25 percent of Viagra mentions in 1999.

## How Does an Erection Occur?

The penis contains two chambers called the corpora cavernosa, which run the length of the organ (see Figure 28.1). A spongy tissue fills the chambers. The corpora cavernosa are surrounded by a membrane, called the tunica albuginea. The spongy tissue contains smooth muscles, fibrous tissues, spaces, veins, and arteries. The urethra, which is the channel for urine and ejaculate, runs along the underside of the corpora cavernosa.

Erection begins with sensory or mental stimulation, or both. Impulses from the brain and local nerves cause the muscles of the corpora cavernosa to relax, allowing blood to flow in and fill the spaces. The blood creates pressure in the corpora cavernosa, making the penis expand. The tunica albuginea helps trap the blood in the corpora cavernosa, thereby sustaining erection. When muscles in the penis contract to stop the inflow of blood and open outflow channels, erection is reversed.

## What Causes ED?

Since an erection requires a precise sequence of events, ED can occur when any of the events is disrupted. The sequence includes nerve impulses in the brain, spinal column, and area around the penis, and response in muscles, fibrous tissues, veins, and arteries in and near the corpora cavernosa.

Damage to nerves, arteries, smooth muscles, and fibrous tissues, often as a result of disease, is the most common cause of ED. Diseases—such as diabetes, kidney disease, chronic alcoholism, multiple sclerosis, atherosclerosis, vascular disease, and neurologic disease—

account for about 70 percent of ED cases. Between 35 and 50 percent of men with diabetes experience ED.

Also, surgery (especially radical prostate surgery for cancer) can injure nerves and arteries near the penis, causing ED. Injury to the penis, spinal cord, prostate, bladder, and pelvis can lead to ED by harming nerves, smooth muscles, arteries, and fibrous tissues of the corpora cavernosa.

In addition, many common medicines—blood pressure drugs, antihistamines, antidepressants, tranquilizers, appetite suppressants, and cimetidine (an ulcer drug)—can produce ED as a side effect.

Experts believe that psychological factors such as stress, anxiety, guilt, depression, low self-esteem, and fear of sexual failure cause 10 to 20 percent of ED cases. Men with a physical cause for ED frequently experience the same sort of psychological reactions (stress, anxiety, guilt, depression).

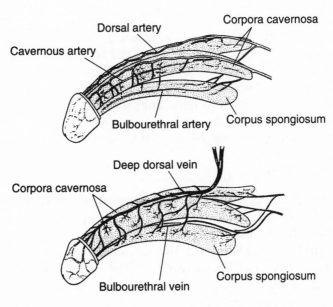

*Figure 28.1. Arteries (top) and veins (bottom) penetrate the long, filled cavities running the length of the penis—the corpora cavernosa and the corpus spongiosum. Erection occurs when relaxed muscles allow the corpora cavernosa to fill with excess blood fed by the arteries, while drainage of blood through the veins is blocked.*

Other possible causes are smoking, which affects blood flow in veins and arteries, and hormonal abnormalities, such as not enough testosterone.

## How Is ED Diagnosed?

### Patient History

Medical and sexual histories help define the degree and nature of ED. A medical history can disclose diseases that lead to ED, while a simple recounting of sexual activity might distinguish between problems with sexual desire, erection, ejaculation, or orgasm.

Using certain prescription or illegal drugs can suggest a chemical cause, since drug effects account for 25 percent of ED cases. Cutting back on or substituting certain medications can often alleviate the problem.

### Physical Examination

A physical examination can give clues to systemic problems. For example, if the penis is not sensitive to touching, a problem in the nervous system may be the cause. Abnormal secondary sex characteristics, such as hair pattern, can point to hormonal problems, which would mean that the endocrine system is involved. The examiner might discover a circulatory problem by observing decreased pulse in the wrist or ankles. And unusual characteristics of the penis itself could suggest the source of the problem—for example, a penis that bends or curves when erect could be the result of Peyronie disease.

### Laboratory Tests

Several laboratory tests can help diagnose ED. Tests for systemic diseases include blood counts, urinalysis, lipid profile, and measurements of creatinine and liver enzymes. Measuring the amount of testosterone in the blood can yield information about problems with the endocrine system and is indicated especially in patients with decreased sexual desire.

### Other Tests

Monitoring erections that occur during sleep (nocturnal penile tumescence) can help rule out certain psychological causes of ED. Healthy men have involuntary erections during sleep. If nocturnal erections do not occur, then ED is likely to have a physical rather than psychological cause. Tests of nocturnal erections are not completely reliable, however. Scientists have not standardized such tests and have not determined when they should be applied for best results.

### Psychosocial Examination

A psychosocial examination, using an interview and a questionnaire, reveals psychological factors. A man's sexual partner may also be interviewed to determine expectations and perceptions during sexual intercourse.

## How Is ED Treated?

Most physicians suggest that treatments proceed from least to most invasive. Cutting back on any drugs with harmful side effects is considered first. For example, drugs for high blood pressure work in different ways. If you think a particular drug is causing problems with erection, tell your doctor and ask whether you can try a different class of blood pressure medicine.

Psychotherapy and behavior modifications in selected patients are considered next if indicated, followed by oral or locally injected drugs, vacuum devices, and surgically implanted devices. In rare cases, surgery involving veins or arteries may be considered.

### Psychotherapy

Experts often treat psychologically based ED using techniques that decrease the anxiety associated with intercourse. The patient's partner can help with the techniques, which include gradual development of intimacy and stimulation. Such techniques also can help relieve anxiety when ED from physical causes is being treated.

### Drug Therapy

Drugs for treating ED can be taken orally, injected directly into the penis, or inserted into the urethra at the tip of the penis. In March 1998, the Food and Drug Administration approved Viagra, the first pill to treat ED. Taken an hour before sexual activity, Viagra works by enhancing the effects of nitric oxide, a chemical that relaxes smooth muscles in the penis during sexual stimulation and allows increased blood flow.

While Viagra improves the response to sexual stimulation, it does not trigger an automatic erection as injections do. The recommended dose is 50 mg, and the physician may adjust this dose to 100 mg or 25 mg, depending on the patient. The drug should not be used more than once a day. Men who take nitrate-based drugs such as nitroglycerin for heart problems should not use Viagra because the combination can cause a sudden drop in blood pressure.

Additional oral medicines may soon be available to treat ED. Vardenafil and Cialis® are being tested for safety and effectiveness. Both of these drugs work like Viagra by increasing blood flow to the penis. A third drug being tested, Uprima®, works on the brain and nervous system to trigger an erection.

Oral testosterone can reduce ED in some men with low levels of natural testosterone, but it is often ineffective and may cause liver damage. Patients also have claimed that other oral drugs—including yohimbine hydrochloride, dopamine and serotonin agonists, and trazodone—are effective, but the results of scientific studies to substantiate these claims have been inconsistent. Improvements observed following use of these drugs may be examples of the placebo effect; that is, a change that results simply from the patient's believing that an improvement will occur.

Many men achieve stronger erections by injecting drugs into the penis, causing it to become engorged with blood. Drugs such as papaverine hydrochloride, phentolamine, and alprostadil (marketed as Caverject®) widen blood vessels. These drugs may create unwanted side effects, however, including persistent erection (known as priapism) and scarring. Nitroglycerin, a muscle relaxant, can sometimes enhance erection when rubbed on the penis.

A system for inserting a pellet of alprostadil into the urethra is marketed as Muse®. The system uses a prefilled applicator to deliver the pellet about an inch deep into the urethra. An erection will begin within eight to 10 minutes and may last 30 to 60 minutes. The most common side effects are aching in the penis, testicles, and area between the penis and rectum; warmth or burning sensation in the urethra; redness from increased blood flow to the penis; and minor urethral bleeding or spotting.

Research on drugs for treating ED is expanding rapidly. Patients should ask their doctor about the latest advances.

### *Vacuum Devices*

Mechanical vacuum devices cause erection by creating a partial vacuum, which draws blood into the penis, engorging and expanding it. The devices have three components: a plastic cylinder, into which the penis is placed; a pump, which draws air out of the cylinder; and an elastic band, which is placed around the base of the penis to maintain the erection after the cylinder is removed and during intercourse by preventing blood from flowing back into the body (see Figure 28.2).

One variation of the vacuum device involves a semirigid rubber sheath that is placed on the penis and remains there after erection is attained and during intercourse.

### *Surgery*

Surgery usually has one of three goals:

- To implant a device that can cause the penis to become erect
- To reconstruct arteries to increase flow of blood to the penis
- To block off veins that allow blood to leak from the penile tissues

Implanted devices, known as prostheses, can restore erection in many men with ED. Possible problems with implants include mechanical breakdown and infection, although mechanical problems have diminished in recent years because of technological advances.

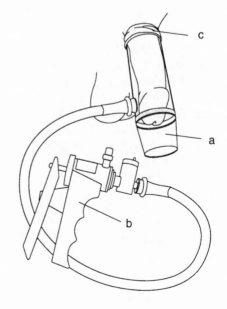

*Figure 28.2.* A vacuum-constrictor device causes an erection by creating a partial vacuum around the penis, which draws blood into the corpora cavernosa. Pictured here are the necessary components: (a) a plastic cylinder, which covers the penis; (b) a pump, which draws air out of the cylinder; and (c) an elastic ring, which, when fitted over the base of the penis, traps the blood and sustains the erection after the cylinder is removed.

Malleable implants usually consist of paired rods, which are inserted surgically into the corpora cavernosa. The user manually adjusts the position of the penis and, therefore, the rods. Adjustment does not affect the width or length of the penis.

Inflatable implants consist of paired cylinders, which are surgically inserted inside the penis and can be expanded using pressurized fluid (see Figure 28.3). Tubes connect the cylinders to a fluid reservoir and a pump, which are also surgically implanted. The patient inflates the cylinders by pressing on the small pump, located under the skin in the scrotum. Inflatable implants can expand the length and width of the penis somewhat. They also leave the penis in a more natural state when not inflated.

Surgery to repair arteries can reduce ED caused by obstructions that block the flow of blood. The best candidates for such surgery are young men with discrete blockage of an artery because of an injury to the crotch or fracture of the pelvis. The procedure is less successful in older men with widespread blockage.

Surgery to veins that allow blood to leave the penis usually involves an opposite procedure—intentional blockage. Blocking off veins (ligation) can reduce the leakage of blood that diminishes the rigidity of

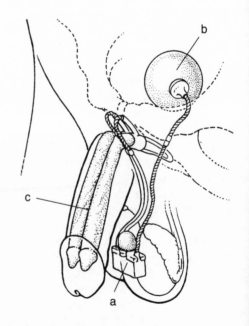

*Figure 28.3.* With an inflatable implant, erection is produced by squeezing a small pump (a) implanted in a scrotum. The pump causes fluid to flow from a reservoir (b) residing in the lower pelvis to two cylinders (c) residing in the penis. The cylinders expand to create the erection.

the penis during erection. However, experts have raised questions about the long-term effectiveness of this procedure, and it is rarely done.

## Hope through Research

Advances in suppositories, injectable medications, implants, and vacuum devices have expanded the options for men seeking treatment for ED. These advances have also helped increase the number of men seeking treatment. Gene therapy for ED is now being tested in several centers and may offer a long-lasting therapeutic approach for ED.

## Points to Remember

Erectile dysfunction (ED) is the repeated inability to get or keep an erection firm enough for sexual intercourse.

- ED affects 15 to 30 million American men.
- ED usually has a physical cause.
- ED is treatable at all ages.
- Treatments include psychotherapy, drug therapy, vacuum devices, and surgery.

# Chapter 29

# *Cancer Treatment and Male Sexuality*

For most people at the time of diagnosis, the words cancer and sexuality do not even fit in the same sentence. The word cancer conjures up fears of disability and death, both of which take center stage and demand immediate attention from the person with cancer. However, loss of sexual functioning and attractiveness can often times become a priority as cancer treatments and their side effects are experienced. For women, losing a breast or ovaries may create fear of losing one's attractiveness or fertility. For men, the idea of nerve damage near the prostate, which might affect erection, or the possibility of a colostomy may trigger similar concerns. Having frank discussions with your health care team about what changes may or may not occur due to cancer treatment will help you make more informed treatment decisions and prepare for possible outcomes that may affect your sexuality.

## *Loss of Sexual Desire: "I just don't feel like it."*

Many people with cancer report a loss in "libido" (sexual desire) as a very common problem. There are many factors, both physical and emotional that can contribute to the loss of sexual desire, and it is often not easy to determine what the cause is.

Cancer and its treatment often leaves one feeling fatigued, nauseous, in pain, or weak. Chemotherapy can produce all of these feelings, as can

---

the drugs that treat nausea associated with chemotherapy. It is important to remember that sexual longings often return when normal energy levels return. Although we don't fully understand the role of the brain in human sexuality, it is possible that cancer treatments have an impact on loss of sexual desire on this level. Prescription medications, including medications for pain, depression, and anxiety may interfere with your sex life. Ask your doctor to provide you with information on the possible side effects of any medication you are taking. If you suspect that medications you are taking are decreasing your sexual desire, talk to your health care team. It is possible that a change in medications or a reduced dosage may help this situation. It is always important to never change your medication or schedule of doses without talking to your doctor.

Changes in sexual desire can also occur when cancer treatments cause an imbalance in sex hormones. Although the cells that produce testosterone are not generally affected by chemotherapy and radiation, sometimes men do experience abnormal changes in hormone levels, characterized by loss of libido, difficulty with erections and orgasms, hot flashes, low threshold for stress, and diminished beard growth. There are several situations that may produce a loss of hormone level. Surgical removal of the testicle, as with testicular cancer, will interfere with sexual desire if both testicles are removed, or if the remaining testicle is not producing enough testosterone. Bone marrow transplants and radiation therapy can sometimes interfere with the production of testosterone. Sometimes this interference is permanent; for others, the damage is temporary.

Hormone therapy for prostate cancer is based on the premise that prostate cancer cells require testosterone to grow; therefore, this treatment (called luteinizing hormone releasing hormone, LHRH agonist) works to shut down the production of testosterone. Men may be given Lupron® or Goserelin® that works on decreasing production of testosterone, or Flutamide® or Casodex® combined with the LHRH agonist that stops testosterone at the cell level. About 80 percent of men on these treatments report little interest in sexual activity, with 20 percent managing to remain sexually active. Erections may take longer, and may be less firm. Orgasm also can take more effort, and may be "dry"; that is, with little or no semen. Sex can still be enjoyed by adjusting one's definitions of what is satisfying, and trying new ways to become aroused, using mental stimulus as much as physical stimulus.

A colostomy may make you feel self-conscious and decrease desire. Body image issues are important considerations as you think of returning to sexual functioning. Counseling to help you adjust to these changes may be useful.

There is no magic pill or cure for loss of sexual desire. Because of this, it becomes necessary for men to find other ways to find an interest in sex again. Some ideas for increasing desire include:

- Help yourself to feel physically vital again through exercise, walking, swimming—any activity or exercise that can help your flexibility and strength. Start slowly. If you used to swim 20 laps, try swimming less, walking instead of jogging, or using a golf cart instead of walking the course.

- Readjust negative feelings about your body. Most people typically have harsh judgments about their bodies and appearance. Find the things to still celebrate about your appearance, and emphasize them. Sometimes having to face thoughts of death can make living all the more precious and exciting. Remember your partner cares for your entire being, not just your body parts.

- Learn to enjoy sensuous pleasures. Using extra mental and physical stimulation (longer time on foreplay, erotic pictures or videos, lubricants, different kinds of oral stimulation, varying positions, or increased hand caressing) may all be helpful to increase desire, leading to a better chance at having an orgasm.

- Talking to a professional about the changes you have experienced due to cancer treatment may be useful.

## Erection and Cancer Treatments

One of the biggest concerns arising from treatment for prostate cancer, and one that is often not discussed, is that it can affect a man's ability to have an erection, or affect his sexual drive. However, there is some good news: In the last twenty years, important advances have been made in treating these problems. It is important to remember that you can still enjoy a satisfying sex life after prostate cancer treatment. Most men can find solutions, either through methods that help with erectile dysfunction or by discovering new ways to achieve intimacy with their partner. This section will review what changes might occur and some ways to cope with the changes.

Here are types of possible side effects specific to particular treatment:

- With a *radical prostatectomy*, a man may have difficulty getting or keeping an erection. This is because the nerves that control the ability to produce an erection may be damaged, causing a weakening or interruption of blood flow. However, these nerves are not the same ones that control orgasm, ejaculation, or sensation. Hence, the desire and ability to enjoy sexual touching usually remains intact, and a person who has had this operation will still have the ability to feel an orgasm. Although they may not have experienced it before, males are physically able to have an orgasm without an erection or ejaculating fluid.

- *Nerve-sparing prostatectomy* was designed to leave the nerve pathways involved in erection undamaged, if possible. Depending on the location and size of the prostate tumor, it may not be possible to spare the nerves on both sides of the prostate. Recovery of erections after nerve-sparing surgery is gradual, and can take from several months up to a year, with improvement sometimes continuing into a second year. Men who are most likely to recover the ability to have strong erections are those who are younger and healthier, those for whom the tumor was such that nerves were spared on both sides, and those who had no problems with erection before surgery.

- *Combination hormonal therapy* will affect sexual activity as long as treatment is being received. Men report that it can take longer and more effort to get an erection during treatment, and ejaculation may contain little or no semen. Sexual desire generally decreases over the duration of the treatment. Again, this happens because hormone treatment decreases male hormones in order to slow the growth of the cancer. These same hormones are responsible for sexual drive, or libido.

- *External beam radiation* can result in gradual changes in sexual functioning. Men who had weak erections prior to radiation therapy are most likely to be affected. Between 25 and 50 percent of men develop new erection problems after radiation therapy. Internal radiation (seed implantation or brachytherapy) has a much lower rate of impeding sexual functioning.

- The experimental treatment *cryosurgery* does carry the possibility of damaging the nerves responsible for erection. About two-thirds of men report having problems becoming erect after having this procedure done. However, the ability to achieve an erection may improve over time.

## Ways to Cope with Sexual Changes

There are several options available to men who have erectile dysfunction or impotence (inability to have or difficulty having an erection), which are discussed below. There are also many strategies for approaching sex that can help, even before beginning cancer treatment. These will also be discussed.

- If you are reading this before you have any treatment, then one of the things you can do to prepare to cope is to provide your doctor honest information about your pre-treatment sexual functioning. You may be asked questions about how often you have sex, detailed information about your erections (including firmness and frequency), and whether you currently have any problems with erections. Although this may not be an easy discussion to have, a clear picture of your sexual functioning before treatment will be helpful in identifying any problems after treatment.

- Before you make any treatment choices to restore erectile functioning, it is important to:

  - Learn about all the treatment options first so you can make an informed choice and choose an option that works best for you.

  - If you have a partner or a spouse, involve him or her in the decision-making process. Whatever method you choose should be compatible with the way you and your partner enjoy sex. Most men and women have difficulty talking openly about these matters; however, it is important that you try. One of the additional benefits of having this discussion may be a closer bond of intimacy with your partner. Counseling may be helpful for you and your partner if talking about sexuality is proving to be uncomfortable.

## Options for Treatment

It is perfectly acceptable for men to choose no treatment to restore erections. You and your partner may make this choice together after exploring all the issues. There is no reason that you cannot enjoy a satisfying sex life in other ways besides having intercourse. For many men and their partners, this is the best choice. However, there are many others:

- Counseling may help you and your partner talk about sexual issues. Counseling can help a man reduce anxiety about sexual functioning and body image issues. It also can help you deal with any depression or sadness you may be experiencing from your cancer diagnosis. Many people seek guidance from a mental heath professional when cancer strikes. Cancer Care offers free professional counseling, information, and referrals for services in your area through our toll free line (call 800-813-HOPE) and e-mail (access through our website at www.cancercare.org). If you do decide to seek sexual counseling, some questions you may wish to explore with your partner are:

- If your erections are no longer firm, are there other ways your partner would be willing to have orgasms, such as oral or hand caressing?

- How would you and your partner feel about a penile implant?

- Do you both feel ready to resume sexual activity? If not, what kinds of affection can you show each other to maintain a level of intimacy during this time? If so, how may any changes present after treatment affect what you do during sex?

- What are different ways you may explore your sexuality, such as rediscovering petting, taking a sensual shower together, or using erotic materials to help?

- A new drug for treating erectile dysfunction (impotence) has been approved by the FDA. It is called Viagra®. You may wish to discuss this medication with your doctor to find out if it is an option for you.

- *Vacuum constriction devices* (VCD, also called vacuum pumps or suction pumps) are a viable, noninvasive option that can be used immediately after a man recovers from radical prostate surgery. It works by inserting the penis into a cylinder and activating the pump (by hand or by battery), which causes a vacuum that draws blood into the shaft of the penis. The penis becomes swollen and erect. An elastic ring is then placed at the base of the penis to retain the blood. This is done each time an erection is desired, and each erection can last 20–30 minutes (the elastic ring must be taken off within 30–40 minutes to restore the normal flow of blood). It tends to work best with men who still achieve some swelling in the penis with sexual stimulation. It generally produces a functional erection in most men. VCDs can cost between $75 and more than $200. Fortunately, the cost is often covered at least partially by insurance and Medicare. Some men find the elastic ring uncomfortable to wear or have difficulty coordinating the process. Using the device can be built into the sexual experience, although some partners report discomfort with the disruption. Again, discussing these issues with your spouse or partner will help you make better choices.

- *Injections of medication* directly into the penile shaft can also stimulate erections, or help maintain them. Despite sounding painful, most men actually report little discomfort after learning the procedure themselves. Partners can also learn to do the injections. The medication most often used is prostaglandin E1 (Caverject®) or a combination of papaverine and phentolamine (Regitine®). Combinations of all three drugs may be the best option for long-term use and decreased risk of side effects. The erections last between 40 and 60 minutes, and most men report no adverse side effects. In a small percentage of men, scar tissue may form at the site of the injection. The cost of injections runs between $50 and $100 per month, and insurance coverage varies; unfortunately, often this is not covered.

- A *penile implant* (also called penile prosthesis) can be surgically implanted into the penis to provide an erection rigid enough for sexual intercourse. Because having an implant will destroy the natural erection reflex, it is important to use this option only when erections are unlikely to improve on their own. Complications from the procedure include mechanical failure of the device and infection (about 10 percent of men have complications). The cost is usually between $15,000 and $20,000, which insurance usually covers when a medical problem has been documented. There are different models available:

  - *Semirigid or malleable rods* are the simplest implants. In this procedure, a semi-rigid (but bendable) rod is surgically implanted, making the penis permanently semierect. The rod can be bent up into an erection, or down into a relaxed position. The implant procedure is simple and there is little risk of infection or other complications.

  - *Inflatable implants* are more complicated. They are made up of a small reservoir, two cylinders on either side of the penis, and a pump that transfers fluid into the cylinders to create an erection. After sex, a valve releases the liquid back into the reservoir. There are several models of inflatable implants that range from simple to more complex.

When dealing with erectile dysfunction, it may make sense to start with the least invasive method first and proceed from there. For example, you may wish to try the vacuum device first, then try injection therapy or an implant if this proves unsatisfactory.

Remember that even if you find a treatment that works for you, your erections will probably not feel the way they did before. Aim for goals that are attainable. A realistic goal is to achieve erections that are firm enough to allow penetration.

## Inability to Reach Orgasm or Dry Orgasm

There are a number of changes in orgasm that can occur due to cancer treatments. You may be slower to reach orgasm, need different kinds of stimulation, or have a dry orgasm (no semen is ejaculated). Some men find it difficult to reach orgasm at all.

You may be surprised to know that it is somewhat uncommon for a man or a woman to develop a new problem in reaching orgasm as a result of cancer treatment. Of all the problems described at M.D. Anderson's Sexual Rehabilitation Clinic, problems with orgasm were reported less often.

There are a number of reasons why cancer treatment may interfere with your ability to have an orgasm:

- Treatment of brain or spinal cord tumors may result in numbness or paralysis that could affect your sense of touch and pleasure from genital stimulation.

- Removal of the penis may cause one to assume sexual activity is completely lost. Often times this occurs in elderly men who prefer to give up sexual activity altogether. Men can learn to reach orgasm through caressing the remaining genital areas.

- Cancer treatment can decrease genital sensation, similar to the changes that may occur when a man ages.

- Medications, such as antidepressant, tranquilizer, or pain medication, may reduce your ability to have an orgasm.

Ways to reach orgasm when you are having difficulty:

- Focus on increasing your desire and enjoying the experience rather than focusing on the orgasm. Increasing your pleasure will help you eventually reach climax.

- Experiment through masturbation to find out what works best. Taking the pressure off you and your partner to find a solution together can often times help. You can then share your results with your partner.

- Using a vibrator to intensify stimulation either at the base or the head of the penis may be effective.

The good news is that premature ejaculation rarely is a problem after cancer treatments, although some men will experience no ejaculations or a "dry" orgasm. There are a number of treatments that can cause this to occur, including radical prostatectomy, radical cystectomy, radiation to the pelvis, and some chemotherapy drugs. The damage occurs to the prostate and seminal vesicles that produce semen. Erection problems may also occur but may be helped by oral and hand stimulation. Orgasm still occurs without semen. Half of men report their climax as pleasurable but weaker than before; many report the orgasm feeling the same. Men have worried that a dry orgasm may be less pleasurable for their partner; however, partners report that lack of semen can in fact increase pleasure during oral sex, and partners do not feel the spurt of semen in vaginal and anal sex so do not miss it. Dry orgasm becomes a larger dilemma for a man wishing to father a child.

## Cancer Treatments and Sperm Count

Male infertility is generally caused by damage to the production of sperm cells. Because cancer treatments target cells that are rapidly dividing (as cancer cells do), they can also harm other rapidly dividing cells in the body, including sperm cells.

The testicles are sometimes a direct target for radiation therapy, as is the case for testicular cancer or some leukemias. A dose of 600 rad to the testicles is enough to permanently destroy stem cells that produce sperm cells. A dose of less than 600 rad to the testicles will slow down or stop sperm cell production. It is possible for sperm cell counts to recover in a matter of months or years. Sheets of lead that are specially molded can be used to protect the testicles; however, sometimes there is an indirect effect. Higher doses cause a greater time for recovery. Younger boys are less susceptible to radiation damage.

Chemotherapy can affect sperm production in similar ways. Combinations of chemotherapy with radiation to the pelvis or abdomen can be especially damaging. For men over age 40, recovery of fertility is less likely than for teenagers or younger adults.

## How Can I Preserve Fertility?

Because once sperm cell production is damaged there is currently no way to fix the damage, the best option is to bank sperm prior to surgery to the pelvis or chemotherapy and radiation therapy. It is a choice that is often hard to make ahead of time, because many men believe they will not lose their fertility or don't know if they want to have children. But it is a decision that one may regret not making later on in life so it is worth consideration. Many cancer centers offer sperm banking, as do most large cities.

The procedure is as follows:

- Usually two weeks are used to collect enough semen samples.

- If time is a problem, men who need to start treatment quickly can sometimes collect enough semen within a couple of days.

- It is requested that the man not ejaculate for 24–48 hours before each sample is taken.

- Three to six samples are requested to bank enough semen to provide a reasonable chance for a couple's conception later.

- The sample is collected through masturbation at the laboratory, as it is important to decrease the risk of contamination through bacteria and sperm can easily die if not quickly frozen. Freezing will damage some of the sperm, making some less active.

- Sperm can be frozen up to 50 years without problem.

- There is usually an annual fee for storage.

Sometimes men with cancer have infertility problems even before treatment. Banking sperm may not be recommended for men with low sperm counts and motility (sperm's ability to move) problems. However, with advances in fertility, any type of sperm cell can be important. Research has shown no increased risk for birth defects from babies conceived from frozen sperm.

You may wish to contact an infertility specialist sooner than normal if you are trying to conceive a child and having difficulty. Infertility treatments are expensive and not often covered by insurance; be sure to check with your health insurance provider to understand your benefits. Find a fertility clinic that specializes in male and female fertility issues, and ask if they have had experience in helping cancer survivors. For more information about finding a specialist in infertility, visit the American Society for Reproductive Medicine website.

Wanting to conceive a child and not being able to can cause immense heartbreak for a couple. When the reasons one cannot conceive are related to cancer, feelings of grief and anger can be especially intense. A man may feel like he is damaged or defective on top of the range of burdensome emotions that a diagnosis of cancer can bring. For a couple that looked forward to having children, the loss of the dream is real and must be mourned. It is important to find emotional support to help you cope with these difficult issues. Try locating a mental health professional through a local infertility clinic. Another good resource is Resolve, a national information and support organization for infertility that has local chapters.

## *Sex after Surgical Removal of Body Parts*

Surgical treatment for men with penile cancer and testicular cancer may result in the removal or partial removal of body parts.

### *Penectomy*

The most common form of treatment for penile cancer is surgical removal of part or all of the penis. If the tumor is limited to the tip of the penis, a partial penectomy (removal of part of penis) is performed, leaving enough of the shaft to direct the urine stream away from the body. The remaining shaft is long enough for penetration of the vagina and is able to become erect upon sexual arousal.

When the shaft of the penis cannot be saved, a total penectomy (removal of the entire penis) is required. A new opening in the perineal area (area between scrotum and anus), called perineal urethrostomy, is created for urination. Many men with penile cancer are elderly and adjust to the loss of the penis by simply giving up sex. However, for those who wish to have a sex life can do so using "outercourse." Outercourse involves deep kissing, sexual massages, and kissing and caressing of sensitive genital areas (such as the scrotum, skin behind scrotum, and the skin around where the penis was removed). Having a sexual fantasy or looking at an erotic video or stories can enhance excitement. Some men are still able to experience sexual pleasure and reach orgasms by engaging in outercourse.

### *Loss of One or Both Testicles*

Orchiectomy, or surgical removal of the testicles, can be compared to a mastectomy (surgical removal of breast) for a woman, in that the operation may make a man feel self-conscious about the loss of his testicles. Testicles can be viewed as a symbol of manhood. Although some men are not affected by the new appearance, others may fear the reaction of their partners, especially single men. In such cases, surgical implantation of prosthesis may be an option to discuss with your doctor.

Men treated for metastatic prostate cancer may have one or both testicles removed to stop the production of testosterone and other male hormones that feed the tumor. In men with testicular cancer, only the testicle with cancer is removed (rarely does a man develop a cancer in the second testicle). According to the American Cancer Society, testicular cancer is one of the most common forms of cancer in young men. Although sexual functioning and fertility often remain unimpaired, a young, single, and dating male may find it emotionally painful and embarrassing to have a testicle missing.

A prosthesis that looks and feels like a testicle could be used to help deal with body image issues.

# Chapter 30

# Sexually Transmitted Diseases

## Chapter Contents

Section 30.1

*STDs:*
*The Basics*

Reprinted from "An Introduction to Sexually Transmitted Diseases," National Institute of Allergy and Infectious Disease, July 1999, http://www. niaid.nih.gov/factsheets/stdinfo.htm. Reviewed by David A. Cooke, M.D., June 29, 2003.

Sexually transmitted diseases (STDs), once called venereal diseases, are among the most common infectious diseases in the United States today. More than 20 STDs have now been identified (see Table 30.1), and they affect more than 13 million men and women in this country each year. The annual comprehensive cost of STDs in the United States is estimated to be well in excess of $10 billion.

Understanding the basic facts about STDs—the ways in which they are spread, their common symptoms, and how they can be treated— is the first step toward prevention. The National Institute of Allergy and Infectious Diseases (NIAID), a part of the National Institutes of Health, has prepared a series of fact sheets about STDs to provide this important information. Research investigators supported by NIAID are looking for better methods of diagnosis and more effective treatments, as well as for vaccines and topical microbicides to prevent STDs. It is important to understand at least five key points about all STDs in this country today:

1.  STDs affect men and women of all backgrounds and economic levels. They are most prevalent among teenagers and young adults. Nearly two-thirds of all STDs occur in people younger than 25 years of age.

2.  The incidence of STDs is rising, in part because in the last few decades, young people have become sexually active earlier yet are marrying later. In addition, divorce is more common. The net result is that sexually active people today are more likely to have multiple sex partners during their lives and are potentially at risk for developing STDs.

3.  Most of the time, STDs cause no symptoms, particularly in women. When and if symptoms develop, they may be confused with those of other diseases not transmitted through sexual contact. Even when an STD causes no symptoms, however, a person who is infected may be able to pass the disease on to a sex partner. That is why many doctors recommend periodic testing or screening for people who have more than one sex partner.

**Table 30.1.** Sexually Transmitted Diseases and the Organisms Responsible

| Disease | Organism(s) |
| --- | --- |
| Acquired immunodeficiency syndrome (AIDS) | Human immunodeficiency virus (HIV) |
| Bacterial vaginosis | *Bacteroides, Gardnerella vaginalis, Mobiluncus* spp., *Mycoplasma hominis, Ureaplasma urealyticum* |
| Chancroid | *Haemophilus ducreyi* |
| Chlamydial infections | *Chlamydia trachomatis* |
| Cytomegalovirus infections | *Cytomegalovirus* |
| Genital herpes | Herpes simplex virus |
| Genital (venereal) warts | Human papillomavirus |
| Gonorrhea | *Neisseria gonorrhoeae* |
| Granuloma inguinale (donovanosis) | *Calymmatobacterium granulomatis* |
| Leukemia-lymphoma/myelopathy | HTLV-I and II |
| Lymphogranuloma venereum | *Chlamydia trachomatis* |
| Molluscum contagiosum | Molluscum contagiosum virus |
| Pubic lice | *Phthirus pubis* |
| Scabies | *Sarcoptes scabiei* |
| Syphilis | *Treponema pallidum* |
| Trichomoniasis | *Trichomonas vaginalis* |
| Vaginal yeast infections | *Candida albicans* |

4. Health problems caused by STDs tend to be more severe and more frequent for women than for men, in part because the frequency of asymptomatic infection means that many women do not seek care until serious problems have developed.

   • Some STDs can spread into the uterus (womb) and fallopian tubes to cause pelvic inflammatory disease (PID), which in turn is a major cause of both infertility and ectopic (tubal) pregnancy. The latter can be fatal.

   • STDs in women also may be associated with cervical cancer. One STD, human papillomavirus infection (HPV), causes genital warts and cervical and other genital cancers.

   • STDs can be passed from a mother to her baby before, during, or immediately after birth; some of these infections of the newborn can be cured easily, but others may cause a baby to be permanently disabled or even die.

5. When diagnosed and treated early, many STDs can be treated effectively. Some infections have become resistant to the drugs used to treat them and now require newer types of antibiotics. Experts believe that having STDs other than AIDS increases one's risk for becoming infected with the AIDS virus.

## HIV Infection and AIDS

AIDS (acquired immunodeficiency syndrome) was first reported in the United States in 1981. It is caused by the human immunodeficiency virus (HIV), a virus that destroys the body's ability to fight off infection. An estimated 900,000 people in the United States are currently infected with HIV. People who have AIDS are very susceptible to many life-threatening diseases, called opportunistic infections, and to certain forms of cancer. Transmission of the virus primarily occurs during sexual activity and by sharing needles used to inject intravenous drugs. If you have any questions about HIV infection or AIDS, you can call the AIDS Hotline confidential toll-free number: 1-800-342-AIDS.

## Chlamydial Infection

This infection is now the most common of all bacterial STDs, with an estimated 4 to 8 million new cases occurring each year. In both men and women, chlamydial infection may cause an abnormal genital discharge and burning with urination. In women, untreated chlamydial infection may lead to pelvic inflammatory disease, one of the most common causes of ectopic pregnancy and infertility in women. Many people with chlamydial infection, however, have few or no symptoms of infection. Once diagnosed with chlamydial infection, a person can be treated with an antibiotic.

## Genital Herpes

Genital herpes affects an estimated 60 million Americans. Approximately 500,000 new cases of this incurable viral infection develop annually. Herpes infections are caused by herpes simplex virus (HSV). The major symptoms of herpes infection are painful blisters or open sores in the genital area. These may be preceded by a tingling or burning sensation in the legs, buttocks, or genital region. The herpes sores usually disappear within two to three weeks, but the virus remains in the body for life and the lesions may recur from time to time. Severe or frequently recurrent genital herpes is treated with one of several antiviral drugs that are available by prescription. These drugs help control the symptoms but do not eliminate the herpes virus from the body. Suppressive antiviral therapy can be used to prevent occurrences and perhaps transmission. Women who acquire genital herpes during pregnancy can transmit the virus to their babies. Untreated HSV infection in newborns can result in mental retardation and death.

## Genital Warts

Genital warts (also called venereal warts or condylomata acuminata) are caused by human papillomavirus, a virus related to the virus that causes common skin warts. Genital warts usually first appear as small, hard painless bumps in the vaginal area, on the penis, or around the anus. If untreated, they may grow and develop a fleshy, cauliflower-like appearance. Genital warts infect an estimated one million Americans each year. In addition to genital warts, certain high-risk types of HPV cause cervical cancer and other genital cancers. Genital warts are treated with a topical drug (applied to the skin), by freezing, or, if they recur, with injections of a type of interferon. If the warts are very large, they can be removed by surgery.

## Gonorrhea

Approximately 400,000 cases of gonorrhea are reported to the U.S. Centers for Disease Control and Prevention (CDC) each year in this country. The most common symptoms of gonorrhea are a discharge from the vagina or penis and painful or difficult urination. The most common and serious complications occur in women and, as with chlamydial infection, these complications include PID, ectopic pregnancy, and infertility. Historically, penicillin has been used to treat gonorrhea, but in the last decade, four types of antibiotic resistance have emerged. New antibiotics or combinations of drugs must be used to treat these resistant strains.

## Syphilis

The incidence of syphilis has increased and decreased dramatically in recent years, with more than 11,000 cases reported in 1996. The first symptoms of syphilis may go undetected because they are very mild and disappear spontaneously. The initial symptom is a chancre; it is usually a painless open sore that usually appears on the penis or around or in the vagina. It can also occur near the mouth, anus, or on the hands. If untreated, syphilis may go on to more advanced stages, including a transient rash and, eventually, serious involvement of the heart and central nervous system. The full course of the disease can take years. Penicillin remains the most effective drug to treat people with syphilis.

Other diseases that may be sexually transmitted include trichomoniasis, bacterial vaginosis, cytomegalovirus infections, scabies, and pubic lice.

STDs in pregnant women are associated with a number of adverse outcomes, including spontaneous abortion and infection in the newborn. Low birth weight and prematurity appear to be associated with STDs, including chlamydial infection and trichomoniasis. Congenital or perinatal infection (infection that occurs around the time of birth) occurs in 30 to 70 percent of infants born to infected mothers, and complications may include pneumonia, eye infections, and permanent neurologic damage.

## What Can You Do to Prevent STDs?

The best way to prevent STDs is to avoid sexual contact with others. If you decide to be sexually active, there are things that you can do to reduce your risk of developing an STD:

• Have a mutually monogamous sexual relationship with an uninfected partner.

- Correctly and consistently use a male condom.

- Use clean needles if injecting intravenous drugs.

- Prevent and control other STDs to decrease susceptibility to HIV infection and to reduce your infectiousness if you are HIV-infected.

- Delay having sexual relations as long as possible. The younger people are when having sex for the first time, the more susceptible they become to developing an STD. The risk of acquiring an STD also increases with the number of partners over a lifetime.

Anyone who is sexually active should:

- Have regular checkups for STDs even in the absence of symptoms, and especially if having sex with a new partner. These tests can be done during a routine visit to the doctor's office.

- Learn the common symptoms of STDs. Seek medical help immediately if any suspicious symptoms develop, even if they are mild.

- Avoid having sex during menstruation. HIV-infected women are probably more infectious, and HIV-uninfected women are probably more susceptible to becoming infected during that time.

- Avoid anal intercourse, but if practiced, use a male condom.

- Avoid douching because it removes some of the normal protective bacteria in the vagina and increases the risk of getting some STDs.

Anyone diagnosed as having an STD should:

- Be treated to reduce the risk of transmitting an STD to an infant.

- Discuss with a doctor the possible risk of transmission in breast milk and whether commercial formula should be substituted.

- Notify all recent sex partners and urge them to get a checkup.

- Follow the doctor's orders and complete the full course of medication prescribed. A follow-up test to ensure that the infection has been cured is often an important step in treatment.

- Avoid all sexual activity while being treated for an STD.

Sometimes people are too embarrassed or frightened to ask for help or information. Most STDs are readily treated, and the earlier a person seeks treatment and warns sex partners about the disease, the less likely the disease will do irreparable physical damage, be spread to others, or, in the case of a woman, be passed on to a newborn baby.

Private doctors, local health departments, and STD and family planning clinics have information about STDs. In addition, the American Social Health Association (ASHA) provides free information and keeps lists of clinics and private doctors who provide treatment for people with STDs. ASHA has a national toll-free telephone number, 1-800-227-8922. The phone number for the Herpes Hotline, also run by ASHA, is 1-919-361-8488. Callers can get information from the ASHA hotline without leaving their names.

## *Research*

STDs cause physical and emotional suffering to millions and are costly to individuals and to society as a whole. NIAID conducts and supports many research projects designed to improve methods of prevention, and to find better ways to diagnose and treat these diseases. NIAID also supports several large university-based STD research centers.

Within the past few years, NIAID-supported research has resulted in new tests to diagnose some STDs faster and more accurately. New drug treatments for STDs are under investigation by NIAID researchers. This is especially important because some STDs are becoming resistant to the standard drugs. In addition, vaccines are being developed or tested for effectiveness in preventing several STDs, including AIDS, chlamydial infection, genital herpes, and gonorrhea.

It is up to each individual to learn more about STDs and then make choices about how to minimize the risk of acquiring these diseases and spreading them to others. Knowledge of STDs, as well as honesty and openness with sex partners and with one's doctor, can be very important in reducing the incidence and complications of sexually transmitted diseases.

# Section 30.2

# *Gonorrhea*

Reprinted from "Gonorrhea," National Institute of Allergy and Infectious Diseases, May 2002, http://www.niaid.nih.gov/factsheets/stdgon.htm.

## *What Is Gonorrhea?*

Gonorrhea is a curable, sexually transmitted disease (STD) caused by a bacterium called *Neisseria gonorrhoeae*. These bacteria can infect the genital tract, the mouth, and the rectum. In women, the opening to the uterus, the cervix, is the first place of infection.

The disease however can spread into the uterus and fallopian tubes, resulting in pelvic inflammatory disease (PID). PID affects more than one million women in this country every year and can cause infertility in as many as 10 percent of infected women and tubal (ectopic) pregnancy.

In 2000, 358,995 cases of gonorrhea were reported to the U.S. Centers for Disease Control and Prevention (CDC). In the United States, approximately 75 percent of all reported cases of gonorrhea are found in younger persons aged 15 to 29 years. The highest rates of infection are usually found in 15- to 19-year-old women and 20- to 24-year-old men. Health economists estimate that the annual cost of gonorrhea and its complications is close to $1.1 billion.

Gonorrhea is spread during sexual intercourse. Infected women also can pass gonorrhea to their newborn infants during delivery, causing eye infections in their babies. This complication is rare because newborn babies receive eye medicine to prevent infection. When the infection occurs in the genital tract, mouth, or rectum of a child, it is due most commonly to sexual abuse.

## *What Are the Symptoms of Gonorrhea?*

The early symptoms of gonorrhea often are mild. Symptoms usually appear within two to 10 days after sexual contact with an infected partner. A small number of people may be infected for several months without showing symptoms.

When women have symptoms, the first ones may include:

- Bleeding associated with vaginal intercourse
- Painful or burning sensations when urinating
- Vaginal discharge that is yellow or bloody

More advanced symptoms, which may indicate development of PID, include cramps and pain, bleeding between menstrual periods, vomiting, or fever.

Men have symptoms more often than women, including:

- Pus from the penis and pain
- Burning sensations during urination that may be severe

Symptoms of rectal infection include discharge, anal itching, and occasional painful bowel movements with fresh blood on the feces.

## How Is Gonorrhea Diagnosed?

Doctors or other health care workers usually use three laboratory techniques to diagnose gonorrhea: staining samples directly for the bacterium, detection of bacterial genes or DNA in urine, and growing the bacteria in laboratory cultures. Many doctors prefer to use more than one test to increase the chance of an accurate diagnosis.

The staining test involves placing a smear of the discharge from the penis or the cervix on a slide and staining the smear with a dye. Then the doctor uses a microscope to look for bacteria on the slide. You usually can get the test results while in the office or clinic. This test is quite accurate for men but is not good in women. Only one in two women with gonorrhea have a positive stain.

More often, doctors use urine or cervical swabs for a new test that detects the genes of the bacteria. These tests are as accurate or more so than culturing the bacteria, and many doctors use them.

The culture test involves placing a sample of the discharge onto a culture plate and incubating it up to two days to allow the bacteria to grow. The sensitivity of this test depends on the site from which the sample is taken. Cultures of cervical samples detect infection approximately 90 percent of the time. The doctor also can take a culture to detect gonorrhea in the throat. Culture allows testing for drug-resistant bacteria.

## How Is Gonorrhea Treated?

Doctors usually prescribe a single dose of one of the following antibiotics to treat gonorrhea:

- Cefixime
- Ciprofloxacin
- Ofloxacin
- Ceftriaxone
- Levofloxacin

If you have gonorrhea and are younger than 18 years old, you should not take ciprofloxacin or ofloxacin. Your doctor can prescribe the best and safest antibiotic for you.

Gonorrhea and chlamydial infection, another common STD, often infect people at the same time. Therefore, doctors usually prescribe a combination of antibiotics, such as ceftriaxone and doxycycline or azithromycin, which will treat both diseases.

If you have gonorrhea, all of your sexual partners should get tested and then treated if infected, whether or not they have symptoms of infection.

## What Can Happen If Gonorrhea Is Not Treated?

In untreated gonorrhea infections, the bacteria can spread up into the reproductive tract or, more rarely, through the bloodstream and infect the joints, heart valves, or the brain.

The most common result of untreated gonorrhea is PID, a serious infection of the female reproductive tract. Gonococcal PID often appears immediately after the menstrual period. PID causes scar tissue to form in the fallopian tubes. If the tube is partially scarred, the fertilized egg may not be able to pass into the uterus. If this happens, the embryo may implant in the tube causing a tubal (ectopic) pregnancy. This serious complication may result in a miscarriage and can cause death of the mother.

Rarely, untreated gonorrhea can spread through the blood to the joints. This can cause an inflammation of the joints which is very serious.

If you are infected with gonorrhea, your risk of getting HIV infection increases (HIV, human immunodeficiency virus, causes AIDS). Therefore, it is extremely important for you to either prevent yourself from getting gonorrhea or get treated early if you already are infected with it.

## Can Gonorrhea Affect a Newborn Baby?

The infection can be passed to a baby as it passes through the birth canal during delivery. A doctor can prevent infection of the baby's eyes by applying silver nitrate or other medications to the eyes immediately after birth. Because of the risks from gonococcal infection, doctors recommend that pregnant women have at least one test for gonorrhea during pregnancy.

## How Can I Prevent Getting Infected with Gonorrhea?

By using latex condoms correctly and consistently during vaginal or rectal sexual activity, you can reduce your risk of getting gonorrhea and its complications.

## What Research Is Going on?

The National Institute of Allergy, Immunology and Infectious Diseases (NIAID) continues to support a comprehensive, multidisciplinary program of research on *N. gonorrhoeae* (gonococci). Researchers are trying to understand how gonococci infect cells while evading human immune defenses (immune response). Studies are ongoing to determine:

1. How this bacterium attaches to host cells

2. How it gets inside them

3. Gonococcal surface structures and how they can change

4. Human response to infection by gonococci

All of these efforts, together, will eventually lead to development of an effective vaccine against gonorrhea. They also have led to, and will lead to, further improvements in diagnosis and treatment of gonorrhea.

Another important area of gonorrhea research concerns antibiotic resistance. This is particularly important because strains of *N. gonorrhoeae* that are resistant to recommended antibiotic therapies have spread from Southeast Asia to Hawaii and are now starting to appear on the West Coast. These events add urgency to NIAID efforts to develop effective microbicides (antimicrobial preparations that can be applied inside the vagina) to prevent infections.

Recently, scientists have determined the sequence of the *N. gonorrhoeae* genome. They are using this information to find promising new leads to help us better understand how the organism causes disease and becomes resistant to antibiotics.

Section 30.3

# *Syphilis*

Reprinted from "Syphilis," National Institute of Allergy and Infectious Diseases, November 2002, http://www.niaid.nih.gov/factsheets/stdsyph.htm.

## *What Is Syphilis?*

Syphilis is a sexually transmitted disease (STD), once responsible for devastating epidemics. It is caused by a bacterium called *Treponema pallidum*. The rate of primary and secondary syphilis in the United States declined by 89.2 percent from 1990 to 2000. The number of cases rose, however, from 5,979 in 2000 to 6,103 in 2001. The U.S. Centers for Disease Control and Prevention reported in November 2002 that this was the first increase since 1990.

Of increasing concern is the fact that syphilis increases by three- to fivefold the risk of transmitting and acquiring HIV (human immunodeficiency virus), the virus that causes AIDS (acquired immunodeficiency syndrome).

## *How Is Syphilis Transmitted?*

The syphilis bacterium is very fragile, and the infection is almost always transmitted by sexual contact with an infected person. The bacterium spreads from the initial ulcer (sore) of an infected person to the skin or mucous membranes (linings) of the genital area, mouth, or anus of an uninfected sexual partner. It also can pass through broken skin on other parts of the body.

In addition, a pregnant woman with syphilis can pass *T. pallidum* to her unborn child, who may be born with serious mental and physical problems as a result of this infection.

## *What Are the Symptoms of Syphilis?*

The initial infection causes an ulcer at the site of infection. The bacteria, however, move throughout the body, damaging many organs over time. Medical experts describe the course of the disease by dividing it into four stages: primary, secondary, latent, and tertiary (late). An infected person who has not been treated may infect others during the first two stages, which usually last one to two years. In its late stages, untreated syphilis, although not contagious, can cause serious heart abnormalities, mental disorders, blindness, other neurologic problems, and death.

## Primary Syphilis

The first symptom of primary syphilis is an ulcer called a chancre ("shan-ker"). The chancre can appear within 10 days to three months after exposure, but it generally appears within two to six weeks. Because the chancre may be painless and may occur inside the body, the infected person might not notice it. It usually is found on the part of the body exposed to the infected partner's ulcer, such as the penis, vulva, or vagina. A chancre also can develop on the cervix, tongue, lips, or other parts of the body. The chancre disappears within a few weeks whether or not a person is treated. If not treated during the primary stage, about one-third of people will go on to the chronic stages.

## Secondary Syphilis

A skin rash, with brown sores about the size of a penny, often marks this chronic stage of syphilis. The rash appears anywhere from three to six weeks after the chancre appears. While the rash may cover the whole body or appear only in a few areas, it is almost always on the palms of the hands and soles of the feet.

Because active bacteria are present in the sores, any physical contact—sexual or nonsexual—with the broken skin of an infected person may spread the infection at this stage. The rash usually heals within several weeks or months.

Other symptoms also may occur, such as mild fever, fatigue, headache, sore throat, patchy hair loss, and swollen lymph glands throughout the body. These symptoms may be very mild and, like the chancre of primary syphilis, will disappear without treatment. The signs of secondary syphilis may come and go over the next one to two years of the disease.

## Latent Syphilis

If untreated, syphilis may lapse into a latent stage during which the disease is no longer contagious and no symptoms are present. Many people who are not treated will suffer from no further signs and symptoms of the disease.

*Tertiary Syphilis*

Approximately one-third of people who have had secondary syphilis go on to develop the complications of late, or tertiary, syphilis, in which the bacteria damage the heart, eyes, brain, nervous system, bones, joints, or almost any other part of the body. This stage can last for years or even for decades. Late syphilis can result in mental illness, blindness, other neurologic problems, heart disease, and death.

## How Is Syphilis Diagnosed?

Syphilis is sometimes called "the great imitator" because its early symptoms are similar to those of many other diseases. Sexually active people should consult a doctor or other health care worker about any rash or sore in the genital area. Those who have been treated for another STD, such as gonorrhea, should be tested to be sure they do not also have syphilis.

There are three ways to diagnose syphilis:

* Recognizing the signs and symptoms
* Examining blood samples
* Identifying syphilis bacteria under a microscope

The doctor usually uses all these approaches to diagnose syphilis and decide upon the stage of infection.

Blood tests also provide evidence of infection, although they may give false-negative results (not show signs of an infection despite its presence) for up to three months after infection. False-positive tests (showing signs of an infection when it is not present) also can occur. Therefore, two blood tests are usually used. Interpretation of blood tests for syphilis can be difficult, and repeated tests are sometimes necessary to confirm the diagnosis.

## How Is Syphilis Treated?

Unfortunately, the early symptoms of syphilis can be very mild, and many people do not seek treatment when they first become infected.

Doctors usually treat patients with syphilis with penicillin, given by injection. They use other antibiotics for patients allergic to penicillin. A person usually can no longer transmit syphilis 24 hours after starting treatment. Some people, however, do not respond to the usual doses of penicillin. Therefore, it is important that people being treated for syphilis have periodic blood tests to check that the infectious agent has been completely destroyed.

People with neurosyphilis may need to be retested for up to two years after treatment. In all stages of syphilis, proper treatment will cure the disease. But in late syphilis, damage already done to body organs cannot be reversed.

## What Are the Effects of Syphilis in Pregnant Women?

A pregnant woman with untreated, active syphilis is likely to pass the infection to her unborn child. In addition, miscarriage may occur in as many as 25 to 50 percent of women acutely infected with syphilis during pregnancy. Between 40 to 70 percent of women with active syphilis will give birth to a syphilis-infected infant.

Some infants with congenital syphilis may have symptoms at birth, but most develop symptoms between two weeks and three months later. These symptoms may include:

- Skin ulcers
- Rashes
- Fever
- Weakened or hoarse crying sounds
- Swollen liver and spleen
- Yellowish skin (jaundice)
- Anemia (low red blood cell count)
- Various deformities

People who care for infants with congenital syphilis must use special cautions because the moist sores are infectious.

Rarely, the symptoms of syphilis go undetected in infants. As infected infants become older children and teenagers, they may develop the symptoms of late-stage syphilis, including damage to their bones, teeth, eyes, ears, and brains.

## Can Syphilis Cause Other Complications?

Syphilis bacteria frequently invade the nervous system during the early stages of infection. Approximately 3 to 7 percent of persons with untreated syphilis develop neurosyphilis, a sometimes serious disorder of the nervous system. In some instances, the time from infection to developing neurosyphilis may be up to 20 years.

Some people with neurosyphilis never develop any symptoms. Others may have headache, stiff neck, and fever that result from an inflammation of the lining of the brain. Some people develop seizures. People whose blood vessels are affected may develop symptoms of stroke with numbness, weakness, or visual problems. Neurosyphilis may be more difficult to treat, and its course may be different, in people with HIV infection or AIDS.

## How Can Syphilis Be Prevented?

The open sores of syphilis may be visible and infectious during the active stages of infection. Any contact with these infectious sores and other infected tissues and body fluids must be avoided to prevent spread of the disease. As with many other STDs, using latex male condoms properly during sexual intercourse may give some protection from the disease.

Screening and treatment of infected individuals, or secondary prevention, is one of the few options for preventing the advanced stages of the disease. Testing and treatment early in pregnancy are the best ways to prevent syphilis in infants and should be a routine part of prenatal care.

## What Research Is Going on?

Developing better ways to diagnose and treat syphilis is an important research goal of scientists supported by the National Institute of Allergy and Infectious Diseases (NIAID). New tests are being developed that may provide better ways to diagnose syphilis and define the stage of infection.

In an effort to stem the spread of syphilis, scientists are conducting research on the development of a vaccine. Molecular biologists are learning more about the various surface components of the syphilis bacterium that stimulate the immune system to respond to the invading organism. This knowledge will pave the way for development of an effective vaccine that can ultimately prevent this STD.

A high priority for researchers is developing a diagnostic test that does not require a blood sample. Saliva and urine are being evaluated to see whether they would work as well as blood. Researchers also are trying to develop other diagnostic tests for detecting infection in babies.

Another high research priority is the development of a safe, effective single-dose oral antibiotic therapy for syphilis. Many patients do not like getting an injection for treatment, and about 10 percent of the general population is allergic to penicillin.

The genome of the bacterium that causes syphilis has been sequenced through NIAID-funded research. The DNA sequence represents an encyclopedia of information about the bacterium. Clues as to how to diagnose, treat, and vaccinate against syphilis have been identified and are fueling intensive research efforts on this ancient but intractable disease.

## Section 30.4

# *Chlamydia*

Reprinted from "Chlamydial Infection," National Institute of Allergy and Infectious Diseases, May 2002, http://www.niaid.nih.gov/factsheets/stdclam.htm.

### What Is Chlamydial Infection?

Chlamydial ("kla-MID-ee-uhl") infection is a curable, sexually transmitted disease (STD), which is caused by a bacterium called *Chlamydia trachomatis.* You can get genital chlamydial infection during oral, vaginal, or anal sexual contact with an infected partner. It can cause serious problems in men and women as well as in newborn babies of infected mothers.

Chlamydial infection is one of the most widespread bacterial STDs in the United States. The U.S. Centers for Disease Control and Prevention (CDC) estimates that more than 4 million people are infected each year. Health economists estimate that chlamydial infections and the other problems they cause cost Americans more than $2 billion a year.

### What Are the Symptoms of This STD?

Because chlamydial infection does not make most people sick, you can have it and not know it. Those who do have symptoms may have an abnormal discharge (mucus or pus) from the vagina or penis or pain while urinating. These early symptoms may be very mild. Symptoms usually appear within one to three weeks after being infected. Because the symptoms may be mild or not exist at all, you might not seek care and get treated.

The infection may move inside the body if it is not treated. There, it can cause pelvic inflammatory disease (PID) in women and epididymitis in men, two very serious illnesses.

*C. trachomatis* can cause inflamed rectum and inflammation of the lining of the eye ("pink eye"). The bacteria also can infect the throat from oral sexual contact with an infected partner.

## How Does the Doctor Diagnose Chlamydial Infection?

Chlamydial infection is easily confused with gonorrhea because the symptoms of both diseases are similar and the diseases can occur together, though rarely.

The most reliable ways to find out whether the infection is chlamydial are through laboratory tests. Usually, a doctor or other health care worker will send a sample of pus from the vagina or penis to a laboratory that will look for the bacteria.

The urine test does not require a pelvic exam or swabbing of the penis. Results from the urine test are available within 24 hours.

## How Is Chlamydial Infection Treated?

If you are infected with *C. trachomatis*, your doctor or other health care worker will probably give you a prescription for an antibiotic such as azithromycin (taken for one day only) or doxycycline (taken for seven days). Or, you might get a prescription for another antibiotic such as erythromycin or ofloxacin.

Doctors may treat pregnant women with azithromycin or erythromycin or sometimes, with amoxicillin. Penicillin, which doctors often use to treat some other STDs, won't cure chlamydial infections.

If you have chlamydial infection:

- Take all of the prescribed medicine, even after symptoms disappear.

- If the symptoms do not disappear within one to two weeks after finishing the medicine, go to your doctor or clinic again.

- It is very important to tell your sex partners that you have chlamydial infection so that they can be tested and treated.

## What Can Happen If the Infection Is Not Treated?

In women, untreated chlamydial infections can lead to PID. In men, untreated chlamydial infections may lead to pain or swelling in the scrotal area, which is a sign of inflammation of a part of the male reproductive system located near the testicles known as the epididymis. Left untreated, these complications can prevent people from having children.

Each year up to one million women in the United States develop PID, a serious infection of the reproductive organs. As many as half of all cases of PID may be due to chlamydial infection, and many of these don't have symptoms. PID can cause scarring of the fallopian tubes, which can block the tubes and prevent fertilization from taking place. Researchers estimate that 100,000 women each year become infertile because of PID.

In other cases, scarring may interfere with the passage of the fertilized egg to the uterus during pregnancy. When this happens, the egg may attach itself to the fallopian tube. This is called ectopic or tubal pregnancy. This very serious condition results in a miscarriage and can cause death of the mother.

## Can Chlamydial Infection Affect a Newborn Baby?

A baby who is exposed to *C. trachomatis* in the birth canal during delivery may develop an eye infection or pneumonia. Symptoms of conjunctivitis or "pink eye," which include discharge and swollen eyelids, usually develop within the first 10 days of life.

Symptoms of pneumonia, including a cough that gets steadily worse and congestion, most often develop within three to six weeks of birth. Doctors can treat both conditions successfully with antibiotics. Because of these risks to the newborn, many doctors recommend that all pregnant women get tested for chlamydial infection.

## How Can I Prevent Getting Chlamydial Infection?

You can reduce your chances of getting chlamydia or of giving it to your partner by using male latex condoms correctly every time you have sexual intercourse.

If you are infected but have no symptoms, you may pass the bacteria to your sex partners without knowing it. Therefore, any doctors recommend that anyone who has more than one sex partner, especially women under 25 years of age, be tested for chlamydial infection regularly, even if they don't have symptoms.

## What Research Is Going on?

Scientists are looking for better ways to diagnose, treat, and prevent chlamydial infections. NIAID-supported scientists recently completed sequencing the genome for *C. trachomatis*. The sequence represents an encyclopedia of information about the organism. This accomplishment will give scientists important information as they try to develop a safe and effective vaccine. Developing topical microbicides (preparations that can be inserted into the vagina to prevent infection) that are effective and easy for women to use is also a major research focus.

# Section 30.5

# *Genital Warts*

Reprinted from "Human Papillomavirus and Genital Warts," National Institute of Allergy and Infectious Diseases, March 2001, http://www.niaid.nih.gov/factsheets/stdhpv.htm.

## What Is Human Papillomavirus?

Human papillomavirus (HPV) is one of the most common causes of sexually transmitted disease (STD) in the world. Health experts estimate that there are more cases of genital HPV infection than of any other STD in the United States. According to the American Social Health Association, approximately 5.5 million new cases of sexually transmitted HPV infections are reported every year. At least 20 million Americans are already infected.

Scientists have identified more than 100 types of HPV, most of which are harmless. About 30 types are spread through sexual contact. Some types of HPV that cause genital infections can also cause cervical cancer and other genital cancers.

Like many STDs, genital HPV infections often do not have visible signs and symptoms. One study sponsored by the National Institute of Allergy and Infectious Diseases (NIAID) reported that almost half of the women infected with HPV had no obvious symptoms. People who are infected but who have no symptoms may not know they can transmit HPV to others or that they can develop complications from the virus.

## What Are Genital Warts?

Genital warts (condylomata acuminata, or venereal warts) are the most easily recognized sign of genital HPV infection. Many people, however, have a genital HPV infection without genital warts.

## Can HPV Cause Other Kinds of Warts?

Some types of HPV cause common skin warts, such as those found on the hands and soles of the feet. These types of HPV do not cause genital warts.

## How Are Genital Warts Spread?

Genital warts are very contagious and are spread during oral, genital, or anal sex with an infected partner. About two-thirds of people who have sexual contact with a partner with genital warts will develop warts, usually within three months of contact.

In women, the warts occur on the outside and inside of the vagina, on the opening (cervix) to the womb (uterus), or around the anus. In men, genital warts are less common. If present, they usually are seen on the tip of the penis. They also may be found on the shaft of the penis, on the scrotum, or around the anus. Rarely, genital warts also can develop in the mouth or throat of a person who has had oral sex with an infected person.

Genital warts often occur in clusters and can be very tiny or can spread into large masses in the genital or anal area.

## How Are Genital Warts Diagnosed?

A doctor or other health care worker usually can diagnose genital warts by seeing them on a patient. Women with genital warts also should be examined for possible HPV infection of the cervix.

The doctor may be able to identify some otherwise invisible warts in the genital tissue by applying vinegar (acetic acid) to areas of suspected infection. This solution causes infected areas to whiten, which makes them more visible, particularly if a procedure called colposcopy is performed. During colposcopy, the doctor uses a magnifying instrument to look at the vagina and cervix. In some cases, the doctor takes a small piece of tissue from the cervix and examines it under the microscope.

A Pap smear test also may indicate the possible presence of cervical HPV infection. In a Pap smear, a laboratory worker examines cells scraped from the cervix under a microscope to see if they are cancerous. If a woman's Pap smear is abnormal, she might have an HPV infection. If a woman has an abnormal Pap smear, she should have her doctor examine her further to look for and treat any cervical problems.

## What Is the Treatment for Genital Warts?

Genital warts often disappear even without treatment. In other cases, they eventually may develop a fleshy, small, raised growth that looks like cauliflower. There is no way to predict whether the warts will grow or disappear. Therefore, if you suspect you have genital warts, you should be examined and treated, if necessary.

Depending on factors such as the size and location of the genital warts, a doctor will offer you one of several ways to treat them.

- Imiquimod, an immune response cream which you can apply to the affected area

- A 20 percent podophyllin antimitotic solution, which you can apply to the affected area and later wash off

- A 0.5 percent podofilox solution, applied to the affected area but shouldn't be washed off

- A 5 percent 5-fluorouracil cream

- Trichloroacetic acid (TCA)

If you have small warts, the doctor can remove them by freezing (cryosurgery), burning (electrocautery), or laser treatment. Occasionally, the doctor will have to use surgery to remove large warts that have not responded to other treatment.

Some doctors use the antiviral drug alpha interferon, which they inject directly into the warts, to treat warts that have returned after removal by traditional means. The drug is expensive, however, and does not reduce the rate that the genital warts return.

Although treatments can get rid of the warts, none gets rid of the virus. Because the virus is still present in your body, warts often come back after treatment.

## How Can HPV Infection Be Prevented?

The only way you can prevent getting an HPV infection is to avoid direct contact with the virus, which is transmitted by skin-to-skin contact. If you or your sexual partner have warts that are visible in the genital area, you should avoid any sexual contact until the warts are treated. Studies have not confirmed that male latex condoms prevent transmission of HPV itself, but results do suggest that condom use may reduce the risk of developing diseases linked to HPV, such as genital warts and cervical cancer.

## Can HPV and Genital Warts Cause Complications?

### Cancer

Some types of HPV can cause cervical cancer. Others, however, cause cervical cancer and also are associated with vulvar cancer, anal cancer, and cancer of the penis (a rare cancer).

Most HPV infections do not progress to cervical cancer. If a woman does have abnormal cervical cells, a Pap test will detect them. It is particularly important for women who have abnormal cervical cells to have regular pelvic exams and Pap tests so that they can be treated early, if necessary.

### Pregnancy and Childbirth

Genital warts may cause a number of problems during pregnancy. Sometimes they get larger during pregnancy, making it difficult to urinate. If the warts are in the vagina, they can make the vagina less elastic and cause obstruction during delivery.

Rarely, infants born to women with genital warts develop warts in their throats (laryngeal papillomatosis). Although uncommon, it is a potentially life-threatening condition for the child, requiring frequent laser surgery to prevent obstruction of the breathing passages. Research on the use of interferon therapy in combination with laser surgery indicates that this drug may show promise in slowing the course of the disease.

## What Research Is Going on?

Scientists are doing research on two types of HPV vaccines. One type would be used to prevent infection or disease (warts or precancerous tissue changes). The other type would be used to treat cervical cancers. Researchers are testing both types of vaccines in people.

# Section 30.6

# *Genital Herpes*

Reprinted from "Genital Herpes," National Institute of Allergy and Infectious Diseases, March 2002, http://www.niaid.nih.gov/factsheets/stdherp.htm.

## *What Is Genital Herpes?*

Genital herpes is an infection caused by the herpes simplex virus or HSV. There are two types of HSV, and both can cause genital herpes. HSV type 1 most commonly infects the lips, causing sores known as fever blisters or cold sores, but it also can infect the genital area and produce sores there. HSV type 2 is the usual cause of genital herpes, but it also can infect the mouth during oral sex. A person who has genital herpes infection can easily pass or transmit the virus to an uninfected person during sex.

Both HSV 1 and 2 can produce sores (also called lesions) in and around the vaginal area, on the penis, around the anal opening, and on the buttocks or thighs. Occasionally, sores also appear on other parts of the body where the virus has entered through broken skin.

HSV remains in certain nerve cells of the body for life, and can produce symptoms off and on in some infected people.

## *How Does Someone Get Genital Herpes?*

Most people get genital herpes by having sex with someone who is having a herpes "outbreak." This outbreak means that HSV is active. When active, the virus usually causes visible sores in the genital area. The sores cast off (shed) viruses that can infect another person. Sometimes, however, a person can have an outbreak and have no visible sores at all. People often get genital herpes by having sexual contact with others who don't know they are infected or who are having outbreaks of herpes without any sores.

A person with genital herpes also can infect a sexual partner during oral sex. The virus is spread only rarely, if at all, by touching objects such as a toilet seat or hot tub.

## What Are the Symptoms?

Unfortunately, most people who have genital herpes don't know it because they never have any symptoms, or they do not recognize any symptoms they might have. When there are symptoms, they can be different in each person. Most often, when a person becomes infected with herpes for the first time, the symptoms will appear within two to 10 days. These first episodes of symptoms usually last two to three weeks.

Early symptoms of a genital herpes outbreak include:

- Itching or burning feeling in the genital or anal area
- Pain in the legs, buttocks, or genital area
- Discharge of fluid from the vagina
- Feeling of pressure in the abdomen

Within a few days, sores appear near where the virus has entered the body, such as on the mouth, penis, or vagina. They also can occur inside the vagina and on the cervix in women, or in the urinary passage of women and men. Small red bumps appear first, develop into blisters, and then become painful open sores. Over several days, the sores become crusty and then heal without leaving a scar. Some other symptoms that may go with the first episode of genital herpes are fever, headache, muscle aches, painful or difficult urination, vaginal discharge, and swollen glands in the groin area.

## Will I Ever Have Outbreaks Again?

If you have been infected by HSV 1 and/or 2, you will probably have symptoms or outbreaks from time to time. After the virus has finished being active, it then travels to the nerves at the end of the spine where it stays for a while. Even after the sores are gone, the virus stays inside the nerve cells in a still and hidden state, which means that it's inactive.

In most people, the virus can become active several times a year. This is called a recurrence. But scientists do not yet know why this happens. When it becomes active again, it travels along the nerves to the skin, where it busies itself by making more viruses near the site of the very first infection. That is where new sores usually will appear.

Sometimes, the virus can become active but not cause any sores that can be seen. At these times, small amounts of the virus may be shed at or near places of the first infection, in fluids from the mouth, penis, or vagina, or from barely noticeable sores. You may not notice this shedding because it often does not cause any pain or feel uncomfortable. Even though you might not be aware of the shedding, you still can infect a sex partner during this time.

After the first outbreak, any future outbreaks are usually mild and last only about a week. An infected person may know that an outbreak is about to happen by feeling a tingling feeling or itching in the genital area, or pain in the buttocks or down the leg. For some people, these early symptoms can be the most painful and annoying part of an episode. Sometimes, only the tingling and itching are present and no visible sores develop. At other times, blisters appear that may be very small and barely noticeable, or they may break into open sores that crust over and then disappear.

The frequency and severity of the recurrent episodes vary greatly. While some people have only one or two outbreaks in a lifetime, others may have several outbreaks a year. The number and pattern of repeat outbreaks often change over time for a person. Scientists do not know what causes the virus to become active again. Although some people with herpes report that their outbreaks are brought on by another illness, stress, or having a menstrual period, outbreaks often are not predictable. In some cases, outbreaks may be connected to exposure to sunlight.

## How Does the Doctor Diagnose Genital Herpes?

Because the genital herpes sores may not be visible to the naked eye, a doctor or other health care worker may have to do several laboratory tests to try to prove that any other symptoms are caused by the herpes virus. A person may still have genital herpes, however, even if the laboratory tests don't show the virus in the body.

A blood test cannot show whether a person can infect another person with the herpes virus. A blood test, however, can show if a person has been infected at any time with HSV. There are also newer blood tests that can tell whether a person has been infected with HSV 1 and/or 2.

## *What Is the Treatment?*

Although there is no cure for genital herpes, your doctor might prescribe one of three medicines to treat it:

- Acyclovir (Zovirax®) treats the first and/or later episodes of genital herpes.

- Famciclovir (Famvir®) treats later episodes of genital herpes and helps prevent future outbreaks.

- Valacyclovir (Valtrex®) treats later episodes of genital herpes.

During an active herpes episode, whether the first episode or a repeat one, you should follow a few simple steps to speed healing and avoid spreading the infection to other places on the body or to other people:

- Keep the infected area clean and dry to prevent other infections from developing.

- Try to avoid touching the sores.

- Wash your hands after contact with the sores.

- Avoid sexual contact from the time you first feel any symptoms until the sores are completely healed, that is, the scab has fallen off and new skin has formed where the sore was.

## *Can Genital Herpes Cause Any Other Problems?*

Usually, genital herpes infections do not cause major problems in healthy adults. In some people whose immune systems do not work properly, genital herpes episodes can last a long time and be unusually severe. (The body's immune system fights off foreign invaders such as viruses.)

If a woman has her first episode of genital herpes while she is pregnant, she can pass the virus to her unborn child and may deliver a premature baby. Half of the babies infected with herpes either die or suffer from damage to their nerves. A baby born with herpes can develop serious problems that may affect the brain, the skin, or the eyes. If babies born with herpes are treated immediately with acyclovir, their chances of being healthy are increased. Therefore, if you are pregnant and infected with genital herpes, you should stay in close touch with your doctor before, during, and after your baby is born.

If a pregnant woman has an outbreak and it is not the first one, her baby's risk of being infected during delivery is very low.

If a woman is having an outbreak during labor and delivery and there are herpes lesions in or near the birth canal, the doctor will do a cesarean section to protect the baby. Most women with genital herpes, however, do not have signs of active infection with the virus during this time, and can have a normal delivery.

## Is Genital Herpes Worse in a Person with AIDS?

Genital herpes, like other genital diseases that produce sores, increases a person's risk of getting HIV, the virus that causes AIDS. Also, prior to better treatments for AIDS, persons with HIV (because of lower protection from their immune systems) had severe herpes outbreaks, which may have helped them pass both genital herpes and HIV infections to others.

## How Can I Protect Myself or My Sexual Partner?

If you have early signs of a herpes outbreak or visible sores, you should not have sexual intercourse or oral sex until the signs are gone and/or the sores have healed completely. Between outbreaks, using condoms during sexual intercourse may offer some protection from the virus.

## Is Any Research Going on?

The National Institute of Allergy and Infectious Diseases (NIAID) supports research on genital herpes and on herpes simplex virus, HSV-1 and HSV-2, the viruses that cause it. Studies are currently under way to develop better treatments for the 67 million people who suffer from genital herpes. While some scientists are carrying out clinical trials to determine the best way to use existing drugs, others are studying the biology of herpes simplex virus. NIAID intramural scientists have identified certain genes and enzymes that the virus needs to survive. They are hopeful that drugs aimed at disrupting these viral targets might lead to the design of more effective therapies.

Meanwhile, other researchers are devising methods to control the virus's spread. Two important means of preventing HSV infection are vaccines and topical microbicides. Several different vaccines are in various stages of development. These include vaccines made from proteins on the HSV cell surface, peptides or chains of amino acids that present important targets to the immune system, and the DNA of the virus itself. Topical microbicides, preparations containing microbe-killing compounds, are also in various stages of development and testing. These include gels, creams, or lotions that a woman could insert into the vagina prior to intercourse to prevent infection in both herself and her partner.

### Where Can I Get Help If I'm Upset about Having Herpes or I Have an Infected Partner?

Genital herpes outbreaks can be distressing, inconvenient, and sometimes painful. Concern about transmitting the disease to others and disruption of sexual relations during outbreaks can affect personal relationships. If you or your partner has genital herpes, you can learn to cope with and treat the disease effectively by getting proper counseling and medicine and by using preventive measures as mentioned above.

## Section 30.7

# Crabs, Scabies, and Other STDs

Reprinted from "Other Important STDs," National Institute of Allergy and Infectious Diseases, June 1998, http://www.niaid.nih.gov/factsheets/stdother.htm. Reviewed by David A. Cooke, M.D., June 29, 2003.

Although some of these diseases are less well-known in the United States than other STDs, they are still important—some are especially significant for pregnant women. Many of these infections are of serious concern for people in other parts of the world, particularly in developing countries.

### Chancroid

Chancroid ("shan-kroid") is an important bacterial infection caused by *Haemophilus ducreyi*, which is spread by sexual contact. Periodic outbreaks of chancroid have occurred in the United States, the last one being in the late 1980s. These outbreaks are usually seen in minority populations in the inner cities, especially in the southern and eastern portion of the country. Globally, this disease is common in sub-Saharan Africa among men who have frequent contact with prostitutes.

The infection begins with the appearance of painful open sores on the genitals, sometimes accompanied by swollen, tender lymph nodes in the groin. These symptoms occur within a week after exposure. Symptoms in women are often less noticeable and may be limited to painful urination or defecation, painful intercourse, rectal bleeding, or vaginal discharge. Chancroid lesions may be difficult to distinguish from ulcers caused by genital herpes or syphilis. A physician must therefore diagnose the infection by excluding other diseases with similar symptoms. People with chancroid can be treated effectively with one of several antibiotics. Chancroid is one of the genital ulcer diseases that may be associated with an increased risk of transmission of the human immunodeficiency virus (HIV), the cause of AIDS.

## Cytomegalovirus Infections

Cytomegalovirus (CMV) is a very common virus that infects approximately one-half of all young adults in the United States. It rarely causes serious consequences except in people with suppressed or impaired immune systems or in infants, whose immune systems are still developing. The virus, a member of the herpesvirus family, is found in saliva, urine, and other bodily fluids. Because it is often found in semen as well as in cervical secretions, the virus can be spread by sexual contact; it also can be easily spread by other forms of physical contact such as kissing. Day-care center staff for children under the age of three are at increased risk of CMV infection and should carefully wash their hands after changing diapers. Like other herpesvirus infections, CMV is incurable; people are infected with it for life. Although the virus usually remains in an inactive state, it can reactivate from time to time.

### Symptoms

In healthy adults, CMV usually produces no symptoms of infection. Occasionally, however, mild symptoms of swollen lymph glands, fever, and fatigue may occur. These symptoms may be similar to those of infectious mononucleosis.

## Diagnosis

The ELISA (enzyme-linked immunosorbent assay) test is commonly used to detect levels of antibodies (disease-fighting proteins of the immune system) in the blood. A number of other blood tests can suggest a diagnosis of CMV infection, but no blood test can reliably diagnose it. Although CMV can be isolated from urine or other body fluids, it may be excreted months or years after an infection; therefore, isolation of the virus from these fluids is not a reliable method of diagnosing recent infection.

## Complications

Babies can be infected with CMV in the uterus if their mothers become infected with the virus or develop a recurrence of a previous infection during pregnancy. Although most babies infected with CMV before birth do not develop any symptoms, CMV is the leading cause of congenital infection in the United States. An estimated 6,000 babies each year develop life-threatening complications of congenital CMV infection at birth or suffer serious consequences later in life, including mental retardation, blindness, deafness, or epilepsy. Investigators supported by NIAID are currently studying how the virus interferes with normal fetal development and at which stages the fetus is most susceptible to infection. Congenital CMV is the most common cause of progressive deafness in children.

When CMV is acquired after birth, or if it reactivates, it can be life-threatening for persons with suppressed immune systems, such as those receiving chemotherapy or persons who have received immunosuppressant drugs for organ transplantation. Persons with HIV infection or AIDS may develop severe CMV infections, including CMV retinitis, an eye disease that can lead to blindness.

## Treatment

NIAID scientists are testing new antiviral drugs that might be effective against CMV infections. The antiviral drugs foscarnet and ganciclovir have been approved for treating people with AIDS-associated CMV retinitis.

## Prevention

There is no intervention to prevent CMV. Use of the male condom may reduce risk, although virus in the saliva would be transmitted by kissing or oral intercourse. Some experts believe that primary or first-time exposure during pregnancy is a major cause of CMV infection in newborns. Infants infected before or just after birth are likely to be shedding CMV in saliva and urine, which can infect others. Handwashing and proper handling of diapers may reduce risk. Scientists are working to develop a vaccine and other methods to provide immunity to CMV and offer protection against severe disease.

## Molluscum Contagiosum

This common viral infection most often affects young children, who pass it to each other through saliva. In adults, however, the virus is transmitted sexually, resulting in lesions on the genitals, lower abdomen, buttocks, or inner thighs. Most people with the infection do not have noticeable symptoms, although sometimes the lesions, which are painless wart-like bumps, may itch or become irritated. The lesions often heal without treatment, although physicians may sometimes scrape them off or treat them with chemical irritants.

## Pubic Lice

Pubic lice (pediculosis pubis, or crab lice) are very tiny insects that infest the pubic hair and survive by feeding on human blood. These parasites are most often spread by sexual contact; in a few cases, they may be picked up through contact with infested bedding or clothing. An estimated 3 million people with new cases of the infestation are treated each year in the United States.

### Symptoms

The primary symptom of infestation is itching in the pubic area. Scratching may spread the lice to other parts of the body; thus, every effort should be made to avoid touching the infected area, although this may be difficult.

### Diagnosis

Pubic lice are diagnosed easily because they are visible to the naked eye. They are pinhead size, oval in shape, and grayish, but appear reddish-brown when full of blood from their host. Nits, the tiny white eggs, also are visible and usually are observed clinging to the base of pubic hair.

## Treatment

Lotions and shampoos that will kill pubic lice are available both over the counter and by prescription. Creams or lotions containing lindane, a powerful pesticide, are most frequently prescribed for the treatment of pubic lice. Pregnant women may be advised not to use this drug, and a physician's recommendations for use in infants and small children should be followed carefully. Itching may persist even after the lice have been eradicated. This is because the skin has been irritated and requires time to heal. A soothing lotion such as calamine may offer temporary relief.

## Prevention

All persons with whom an infested individual has come into close contact, including family and close friends as well as sex partners, should be treated to ensure that the lice have been eliminated. In addition, all clothing and bedding should be dry-cleaned or washed in very hot water (125° F), dried at a high setting, and ironed to rid them of any lice. Pubic lice die within 24 hours of being separated from the body. Because the eggs may live up to six days, it is important to apply the treatment for the full time recommended.

## Scabies

Scabies is a skin infestation with a tiny mite, *Sarcoptes scabiei*. Scabies has become relatively common throughout the general population. It is highly contagious and is spread primarily through sexual contact, although it also is commonly transmitted by contact with skin, infested sheets, towels, or even furniture.

### Symptoms

Scabies causes intense itching, which often becomes worse at night. Small red bumps or lines appear on the body at sites where the female scabies mite has burrowed into the skin to lay her eggs. The areas most commonly affected include the hands (especially between the fingers), wrists, elbows, lower abdomen, and genitals. The skin reaction may not develop until a month or more after infestation. During this time, a person may pass the disease unknowingly to a sex partner or to another person with whom he or she has close contact.

## Diagnosis

Scabies may be confused with other skin irritations such as poison ivy or eczema. To make an accurate diagnosis, a doctor takes a scraping of the irritated area and examines it under a microscope to reveal the presence of the mite.

## Treatment

As with pubic lice, lindane is an effective treatment for scabies. Pregnant women should consult a doctor before using this product. Nonprescription remedies such as sulfur ointment also are available. Sulfur is fairly effective but may be objectionable because of its odor and messiness. Itching can persist even after the infestation has been eliminated because of lingering skin irritation. A hydrocortisone cream or ointment or a soothing lotion may provide relief from itching.

## Prevention

Family members and sex partners of a person with scabies are advised to undergo treatment. Twenty-four hours after drug therapy, a person with scabies infestation is no longer contagious to others, even though the skin irritation may persist for some time. As with pubic lice, special care must be taken to rid clothing and bedding of any mites.

## Human T-Cell Lymphotropic Virus

The human T-cell lymphotropic viruses (retroviruses), HTLV-I and HTLV-II, are uncommon in the general U.S. population. They appear to be most prevalent among IV drug users and persons who have multiple sex partners, genital ulcers, or a history of syphilis. The virus can be transmitted by blood or intimate sexual contact, and can be passed from mother to child during pregnancy and through breast milk.

Most infected persons remain healthy carriers of the virus. In rare cases, however, HTLV-I can cause adult T-cell leukemia/lymphoma (ATL), a rare and aggressive cancer of the blood. Infected persons also may develop myelopathy, a neurologic disorder that affects the muscles in the legs. In addition, researchers think that HTLV-I plays a role in the development of B-cell chronic lymphocytic leukemia. HTLV-II can cause another rare cancer called hairy-cell leukemia. Because the chances of curing ATL rely on early detection, scientists are studying protein in the blood of HTLV-I-infected persons that may help predict who will develop the disease.

Blood donations are screened routinely for HTLV-I. Because lab tests cannot easily distinguish between HTLV-I and HTLV-II, experts believe many cases of HTLV-II are eliminated from the blood supply as well.

## Research

STD research that is supported and conducted by NIAID will help in the search for new ways to diagnose, treat, and prevent these infections. This is important not only for the well-being of our adult population but also for the health of future generations.

# Chapter 31

# *Preventing the Spread of STDs*

## *What are STDs?*

STDs are diseases that are usually passed through sexual contact with an infected partner. STDs include many diseases, such as AIDS/HIV, chlamydia, gonorrhea, genital herpes, genital warts, and syphilis. STDs are widespread; more than 12 million people in the U.S. are infected each year.

## *Why should I learn about STDs?*

STDs are a danger to everyone who has sex, even *once*. Unborn children are at risk, too. If left untreated, STDs can have serious side effects, including:

- Sterility (being unable to have a child)
- Brain damage
- Heart disease
- Birth defects
- Increased risk for some types of cancer
- Death

Reprinted with permission from the New York City Department of Health and Mental Hygiene Sexually Transmitted Disease Control Program, updated July 2003.

All STDs can be prevented and most can be cured. But first, you need to know the facts.

### *How are STDs spread?*

STDs are spread through contact with:

- Infected body fluids, such as blood, vaginal secretions, or semen
- Infected skin or mucous membranes—for example, sores in the mouth

Activities that expose you to infected body fluids or skin include:

- Vaginal, anal, or oral sex *without* proper use of a latex condom. Anal sex is especially risky because it often causes bleeding.
- Sharing needles or syringes for drug use, ear piercing, tattooing, etc.

Having an STD may increase your risk of getting HIV. Certain STDs cause sores. These sores may provide a way for the HIV virus to get into the body.

Most activities don't spread STDs!

You cannot get an STD from everyday, nonsexual activities, such as:

- Giving blood
- Sitting next to an infected person
- Sitting on toilet seats
- Sharing eating utensils
- Touching doorknobs
- Using swimming pools

### *How can you avoid STDs?*

There are safe alternatives to vaginal, anal, or oral sex. For example:

- Don't have sex. Abstinence is the only sure way to avoid getting an STD.
- Masturbation. Masturbation with your partner (on unbroken skin), or alone, can provide sexual pleasure safely.

- Massage. Caressing and stroking can express affection and give pleasure.

- Kissing. This can be a safe way to be physically close, as long as both partners are free of cuts and sores in the mouth.

- Fantasy. The brain is one of the most powerful sex organs. Use your imagination for satisfying sexual pleasure.

If you have sex, have sex only with one partner who:

- Has sex with you only (monogamy)
- Has never injected drugs

If you are not in a monogamous relationship, be sure to:

- Use latex condoms. Condoms are your best protection from STDs during intercourse. But remember, even condoms are not 100 percent effective.

- Limit the number of partners you have. The more partners you have, the greater the risk of being exposed to an STD. Remember, you can't tell if someone has an STD just by looking at him or her.

- Have regular physical exams. Ask you physician to test for STDs if you think you've been exposed. Regular tests help find STDs early, when treatment can be most effective.

Condoms help protect both partners from STDs and unwanted pregnancy. To use a condom properly, you'll need:

- A latex condom ("rubber"). The HIV virus and other STDs may pass through "natural" or "skin" condoms.

- A spermicide. Note: Results of a recent study indicated that nonoxynol-9(N-9) did not protect against HIV infection and may have in fact caused more transmission. While the NYC Department of Health awaits the Center for Diseases Control's reevaluation regarding the use of N-9 lubricated condoms, we recommend the following: Individuals engaging in sexual activity where bodily fluids may be exchanged should use condoms (whether or not they are lubricated with nonoxynol-9) as an effective means of reducing the risk of HIV transmission. To prevent breakage, condoms should be used with a water-based lubricant.

401

- A water-based lubricant. This helps keep the condom from breaking. Never use products that contain oil or fat, like petroleum jelly or cooking oil. These products weaken latex and may cause the condom to break.

- A new condom. Use one every time you have sex, even oral or anal. Discard any "new" condom that's damaged, sticky, or brittle.

To use condoms correctly:

- Put the condom on *before* any sexual contact. Put a drop of spermicide in the tip of the condom.

- Leave a 1/2-inch space at the tip to collect semen. Cover the penis completely.

- Smooth out any air bubbles to reduce stress on the condom and to increase feeling. Apply spermicide to the outside of the condom.

- Check the condom during sex to make sure it's unbroken and still on properly.

- Withdraw slowly right after climax. Hold the condom by its base so it doesn't slip off. Dispose of properly.

To help further reduce the risk of contracting an STD:

- Don't inject drugs. Sharing needles or syringes can expose you to infected blood. Not injecting drugs is an essential part of protecting yourself from STDs.

- Avoid alcohol and other drugs. They can make you more likely to take chances when having sex.

- Don't douche. You may force germs farther into the vagina.

- Urinate after sex. For women, this can help reduce the risk of getting a bladder infection called cystitis. Urinating after sex does *not* replace the need to use a condom.

The symptoms of STDs may include:

- Sores or blisters on or around the sex organs or mouth
- Pain or burning during urination
- Discharge from the penis or vagina that smells or looks unusual

- Itching, swelling, or pain in or around the sex organs

Get tested right away by a physician or STD clinic if you think you have any symptoms, or think you've been exposed to an STD (even if you don't have any of the symptoms). Remember, many STDs don't have any symptoms, especially in women.

If you have an STD, start proper medical treatment immediately. Home remedies don't work.

If you have an STD, be sure to:

- Talk to all sex partner(s) who may have been exposed. Encourage them to get tested. Both partners need to be treated to avoid reinfection.

- Avoid sexual intercourse until your physician says it's okay so you don't get reinfected or spread the disease to others.

- Follow your treatment plan and finish all medications, even if you feel well. Follow-up exams can make sure treatment was effective.

- Get counseling if you're worried or upset about having an STD. Your physician or STD clinic can recommend a counselor.

### What other types of birth control help protect against STDs?

Only latex condoms are considered effective protection against STDs. Birth control pills, diaphragms, sponges, and other contraceptives do not prevent STDs.

### A lot of men carry condoms in their wallets. Is this a good idea?

No. Exposure to body heat, sunlight, and extreme cold can all damage condoms and make them more likely to break.

### Once I've had an STD, I can't get it again, can I?

You *can* get the same STD again if you have sex without a latex condom. You can also have more than one STD at a time.

Chapter 32

# Family Planning

## Chapter Contents

# Section 32.1

# *The Truth about Condoms*

Reprinted with permission of SIECUS, the Sexuality Information and Education Council of the United States (SIECUS). © 2002 SIECUS. For additional information, visit http://www.siecus.org or contact SIECUS at 130 West 42nd Street, Suite 350, New York, NY 10036-7802; phone: 212-819-9770; fax: 212-819-9776; e-mail: siecus@siecus.org.

Condoms are a barrier method of contraception that, when used consistently and correctly, can prevent pregnancy by blocking the passage of semen into the vaginal canal. Condoms can also prevent the exchange of blood, semen, and vaginal secretions, which are the primary routes for the spread of sexually transmitted diseases (STDs).

In recent years, as a result of misinformation and insufficient research, the efficacy of condoms, especially in terms of STD prevention, has been debated in many forums. Research continues to show that condoms are one of the best methods of preventing unwanted pregnancy and are one of the only methods for sexually active individuals to protect themselves against STDs, including HIV.

This updated chapter includes information on both the male and female condom; on their effectiveness in protecting against unplanned pregnancies and STDs, including HIV; and on condom breakage and slippage, regulations and tests, and consistent and correct use.

This chapter is designed to provide the most recent information about condoms and to clear up confusion and misunderstandings.

## Male Condom

The male condom is a barrier method of contraception that is placed over the glans and shaft of the penis. Male condoms are available in latex, lambskin, and polyurethane.

Condoms manufactured from latex are the most popular, and studies conducted on the ability of condoms to prevent the transmission of STDs and HIV most often involve latex condoms. Condoms manufactured from lambskin, also known as "natural skin," or "natural membrane," are made from the intestinal lining of lambs. While these condoms can prevent pregnancy, they contain small pores that may permit passage of some STDs, including HIV, the hepatitis B virus, and the herpes simplex virus.

Condoms manufactured from polyurethane are thinner and stronger than latex condoms, provide a less constricting fit, are more resistant to deterioration, and may enhance sensitivity. Polyurethane condoms are also recommended for those who have latex allergies. Polyurethane condoms have not been studied for their effectiveness in the prevention of STD transmission. In addition, condoms made of polyurethane are compatible with oil-based lubricants, unlike latex condoms which must be used with water-based lubricants.

## Female Condom

Available under the brand name Reality®, the female condom is made of polyurethane and provides protection against pregnancy and STDs, including HIV. It consists of a tube-like sheath with one flexible polyurethane ring at each end. One ring is placed inside the vaginal canal and is closed off by polyurethane, collecting the ejaculate. The other ring remains outside the vagina, and the penis enters the vagina through this ring. The female condom is coated with a silicone-based lubricant. Additional lubricant can be added as necessary. The female and male condom should not be used together as they can adhere to each other, causing slippage or displacement.

Facts in brief:

- The first-year effectiveness rate of preventing pregnancy among typical condom users averages about 79 percent for female (Reality®) condoms. This includes pregnancies resulting from errors in condom use.

- The female condom Reality® is estimated to reduce the risk of HIV infection for each act of intercourse by 97.1 percent when used consistently and correctly.

- Laboratory studies have shown Reality® to be an effective barrier to microorganisms including HIV and a bacteriophage smaller than hepatitis B, the smallest virus known to cause an STD.

## Pregnancy Prevention

Studies have shown that condoms are one of the most reliable methods for preventing unwanted pregnancy. In addition to being effective, condoms are also inexpensive and are available without a prescription.

Facts in brief:

* Condoms are 98 percent effective in preventing pregnancy when used consistently and correctly.

* The first-year effectiveness rate in preventing pregnancy among typical condom users on average is 86 percent. This includes pregnancies resulting from errors in condom use.

## Condoms and Pregnancy: Understanding Condom Effectiveness

To fully understand research on condom effectiveness, one must understand the difference between method failure and user failure. Method failure refers to failure that results from a defect in the product. User failure refers to failure that results from incorrect or inconsistent use. In its fact sheet on condoms, the U.S. Centers for Disease Control and Prevention explains that the term condom failure often imprecisely refers to the percentage of women who become pregnant over the course of a year in which they reported using condoms as their primary method of birth control—even if they did not use condoms every time they had intercourse. The CDC concluded that "clearly these statistics don't report condom failure but user failure."

Method failure of male condoms is uncommon. In fact, it is estimated to occur among only 3 percent of couples using condoms consistently and correctly during the first year of use. To help individuals understand this estimate, Contraceptive Technology explains that "only three of 100 couples who use condoms perfectly for one year will experience an unintended pregnancy."

It goes on to say that "if each [of these 100 couples] had intercourse at the average coital frequency of 83 acts per year, then 100 couples would have intercourse a combined 8,300 times a year. Three pregnancies resulting from 8,300 acts of condom use is a remarkably low pregnancy rate (.04 percent) when calculated on a per-condom basis."

In truth, condom failures are most often caused by errors in use, "most notably the failure of couples to use condoms during every act of sexual intercourse." It is therefore important to look at the data on typical condom use or user failure.

Among those couples using condoms as their primary method of contraception, approximately 14 percent will experience an unintended pregnancy during the first year. It is important to remember that they may not have used a condom or may have used one incorrectly during the act of intercourse that resulted in pregnancy.

To put this in perspective, individuals need to understand that 85 percent of women using no method of birth control will become pregnant in the first year, as will 25 percent of women using periodic abstinence.

## HIV Prevention

Latex condoms, when used consistently and correctly, are highly effective in preventing transmission of HIV, the virus that causes AIDS. Facts in brief:

- Using a latex condom to prevent transmission of HIV is more than 10,000 times safer than not using a condom.

- A study published in *The New England Journal of Medicine* observed heterosexual couples where one was HIV-positive and the other was HIV-negative, for an average of 20 months. (These couples are referred to as sero-discordant.) Findings included:

  - No sero-conversion occurred among the 124 couples who used latex condoms consistently and correctly for vaginal or anal intercourse.

  - Ten percent of the HIV-negative partners (12 of 121) of couples became infected when condoms were used inconsistently for vaginal or anal intercourse. In contrast, 15 percent of HIV-negative partners became infected when condoms were not used.

- A study published in *The Journal of Acquired Immune Deficiency Syndromes* observed sero-discordant heterosexual couples and showed that only three out of 171 who consistently and correctly used condoms became HIV infected; eight out of 55 who used condoms inconsistently became HIV infected; and eight out of 79 who never used condoms became HIV infected.

## Update on Nonoxynol-9

In the past, public health experts recommended using condoms combined with Nonoxynol-9 (N-9), a spermicide, for increased protection against pregnancy, HIV, and STDs. Two recent studies, however, call into question the effectiveness and safety of N-9.

A study published by UNAIDS found that N-9 used without condoms was ineffective against HIV transmission. This study actually showed some evidence that N-9 increased the risk of HIV-infection.

Researchers note that this study was conducted among commercial sex workers in Africa who are at increased risk and used a N-9 gel on a frequent basis. The adverse affects might not be seen at the same level among women who are using N-9 less frequently or in a different formulation.

As a result of this study, however, the CDC concluded that "given that N-9 has been proven ineffective against HIV transmission, the possibility of risk, with no benefit, indicates that N-9 should not be recommended as an effective means of HIV-prevention."

A similar study published in the *Journal of the American Medical Association* found that N-9, when used with condoms, did not protect women from the bacteria that causes gonorrhea and chlamydial infection any better than condoms used alone.

## STD Prevention

Condoms can be expected to provide different levels of risk reduction for different STDs. There is no definitive study about condom effectiveness for all STDs. Definitive data are lacking on the degree of risk reduction that latex condoms provide for some STDs; for others, the evidence is considered inconclusive.

The U.S. Centers for Disease Control and Prevention (CDC) states, "It is important to note that the lack of data about the level of condom effectiveness indicates that more research is needed—not that latex condoms do not work."

Facts in brief:

- Several studies have demonstrated that condoms can protect against the transmission of chlamydia, gonorrhea, and trichomoniasis, and may protect against genital herpes and syphilis.

## Condom Breakage and Slippage

Although people fear that condoms may break or fall off during use, studies indicate this rarely occurs when condoms are properly used. It is also important to note that not all condom breaks are equally risky. As many as 24 to 65 percent occur before intercourse and pose no biological risk of pregnancy or infection if a new condom is used for intercourse.

Facts in brief:

- A study published in the *American Journal of Public Health* observed female sex workers in Nevada brothels, where condom use is required by law, and found that of 353 condoms used by the sex workers during the study, none broke or fell off during intercourse, and only two (0.6 percent) slipped off during withdrawal.

• Studies have reported breakage rates during vaginal intercourse ranging from zero percent to 6.7 percent. Most studies report that condoms break less than 2 percent of the time during intercourse or withdrawal.

• Condoms fall off the penis in 0.6 percent to 5.4 percent acts of vaginal intercourse and may slip down the penis without falling off in 3.4 percent to 13.1 percent of acts of vaginal intercourse.

• Breakage rates during anal sex for gay men in four prospective studies ranged from 0.5 percent to 12 percent, with rates less than 2 percent in three of the studies.

## Condom Use

Research shows that consistent condom use among sexually active individuals has increased.

Facts in brief:

• In 2001, the Centers for Disease Control and Prevention Youth Risk Behavior Surveillance Summaries found that among currently sexually active students in grades nine through 12 nationwide, 57.9 percent reported that either they or their partner had used a condom during last sexual intercourse compared to 58.0 percent in 1999, 56.8 percent in 1997, 54.4 percent in 1995, and 52.8 percent in 1993.

• The National Survey of Family Growth reported that 20 percent of American women 15 to 44 years of age reported using a condom in 1995 compared to 15 percent in 1988 and 12 percent in 1982.

## Consistent and Correct Condom Use

In order to benefit from the protection that condoms provide, individuals must use them consistently and correctly. This means they must use a condom with every act of sexual intercourse, from start to finish, including penile-vaginal intercourse as well as oral and anal intercourse. In addition, individuals must understand how to properly use a condom. Studies of hundreds of couples show that consistent condom use is possible when sexual partners have the skills and motivation to use them.

### *Correct Use of the Male Condom*

- Store condoms in a cool place out of direct sunlight (not in wallets or glove compartments). Latex will become brittle from changes in temperature, rough handling, or age. Don't use damaged, discolored, brittle, or sticky condoms.

- Check the expiration date.

- Carefully open the condom package; teeth or fingernails can tear the condom.

- Use a new condom for each act of sexual intercourse.

- Put on the condom before it touches any part of a partner's body.

- Hold the condom over an erect penis.

- If a penis is uncircumcised, pull back the foreskin before putting on the condom.

- Put on the condom by pinching the reservoir tip and unrolling it all the way down the shaft of the penis from head to base. If the condom does not have a reservoir tip, pinch it to leave a half-inch space at the head of the penis for semen to collect after ejaculation.

- In the event that the condom breaks, withdraw the penis immediately and put on a new condom before resuming intercourse.

- Use only water-based lubrication. Do not use oil-based lubricants such as cooking/vegetable oil, baby oil, hand lotion, or petroleum jelly—these will cause the condom to deteriorate and break.

- Withdraw the penis immediately after ejaculation. While the penis is still erect, grasp the rim of the condom between the fingers and slowly withdraw the penis (with the condom still on) so that no semen is spilled.

- Remove the condom, making certain that no semen is spilled.

- Carefully dispose of the condom. Do not reuse it.

- Do not use a male condom along with a female condom. If the two condoms rub together, the friction between them can cause the male condom to be pulled off or the female condom to be pushed in.

### Correct Use of the Female Condom

- Do not use damaged, discolored, brittle, or sticky condoms.

- Check the expiration date.

- Carefully open the condom package—teeth or fingernails can tear the condom.

- Use a new condom for each act of sexual intercourse.

- First, inspect the condom and make certain it is completely lubricated on the outside and the inside.

- The female condom is inserted into the vagina with fingers, much like a tampon that has no applicator. To do so:

  - Hold the condom at the closed end and squeeze the flexible inner ring with thumb and middle finger so it becomes long and narrow. With the other hand, separate the outer lips of the vagina.

  - Gently insert the inner ring end as far into the vagina as possible, using the index finger to push up the inner ring until the finger reaches the cervix (similar to how a diaphragm would be inserted).

  - Before having intercourse, make certain the condom is in place. When in place, it will cover the opening of the cervix and line the vaginal walls. A general indicator of correct insertion is that the individual will no longer feel the ring. The open end of the condom must always remain outside the vaginal opening. Before having intercourse, make certain that the condom is straight and not twisted.

  - Add water-based lubricant onto the penis and/or the inside of the female condom to increase comfort and decrease noise. It is important to use enough lubricant so that the condom stays in place during sex. If the condom is pulled out or pushed in, that is an indicator that there is not enough lubricant.

  - Be sure that the penis is not entering the vaginal canal outside of the condom before intercourse.

- To remove the condom, twist the outer ring and gently pull the condom out to avoid any spillage.

413

- Carefully dispose of the condom. Do not reuse it.

- Do not use a male condom along with a female condom. If the two condoms rub together, the friction between them can cause the male condom to be pulled off or the female condom to be pushed in.

## Regulations and Tests

The U.S. Food and Drug Administration (FDA) regulates manufacturers who sell condoms in the United States.

As a quality assurance step, condom manufacturers sample each lot of finished packaged condoms and examine them for holes using a water leak test. The FDA recognizes domestic and international standards that specify that the rate of sampled condoms failing the water leak test, for each manufactured lot of condoms, must be less than one in 400.

Manufacturers also test lots for physical properties using the air burst test and the tensile (strength) property test.

In order to test condoms' ability to prevent the passage of viruses, FDA researchers developed a test using high concentrations of a laboratory created "virus" that is the same size as STD pathogens.

They tested many different types of male condoms and showed that they are highly effective barriers to virus passage with a very small chance of leakage. Intact condoms (those that pass the water leak test) are essentially impermeable to particles the size of STD pathogens. Moreover, these studies show that fluid flow, not virus size, is the most important determinant of viral passage through a hole.

# Section 32.2

# *Vasectomy*

The decision to proceed with a vasectomy is a very personal one. So it is important that you have a clear understanding of what a vasectomy is and what it is not. The following will provide you with information that will assist you in deciding whether or not a vasectomy is an appropriate form of contraception for you.

### *What happens under normal conditions?*

The testicles produce sperm and testosterone and are located in the scrotum at the base of the penis. Once produced, the sperm exit the testicle through a delicate, coiled tube called the epididymis, where they stay until they are fully matured. Each epididymis is connected to the prostate by a tube called the vas deferens. This muscular tube generally extends from the lower portion of the scrotum into the inguinal canal (site of most hernias) and then into the pelvis continuing behind the bladder. It is at this point that the vas deferens joins with the seminal vesicles and forms the ejaculatory duct. During ejaculation, seminal fluid produced by the prostate mixes with sperm to form semen.

### *What is a vasectomy?*

A vasectomy is a minor surgical procedure designed to interrupt the sperm transportation system between the testicle and the penis.

### *How is a vasectomy performed?*

In general, vasectomies are performed in the urologist's office. However, the procedure may be done at an ambulatory surgery center or in a hospital setting if the patient and urologist have determined that intravenous sedation is preferable. The decision to proceed in that type of setting may be based upon the patient's anatomy, anxiety, or the need for associated surgical procedures.

On the day of the procedure, the patient will be asked to sign a surgical consent form. Certain states have regulations regarding the type and timing of the surgical consent for permanent sterilization.

Once the patient has signed the consent form and has been brought into the procedure room, his scrotal area will be shaved. Some urologists will have the patient shave this area at home. The area will then be washed with an antiseptic solution. Local anesthesia will be injected to numb the area but the patient will be aware of touch, tension, and movement during the procedure. However, the local anesthetic should eliminate any sharp pain. The patient is awake during the procedure so, if necessary, he can let the urologist know if he is experiencing pain so more local anesthesia can be given.

With a conventional vasectomy, a urologist makes one or two small cuts in the skin of the scrotum. The vas deferens is cut, and a small piece may be removed, leaving a short gap between the two remaining ends. Next, the urologist ties the cut ends with suture material and closes up the scrotal incision with dissolvable stitches. The entire procedure is then repeated on the other side.

During a no-scalpel vasectomy, the urologist feels for the vas under the skin of the scrotum and holds it in place with a small clamp. A special instrument is then used to make a tiny puncture in the skin and stretch the opening so the vas deferens can gently be lifted out, cut, then tied or cauterized and put back in place.

## What should the patient expect after a vasectomy?

Your urologist should provide you with specific recommendations for your care after a vasectomy. It is generally wise to return home immediately after the procedure and avoid strenuous or sexual activity. Swelling and discomfort can be minimized by placing an ice pack on the scrotum. Most patients can expect to recover completely in less than a week, and many are able to return to their job as early as a day after the procedure. Sexual activity can usually be resumed within a few days following a vasectomy. However, it is important that all patients recognize that a vasectomy, even though successful, is not effective immediately. The effectiveness of the vasectomy must be proven by having the patient submit at least one semen analysis, which demonstrates that there are no sperm in the ejaculate. The time until disappearance of sperm from the ejaculate varies from patient to patient. Most urologists do not recommend checking the semen for sperm for at least two months or 12 ejaculates, whichever comes first. If sperm continue to be present in the ejaculate, that patient must continue to use contraception. The patient should not assume that the vasectomy is effective until semen analysis demonstrates the absence of sperm.

### *Are there any risks associated with a vasectomy?*

In the immediate postoperative period there is the risk of bleeding into the scrotum. If the patient notices a significant increase in the size of their scrotum or significant scrotal discomfort, he should contact the urologist immediately. A patient experiencing fever, scrotal redness, or tenderness should also be evaluated by the surgeon as this may indicate an infection. Discomfort is usually minimal and should respond to mild analgesics. More severe pain may indicate infection or other complications. Patients will often complain of mild lower abdominal discomfort similar to what one would experience from getting hit in the genitalia. A benign lump or granuloma, may develop because there is a leakage of sperm from the cut end of the vas into the scrotal tissues. It may occasionally be painful or sensitive to touch or pressure. Postvasectomy pain syndrome is a chronic pain syndrome that follows vasectomy. The cause of this syndrome and its incidence are unclear. It is generally treated with anti-inflammatory agents. Occasionally, patients will elect to undergo vasectomy reversal in an attempt to alleviate this syndrome. Unfortunately, the response to surgical intervention is unpredictable. Lately, there has been some debate as to whether vasectomies predispose a man to any future health problems. However, there is no conclusive evidence that men who have undergone a vasectomy have a higher risk of cardiovascular disease, prostate cancer, testicular cancer, or other health problems.

### *Can my partner tell if I have had a vasectomy?*

There is no significant change in one's ejaculate after a vasectomy since the sperm contributes a small amount to the overall ejaculate volume. Your partner may on occasion be able to feel the vasectomy site. This is particularly true if you have developed a granuloma.

### *Will my sense of orgasm be altered by having a vasectomy?*

Ejaculation and orgasm are generally not affected by vasectomy. The only exception to this is the occasional patient who has developed postvasectomy pain syndrome.

### Can I become impotent after a vasectomy?

An uncomplicated vasectomy cannot cause impotence.

### Can a vasectomy fail?

First, it is important to be certain that a vasectomy has been successful and that all sperm are absent from the ejaculate prior to stopping other forms of contraception. Even if the vasectomy has been demonstrated to be effective, there is a small chance that a vasectomy may fail. This occurs as a result of sperm leaking from one end of the cut vas deferens (the testicular end) and finding a channel to the other end (the abdominal end). Because of this phenomenon, some urologists recommend having a repeat semen analysis on the anniversary of one's vasectomy.

### Can something happen to my testicles?

Rarely, the testicles may be injured during a vasectomy as a result of injury to the testicular artery. Other complications such as a mass of blood (hematoma) or infection may also affect the testicles.

### Can I have children after my vasectomy?

Yes, but if you have not stored frozen sperm, you will require an additional procedure. The vas deferens can be microsurgically reconnected (in a procedure called a vasectomy reversal) to allow normal conception to occur. Alternatively, sperm can be extracted from the testicle or the epididymis and utilized for in vitro fertilization. These procedures are costly and may or may not be covered by insurance. Additionally, they are not successful 100 percent of the time. Therefore, one should carefully consider nonsurgical alternatives prior to deciding to proceed with a vasectomy.

# Section 32.3

## *Vasectomy Reversal*

There are many reasons to reverse a vasectomy like remarriage following a divorce or starting over after the loss of a wife or child. Regardless of your reason, there are now first-rate methods to restore fertility to you. But how do you know the options that are right for you? By arming yourself with the latest information, you can make informed decisions with your doctor.

### *What is a vasectomy reversal?*

A vasectomy reversal restores fertility by reconnecting the severed sperm duct, or vas, which is located on each side of the scrotum. The procedure, which can be accomplished through various approaches, including microsurgery, clears the way for sperm to reach a female egg.

### *What are the different types of vasectomy reversals?*

Reversals are generally performed in an outpatient area of a hospital or ambulatory surgery center setting. The operation may be performed with local, epidural ("saddle block"), spinal, or general anesthesia. The choice will depend on the preference of the surgeon, patient, and anesthesiologist.

Once the patient is anesthetized, the urologist will make small incisions (cuts) on each side of the scrotum and first remove the two scarred ends of the vas at the point of blockage created by the vasectomy. The urologist will then extract a fluid sample from the end closest to the testicle to examine the fluid to see if it contains sperm.

The presence of sperm is an indication that there is no obstruction between the testicle and the location in the tube from which the fluid was obtained, and particularly that there is no blockage in the tube in the epididymis. When sperm are present in the fluid, the passage can be reestablished by reconnecting the ends of the vas. The medical term for reconnecting the ends of the vas is vasovasostomy. This may be accomplished with one of several methods.

If the urologist uses a "modified one-layer" method, he/she actually places a series of tiny stitches through the entire thickness of the vas (from the exterior into the central canal) to join the ends. Once these full thickness stitches are tied, a second set of stitches that only pierce the outer layer of the vas is placed between each adjacent pair of full thickness stitches. The modified one-layer method is used by surgeons who reconnect the ends of the vas without microsurgery, as well as by some surgeons who use microsurgery.

Urologists who use microsurgery believe they can produce better results using high-powered microscopes that magnify structures from five to 20 times their actual size. The scope allows the urologist to manipulate stitches smaller in diameter than an eyelash to join the ends of the vas. The "two-layer" vasovasostomy method, preferred by many urologists who use microsurgical techniques, involves placing six to eight tiny stitches through the inner portion of the vas. Then, another series of stitches is placed through the outer layer of the two cut ends of the vas.

Which vasovasostomy method actually produces better results? Several reports have shown no difference in outcomes between the modified one-layer and two-layer microsurgical methods of vasovasostomy. When microsurgery is used, both methods result in return of sperm to the semen in 75 percent to 97 percent of patients and pregnancy in 30 percent to 75 percent of female partners, depending upon the time from the vasectomy until the reversal (see next section).

If the urologist does not find sperm in the fluid sample, it may be because the original vasectomy created back pressure that caused a break in the tube in the epididymis. Because any break in this single, continuous tube can result in a blockage, the urologist will have to employ a more complicated reversal technique called a vasoepididymostomy. In this procedure, the urologist must bypass the blockage in the epididymis by connecting the upper end of the vas to the tube in the epididymis above the point of the blockage. This approach was formerly performed without magnification.

Surgeons have since improved upon the low success rates of that method with a microsurgical method of vasoepididymostomy. It allows the surgeon actually to see the opening that he or she creates in the tiny tube in the epididymis. The ability to see the opening permits the surgeon to join the inner lining of the vas to the edge of the opening in the tube of the epididymis, and then to stitch the outer layers separately. With this method, 60 percent to 80 percent of patients have sperm return to their semen, and 20 percent to 40 percent of their partners experience a pregnancy.

When performed under appropriate circumstances, vasovasostomy yields better results than vasoepididymostomy. However, you may need a combination of the two techniques, with a vasovasostomy done on one side and a vasoepididymostomy on the other side.

### *What can be expected after a vasectomy reversal?*

Recovery from a vasectomy reversal should be relatively swift and fairly comfortable. Any pain that might be experienced after surgery can be controlled with oral medications. About 50 percent of men experience discomfort that is similar to the level they had after the original vasectomy. Another quarter report less pain than accompanied the vasectomy. A final 25 percent say it is somewhat increased. The reassuring news is that any pain severe enough to require medication rarely lasts longer than a few days to a week.

Most patients are back to normal routine and light work within a week. Urologists usually want their patients to refrain from heavy physical activity for about four weeks. If your job requires strenuous work, you should discuss with your surgeon the earliest time you can return to work. You will be advised to wear a jockstrap for support for several weeks. You will also be restricted from having sex for at least two weeks.

It takes on average one year to conceive after a vasectomy reversal. Some pregnancies occur in the first few months after the reversal procedure, while others do not occur until several years later.

One of the main factors influencing conception is the obstructive interval, which is the duration of time between your original vasectomy and the reversal. As Table 32.1 shows, rates of both return of sperm to semen and subsequent pregnancy are highest when the reversal is performed relatively shortly after the vasectomy.

The urologist will request a semen analysis every two to three months after surgery until your sperm count either stabilizes or pregnancy occurs. Unless a pregnancy occurs, a sperm count is the only way to determine surgical success. While sperm generally appear in the semen within a few months after a vasovasostomy, it may take from three to 15 months after a vasoepididymostomy.

In either case, if the reversal works, the patient should remain fertile for many years. The possibility of subsequent pregnancies is an important advantage of this procedure over sperm retrieval techniques for in vitro fertilization. Only approximately 5 percent of patients who have sperm appear in the semen after a vasectomy reversal later develop scarring in the reconnected area, which could block the passage of sperm again.

**Table 32.1.** Correlation between Time after Vasectomy and Successful Reversal

| Obstructive Interval | Patients with Sperm in Semen | Pregnancies |
|---|---|---|
| Under 3 years | 97% | 76% |
| 3–8 years | 88% | 53% |
| 9–14 years | 79% | 44% |
| 15 years or longer | 71% | 30% |

## Who performs vasectomy reversals?

Urologists are the surgical specialists who most frequently perform vasectomy reversals. Since not everyone focuses on this procedure, make sure to ask your urologist how many he or she has done—and to what level of success. Also, if your urologist recommends a microsurgical approach, you have the right to ask about experience and success rates with this technique especially since this is a technique that requires additional training.

## Can all vasectomies be reversed?

Almost all vasectomies can be reversed. However, if the vasectomy was performed during the repair of a hernia in the groin, there may be more difficulty reconnecting the ends of the vas. Rarely, reconnection of the ends of the vas is not possible because such a long segment of the vas was removed during the vasectomy procedure.

## Is age a factor in conceiving after a vasectomy reversal?

Your age should not influence the result of your vasectomy reversal. Most men continue to produce sperm from their testicles for many years after their partners have entered menopause and are no longer ovulating, or producing eggs. In fact, a woman's fertility starts declining in her mid-30s, with significant impairment beginning around age 37.

If female age is a factor, your partner should check with her gynecologist to see if she is still ovulating before you agree to a reversal. Abnormal results from a simple blood test measuring hormone levels on the third day of menstruation indicate a significantly lowered chance of fertility. But do not be deceived by a normal reading. It does not always guarantee that she will be able to get pregnant.

## *Are there alternatives to vasectomy reversal?*

Yes. Your doctor can obtain sperm from the testicle or epididymis by either a needle aspiration or surgery. But the sperm may not be useful for simple, inexpensive office artificial inseminations. Instead, the sperm that are obtained by such methods require the more complex, expensive ($5,000 to $15,000) in vitro fertilization (IVF) techniques using intracytoplasmic sperm injection (ICSI).

Most centers report a 30 percent to 35 percent pregnancy rate each time IVF with ICSI is performed if the female partner is younger than 37, but much lower rates if she is older. Since studies consistently show that vasectomy reversals are more cost-effective in achieving pregnancy than obtaining sperm for IVF with ICSI, your better option is with the reversal.

## *If a vasectomy reversal fails, should I consider another surgery?*

The success rates for repeat reversals are generally 8 percent to 10 percent lower than for first reversals. In making a recommendation, your urologist will no doubt review the record of your previous procedure. If sperm were present in fluid obtained from the lower end of the vas during that operation, he or she will probably perform a repeat vasovasostomy, a less complicated procedure than a vasoepididymostomy, but more likely to produce success.

## *How expensive is a vasectomy reversal?*

Costs vary widely, ranging between about $3,500 and $10,000. Those amounts include fees for the surgeon and anesthesiologist as well as costs for the hospital or outpatient facility. Since most insurance companies do not pay for this procedure, you should discuss the finances of your operation early to see if you might just be the exception to the rule.

### Will a vasectomy reversal relieve pain in the testicle that developed after my vasectomy?

It is fortunate that only a very small percentage of men develop pain in the testicle after a vasectomy that is sufficiently severe for them to inquire about treatment to relieve pain. Because such situations are rare, there are few reports of groups of patients who undergo vasectomy reversals to relieve pain in the testicle. Most of these reports indicate that the majority of patients who undergo a vasectomy reversal for relief of pain in the testicles indeed are relieved of their pain. However, your urologist cannot determine in advance that your pain definitely will be relieved if you undergo a reversal.

## Section 32.4

## *Male Infertility*

Some 15 to 20 percent of couples are still trying to conceive a baby after a year of unprotected intercourse. While many people put most of the blame on women, statistics show that this is a shared problem, with male factors involved in more than 50 percent of these infertility cases.

The reassuring news for men is that urologists have a variety of tools and techniques to correct many infertility problems, including hormone manipulation to raise testicular testosterone levels, artificial insemination, medications to counter retrograde ejaculation, and microsurgical techniques to undo damage caused by blockages in the epididymis or vas deferens—not to mention correction of swollen veins in the scrotum called varicoceles.

But which problem affects you? More importantly, which treatment will work? The information below should help you discuss male infertility with your urologist and partner.

## *What occurs under normal conditions?*

The male reproductive system is designed to manufacture, store, and transport sperm—the microscopic genetic cells that fertilize a woman's ovum. A number of hormones, the most important of which are testosterone and follicle-stimulating hormone (FSH), regulate that process. Like sperm, testosterone is produced in both testicles, organs suspended in a pouch-like skin sac—the scrotum—below the penis.

Sperm production begins when immature cells grow and develop within a network of delicate ducts—microscopic seminiferous tubules—inside the testicles. Because these new sperm cannot move initially on their own, they are dependent on adjacent organs to become functional. They mature while traveling through the epididymis, a coiled channel located behind each testicle.

When climax, or orgasm, occurs, sperm are carried out of the body via semen, a fluid composed of secretions from various male reproductive glands, most notably the prostate and paired seminal vesicles.

## *What are the causes of male infertility?*

Developing and transporting mature, healthy, functional sperm depends on a specific sequence of events occurring in the male reproductive tract. Many disturbances can occur along that path, preventing cells from maturing into sperm production or reaching the woman's fallopian tube where fertilization occurs.

For starters, your infertility may be caused by a diminished output of sperm by your testicles. Abnormal sperm production can also be triggered by genetic factors and a number of life-style choices (e.g., smoking, alcohol, and certain medications), all of which impair the normal production of sperm cells, which, in turn, decreases their number. Long-term illnesses (e.g., kidney failure), childhood infections (e.g., mumps), and hormonal or chromosomal deficiencies (e.g., insufficient testosterone) can also account for abnormal sperm numbers.

Perhaps the most prevalent sperm production problem, however, is linked to structural abnormalities, most notably varicoceles. A snake-like bundle of enlarged or dilated varicose veins around the testicles, varicoceles are the most common identifiable cause of male infertility. They are found in about 15 percent of normal males and in approximately 40 percent of infertile men, most often on the left side or simultaneously on both sides. A single, right-sided varicocele is rare. Evidence suggests that by creating an abnormal backflow of blood from the abdomen into the scrotum, triggering a rise in testicular temperature, varicoceles hinder sperm production and cause oligospermia.

Your chances of fathering a child are nonexistent if your semen has no sperm to transport. Azoospermia, which accounts for 10 to 15 percent of all male infertility, refers to a complete absence of such sperm cells in your ejaculate. In its "nonobstructive" form, azoospermia can be triggered by various hormonal or chromosomal deficiencies often linked to testicular failure. But just as likely, it is the result of damage to some portion—the epididymis, vas deferens, or ejaculatory duct—of the reproductive delivery system. In fact, 40 percent of azoospermia sufferers are diagnosed with an "obstructive" form, caused by either congenital or acquired problems like infections. Vasectomy, the chief contraceptive method available to men today, is a primary example of an acquired factor. By cutting and sealing the vas deferens to stop sperm from moving through the reproductive tract, pregnancy is prevented. Vasectomies can often be reversed by use of a vasovasotomy in the hands of an experienced urologic microsurgeon. The blockage may be permanent, however, if the extent of the damage is great and the doctor is unskilled. While vasectomies are a formidable factor, there are other potential disturbances within the reproductive tract that can impede sperm. Because a proper erection is essential in impregnating any partner, it is not surprising that impotence or erectile dysfunction (ED), the inability to sustain an erection, is the most easily identified sexual problem linked to male infertility. Retrograde ejaculation, a lesser known issue, involves the improper deposit of sperm and semen. In this case, your ejaculate content may be normal, but instead of leaving the penis for the vagina, it flows backwards into the bladder due to an improperly functioning bladder neck.

### How is male infertility diagnosed?

Unlike female infertility, the cause of which is often easily identified, diagnosing male factors can be difficult. The problems, however, usually fall in one of two areas—sperm production and/or delivery.

Because male infertility results from such varied factors, you will need to see your physician to sort out the possibilities. A primary care doctor can often locate the problem, correctable or not, by completing an initial evaluation. You will probably need further evaluation by a urologist or reproductive specialist if you and your partner have been trying unsuccessfully for a year to get pregnant or if you have a known male factor, such as an undescended testicle.

In any case, the evaluation usually includes medical and surgical histories. The doctor will want to know about childhood diseases (e.g., mumps), current health problems (e.g., diabetes), or even medications (e.g., anabolic steroids) that might interfere with the formation of sperm. He or she will also ask about your use of alcohol, marijuana, and other recreational drugs, as well as your exposure to the occupational hazards of ionizing radiation, heavy metals, and pesticides. All of these factors can affect fertility.

Every evaluation will also include an assessment of your sexual performance, along with your and your partner's joint efforts to achieve pregnancy. For instance, your doctor will investigate whether you have had difficulty with erections and if your ejaculate has sufficient quality and volume. Such factors can adversely affect your sperm's effectiveness for pregnancy.

In addition to conducting a general exam, your doctor will look for any abnormalities of the penis, epididymis, vas deferens, and testicles. He or she will focus specifically on varicoceles, which can be identified easily in the scrotum when the patient is standing because they feel like a "bag of worms."

Semen analysis is a routine test that is the single most important lab indicator for male infertility. Completed twice, it helps urologists define each factor and its severity. Performed by examining ejaculate within a few hours of masturbation, a semen analysis provides important information about semen volume and content. It also measures the amount, motility (movement), and appearance (shape) of individual sperm. Each factor tells you and your doctor much about your ability to conceive. Your semen is normal, for instance, if it liquefies from a pearly gel into a liquid within 20 minutes. A breakdown in this sequence may indicate a problem with your seminal vesicles. Likewise, a lack of fructose (sugar) in a sperm-free specimen may indicate a congenital absence of the seminal vesicles, or your ejaculatory duct may be entirely blocked.

In addition to the above screens, your doctor may order other tools to assess fertility, including transurethral ultrasonography, which detects ejaculatory duct obstructions, and testicular biopsies, which confirm any reproductive blockages. Getting a complete evaluation should help you and your partner understand your infertility issues, not to mention make better decisions about treatment.

## What are some treatment options?

Your treatment options will depend entirely on the factors causing your infertility. The good news is that few medical fields have changed as dramatically during the past decades as reproductive medicine, particularly as it pertains to men.

Today, many conditions can be corrected with drugs or surgery, thus enabling conception to occur through normal intercourse.

## What is varicocele repair?

Among the most exciting treatment developments are microsurgical approaches to repair dilated varicose scrotal veins to improve semen quality. You should consider treatment if you meet the following criteria:

- You and your partner are trying to conceive a child, but thus far have been unsuccessful.

- You have been diagnosed with a varicocele that can be felt.

- Your semen analysis or sperm function tests are abnormal.

- Your partner has normal fertility or treatable infertility.

- You are contending with a varicocele and abnormal semen.

- You are an adolescent male with a varicocele and reduced testicle size.

If you fit the profile, your doctor can correct your varicocele with any number of surgical options, all of which can be performed in an outpatient center under anesthesia.

**Retroperitoneal (or abdominal) approach.** This conventional "open" varicocelectomy is best suited to men whose previously attempted varicocele or hernia repair resulted in significant groin scarring. Complications, which occur at a rate of 5 to 30 percent, include hydroceles, testicular atrophy, and injury to the vas deferens.

**Laparoscopic varicocelectomy.** While this minimally invasive technique can be used successfully to isolate and repair vessels, it is accompanied by a 6 to 15 percent recurrence rate due, in part, to the preservation of a series of fine veins that may dilate with time and cause recurrence. Also, events such as intestinal injuries or infection give it an 8 to 12 percent complication rate. In addition, laparoscopy must be performed by a urologist experienced in the procedure, which is a limitation.

**Microsurgical varicocelectomy.** Cited by many specialists as their preferred approach, this operation uses the optical magnification of a high-powered microscope to provide direct visual access to veins and arteries. Through a mini-incision in the groin, the doctor can reliably separate and preserve testicular arteries, while identifying and ligating both large and small veins that could dilate in the future. Also, while technically demanding, microsurgical varicocelectomy virtually eliminates hydroceles, the most common surgical complications. In fact, microsurgical techniques have significantly reduced recurrence rates to less than 2 percent and complications rates to less than 5 percent while increasing fertility. The effectiveness of this procedure has been reported in the scientific literature to be as high as a 43 percent pregnancy rate for couples after one year and 69 percent after two years.

**Percutaneous embolization.** This nonsurgical approach is aimed at occluding the varicocele after it is viewed with a specialized x-ray technique. The procedure itself uses a flexible tube inserted into the groin to place a blocking agent that helps obstruct the center of the vessel. This minimally invasive technique is often less painful than surgery, but it requires a physician with experience in interventional radiologic techniques. As such, it is performed in the radiology department.

There is no evidence to suggest that any approach is the best for correcting varicoceles. While surgery removes more than 90 percent of the swollen vein, percutaneous embolization gets rid of 80 to 85 percent. After repair, about 60 percent of men show improved sperm counts and/or motility. The effects of either treatment on fertility, however, are much less clear. While some studies show improvement, others suggest no significant change. Regardless, many infertile couples still choose varicocele repair because it improves semen in many men and may improve fertility, both at little risk.

### What is azoospermia treatment?

If your semen lacks sperm (azoospermia) as a result of blockage, there are several surgical treatment options at your disposal.

**Microsurgical vasovasostomy.** This procedure is designed to restore fertility by reconnecting the severed vas deferens in each testicle. The procedure, which should clear the way for sperm to leave the body, can be accomplished through various approaches, all performed in outpatient hospital or ambulatory surgical settings under general anesthesia, spinal epidurals, or sometimes with localized numbing and sedation. In more than 90 percent of patients, sperm returns in the semen, yielding pregnancy in more than 50 percent of cases.

**Transurethral resection of the ejaculatory duct (TURED).** When properly diagnosed, ejaculatory duct obstructions can be managed surgically by passing a cystoscope into the urethra and opening the offending blockages. Resecting the duct triggers release of sperm into the ejaculate in about 50 to 75 percent of men. But there can be complications—recurrent blockages, incontinence, and even retrograde ejaculation due to bladder injuries. Also, pregnancy rates are only about 25 percent.

**Vasoepididymostomy.** The most common microsurgical procedure for treating epididymal obstructions, vasoepididymostomy is also one of the most difficult of all treatments for male infertility. Surgeons must have excellent skills and extensive experience to perform this procedure, a surgical joining of the vas deferens and epididymis to facilitate the transport of fluid. The approach relies on the precise positioning and tying of sutures to secure tissue layers between the structures. When successful, however, an opened channel is restored in 50 to 70 percent of cases; pregnancy rates vary from 25 to 57 percent.

### What can I expect after treatment?

Male infertility factors can usually be corrected in an outpatient procedure using general anesthesia or intravenous sedation. While postoperative pain is usually mild, postoperative recovery and follow-up varies.

After varicocele repair, your doctor should perform a physical examination to see if the vein is completely gone. Semen should be tested about every three months for at least one year or until pregnancy. If your varicocele returns, or you remain infertile after the repair, ask your doctor about assisted reproductive techniques (ART). These high-tech procedures are often successful in circumventing the same problem to produce a pregnancy.

While vasectomy reversals cause only mild postoperative pain, expect an out-of-work recovery of four to seven days. The chance for pregnancy depends on many factors, most importantly, the age and fertility status of your female partner and the number of years between your original vasectomy and this procedure. The longer you wait, the less likely you will have a successful reversal.

### How are specific male infertility conditions treated without surgery?

**Anejaculation.** A relatively uncommon disorder, anejaculation—or the absence of any semen—can occur as a result of spinal cord injury, previous surgery, diabetes, or multiple sclerosis. It may also be caused by abnormalities present at birth as well as other mental, emotional, or unknown problems. Medical therapy with drugs is usually the first line of treatment, but if that fails, the next step is either rectal probe electroejaculation (RPE) or penile vibratory stimulation (PVS). PVS consists of rhythmic vibratory stimulation of the tip and shaft of the penis to encourage a natural climax. While relatively noninvasive, it is less successful than RPE, particularly in severe cases. RPE, except in the spinal cord injured patient, is usually performed under anesthesia and retrieves sperm in 90 percent of patients. While cell density with this procedure is excellent, sperm movement and shape are still limiting fertility factors. Assisted reproductive techniques, such as in vitro fertilization (IVF) and intracytoplasmic sperm injection (ICSI), have become increasingly important to patients with anejaculation.

**Congenital adrenal hyperplasia (CAH).** A rare cause of male factor infertility, CAH involves congenital deficiencies in certain enzymes, resulting in abnormal hormone production. CAH is usually diagnosed by demonstrating excess steroids in the blood and urine. When treated successfully with hormone replacement, sperm production increases.

**Genital tract infection.** It is rare that acute genital tract infections can be linked to infertility, but it does happen in approximately 2 percent of men suffering from reproduction problems. The problem is usually picked up following a simple semen analysis where white blood cells are found. White blood cells generate excess oxidants—reactive oxygen species (ROS)—known to harm the fertilizing potential of sperm. But an infection need not be acute to cause reproductive problems. For instance, testicular atrophy, along with epididymal duct obstruction, may occur following severe infection of the epididymis and testes. Chronic prostatitis, on rare occasions, may also cause obstruction by occluding the ejaculatory ducts. While antibiotics are generally prescribed for full-blown infections, they are not warranted for lesser inflammations since they can be occasionally harmful to sperm production. In those cases, nonsteroidal anti-inflammatories are usually recommended.

**Hyperprolactinemia.** This condition of excessive production of the hormone prolactin by the pituitary gland has been implicated in both infertility and erectile dysfunction. Treatment of hyperprolactinemia is based on the cause of the increased secretion. If medications are the root, they should be discontinued immediately. Medical therapy may consist of medications to bring prolactin levels to normal.

**Hypogonadotropic hypogonadism.** Hypogonadotropic hypogonadism refers to the failure of the testicles to produce sperm due to a hypothalamic or pituitary disorder. It is the cause of infertility in a small percentage of patients and can exist at birth or be acquired. Known also as Kallmann's syndrome, the congenital form results from an abnormal production of gonadotropin-releasing hormone (GnRH), a hormone produced by the hypothalamus. Acquired hypogonadotropic hypogonadism can be triggered by a variety of other conditions, including pituitary tumors, head trauma, and anabolic steroid use.

When hypogonadotropic hypogonadism is suspected, doctors usually order an MRI along with serum prolactin concentrations to rule out pituitary tumors. If levels of the prolactin are excessive but there is no mass, treatment will consist of lowering prolactin concentrations before proceeding with gonadotropin replacement therapy. During treatment, blood testosterone levels and semen analyses are obtained. Chances for pregnancy are excellent, since resultant sperm are essentially normal.

**Immunologic infertility.** Since the early 1950s, when scientists first demonstrated that some cases of infertility were linked to immunologic causes, much research has focused on this area. While oral steroids to decrease significant antisperm antibody have been advocated, this treatment is rarely successful. In vitro fertilization with ICSI is now the treatment of choice for immunological male factor problems.

**Reactive oxygen species (ROS).** A relatively new interest area in male infertility, ROS refers to small molecules present in many bodily fluids, such as seminal white blood and sperm cells. When in appropriate concentrations, ROS can help prepare the sperm for fertilization. However, if in excess, ROS can be harmful to other cells. Because of their already high polyunsaturated fatty acid content, human sperm membranes are particularly sensitive to ROS-related damage. Recent studies have demonstrated an increase in presence of these molecules in the semen of infertile men. Several compounds have been used to detoxify or "scavenge" ROS. The most effective of these, vitamin E (400 IU twice daily), is a very effective antioxidant. Pentoxifylline, a medication employed occasionally to decrease the thickness of blood, has also been shown to decrease sperm oxidant production, but is used much less frequently than vitamin E.

**Retrograde ejaculation.** Defined as an abnormal backward flow of semen into the bladder with ejaculation, it can be caused by problems that are: anatomic (e.g., previous prostate or bladder neck surgeries); neurogenic (e.g., diabetes, spinal cord injury, and previous surgery); pharmacologic (e.g., antidepressants, certain antihypertensives, and medication used to treat prostatism, prostate enlargement); and idiopathic (other unknown problems). Retrograde ejaculation is diagnosed by the patient urinating immediately following ejaculation to produce a sample that is evaluated microscopically for sperm. Initial treatment for retrograde ejaculation consists of commonly used medications (e.g., Sudafed®). If medical therapy should fail, however, doctors may try to recover sperm from the bladder after ejaculation in conjunction with intrauterine insemination.

### How are nonspecific (idiopathic) male infertility conditions treated without surgery?

Nonspecific male infertility factors are often unexplained or ill defined, unlike specific conditions such as retrograde ejaculation or genital tract infection. However, because these procedures often involve the body's hormonal activities, they are just as troublesome to both the treating physician and the patient. In many cases, empiric therapy—designed to address hormonal imbalances—is used.

Empiric therapies generally involve hormonal manipulation. Assessing the impact of empiric treatments is very difficult, given variations in patients as well as dosing regimens, treatment durations, and outcome definitions. As such, treatment decisions chosen by individual physicians are often based on their own personal philosophies.

### *What are assisted reproductive techniques (ART)?*

ART refers to a series of high-tech procedures used to join a sperm with eggs when sexual intercourse cannot accomplish the task. Your doctor may recommend one or a combination of these techniques, particularly if you are among the many men who fail to achieve natural pregnancy, despite a return of sperm to the ejaculate. Intrauterine insemination (IUI)—placing retrieved and processed sperm into the uterus via a catheter—or in vitro fertilization (IVF)/intracytoplasmic sperm injection (ICSI)—may be the best and only route to pregnancy. IVF, fertilizing an egg outside the body in a laboratory setting and implanting the resulting embryo into the uterus, and ICSI, injecting a single retrieved sperm into a mature egg, are also indicated in men who choose not to have reconstructive surgery or whose duct obstruction cannot be fixed.

### *How are sperm surgically retrieved?*

Sperm blocked by obstructive azoospermia can be removed by various microsurgical approaches. In each case, the goal is to obtain the best quality and number of cells, not to mention minimizing damage to the reproductive tract so future attempts at retrieval or surgical reconstruction are not jeopardized. Often known by their acronyms, these procedures include:

- *Testicular sperm extraction* (TESE). A most common technique to not only diagnose the cause of azoospermia, but also to obtain sufficient tissue for sperm extraction to be used either fresh or as a cryopreserved (frozen) specimen. It involves one or multiple small biopsies often performed in the office.

- *Testicular fine needle aspiration* (TFNA). Initially a diagnostic procedure in azoospermic men, it is now sometimes used to recover sperm from the testicles. A needle and syringe puncture the skin to aspirate a sperm specimen.

- *Percutaneous epididymal sperm aspiration* (PESA). Advocated because it can be performed repeatedly at low cost, PESA, like TFNA, can be completed without a surgical incision. Because it does not require a high-powered microscope, it also does not necessitate microsurgical expertise. Instead, it is done under local or general anesthesia with the physician inserting a needle attached to a syringe into the epididymis, then gently withdrawing fluid. Sperm may not always be obtained, and the surgeon must be prepared to perform an open procedure.

- *Microsurgical epididymal sperm aspiration* (MESA). Performed under a microscope, MESA involves direct retrieval of sperm from individual epididymal tubules. It is completed by isolating the tubes and then aspirating the fluid. Designed to limit damage to the epididymis, while avoiding blood contamination of its fluid, MESA yields high quantities of motile sperm that can be readily frozen and thawed for subsequent IVF treatments. While general anesthesia and microsurgical skill could be considered disadvantages to this process, a lower complication rate, better sperm motility, and the ability to consistently have sufficient sperm for banking make MESA a simple and safe sperm recovery technique.

### If I am suffering from obstructive azoospermia, when should my partner and I consider sperm retrieval with an assisted reproductive technique rather than surgery?

Intracytoplasmic sperm injection (ICSI), a form of IVF, must be used in virtually all obstructive azoospermia cases when sperm are removed from the testicle or epididymis. This technique is employed because the number of motile sperm that can be obtained is frequently limited and the functional capacity of the sperm impaired.

Retrieving sperm cells for ICSI involves several methods (described above), the choice of which will be up to you and your urologist. It can be performed prior to or simultaneously with your partner's egg retrieval. While many reproductive centers prefer to use the "fresh" sperm obtained on the same day as the retrieval, others prefer previously harvested and frozen cells. As stated, sperm retrieval can often be accomplished by either a needle aspiration or microsurgical techniques.

### If I am suffering from a varicocele, when should my partner and I consider an assisted reproductive technique (ART) rather than surgery?

If you and your partner both have fertility factors where the female cannot conceive naturally, then you may benefit from any one of several ART procedures—intrauterine insemination (IUI), in vitro fertilization (IVF)/intracytoplasmic injection (ICSI)—rather than surgical treatment of the male. The choice is not always clear, however. Since so many factors come into play, you and your doctor will want to consider the following:

- The wife's age and assessment of ovarian function

- The possibility that a varicocele repair will not definitely restore your infertility

- The fact that ART is needed for each try at pregnancy

Varicocele repair should remain the treatment of choice, however, if you do not have ideal semen but your partner is normal. Conversely, IVF, with or without ICSI, should be considered the primary option when there is a special need for such methods to treat a female factor.

### Are there risks associated with IVF/ICSI?

Yes, some risks exist, especially for women. For instance, ovarian hyperstimulation, due to the hormones used in the IVF/ICSI process, can result in high blood pressure, fluid accumulation, malaise, weakness, and other symptoms. Mild stimulation, usually tolerated easily by women, occurs in up to 20 percent of patients. Moderate hyperstimulation shows up in 5 percent of women undergoing IVF. Only one percent of women undergoing IVF suffer from severe ovarian hyperstimulation, the form that can cause severe medical problems. Multiple births present another potential issue for IVF/ICSI couples. In the United States, following IVF there is a 30 to 35 percent risk for twin gestations and 5 to 10 percent for triplets (or higher).

### Are the pituitary tumors that cause low gonadotropin or elevated prolactin levels malignant tumors?

No. These are usually benign lesions of the pituitary gland. If the tumor is large enough, you should consult a neurosurgeon to possibly remove the growth. Removal is usually performed through the nasal passages.

### Should I try empiric hormonal therapy if I also have a varicocele?

The general rule of thumb is that unproven empiric therapies should not be tried until known reversible causes of male infertility are addressed. Varicocele remains the leading cause of impaired sperm production in the United States. Serious consideration should be given to any such repair prior to any empiric hormonal therapy.

### *In light of the detrimental effects of oxidants on sperm function, should all infertile men take the antioxidant vitamin E?*

Vitamin E is a safe, well-tolerated supplement that has been shown in studies to reduce the risk of heart disease. Ingestion of 400 IU twice daily is also an inexpensive, effective way to treat any oxidants that maybe affecting fertility. This treatment course, however, does not replace careful examination of other known infertility causes in either men or women.

# Part Four

# Mental and Emotional Health

# Chapter 33

# *Stress*

Stress is a natural part of life. The expressions are familiar to us: "I'm stressed out," "I'm under too much stress," or "Work is one big stress."

Stress is hard to define because it means different things to different people; however, it's clear that most stress is a negative feeling rather than a positive feeling.

## *Both Physical and Mental*

You may feel physical stress which is the result of too much to do, not enough sleep, a poor diet, or the effects of an illness. Stress can also be mental: When you worry about money, a loved one's illness, retirement, or experience an emotionally devastating event, such as the death of a spouse or being fired from work.

However, much of our stress comes from less dramatic every-day responsibilities. Obligations and pressures which are both physical and mental are not always obvious to us. In response to these daily strains your body automatically increases blood pressure, heart rate, respiration, metabolism, and blood flow to your muscles. This response, is intended to help your body react quickly and effectively to a high-pressure situation.

However, when you are constantly reacting to stressful situations without making adjustments to counter the effects, you will feel stress which can threaten your health and well-being.

It is essential to understand that external events, no matter how you perceive those events which may cause stress. Stress often accompanies the feeling of "being out of control."

## How Do I Know If I Am Suffering from Stress?

Remember, each person handles stress differently. Some people actually seek out situations which may appear stressful to others. A major life decision, such as changing careers or buying a house, might be overwhelming for some people, while others may welcome the change. Some find sitting in traffic too much to tolerate, while others take it in stride. The key is determining your personal tolerance levels for stressful situations.

Stress can cause physical, emotional, and behavioral disorders which can affect your health, vitality, and peace of mind, as well as personal and professional relationships. Too much stress can cause relatively minor illnesses like insomnia, backaches, or headaches, and can contribute to potentially life-threatening diseases like high blood pressure and heart disease.

## Tips for Reducing or Controlling Stress

As you read the following suggestions, remember that success will not come from a half-hearted effort, nor will it come overnight. It will take determination, persistence and time. Some suggestions may help immediately, but if your stress is chronic, it may require more attention and/or life-style changes. Determine *your* tolerance level for stress and try to live within these limits. Learn to accept or change stressful and tense situations whenever possible.

**Be realistic.** If you feel overwhelmed by some activities (yours and/ or your family's), learn to say *no*! Eliminate an activity that is not absolutely necessary. You may be taking on more responsibility than you can or should handle. If you meet resistance, give reasons why you're making the changes. Be willing to listen to other's suggestions and be ready to compromise.

**Shed the "superman/superwoman" urge.** No one is perfect, so don't expect perfection from yourself or others. Ask yourself, "What really needs to be done? How much can I do? Is the deadline realistic? What adjustments can I make?" Don't hesitate to ask for help if you need it.

**Meditate.** Just 10 to 20 minutes of quiet reflection may bring relief from chronic stress as well as increase your tolerance to it. Use the time to listen to music, relax, and try to think of pleasant things or nothing.

**Visualize.** Use your imagination and picture how you can manage a stressful situation more successfully. Whether it's a business presentation or moving to a new place, many people feel visual rehearsals boost self-confidence and enable them to take a more positive approach to a difficult task.

**Take one thing at a time.** For people under tension or stress, an ordinary workload can sometimes seem unbearable. The best way to cope with this feeling of being overwhelmed is to take one task at a time. Pick one urgent task and work on it. Once you accomplish that task, choose the next one. The positive feeling of "checking off" tasks is very satisfying. It will motivate you to keep going.

**Exercise.** Regular exercise is a popular way to relieve stress. Twenty to 30 minutes of physical activity benefits both the body and the mind.

**Pursue hobbies.** Take a break from your worries by doing something you enjoy. Whether it's gardening or painting, schedule time to indulge your interest.

**Live a healthy life-style.** Good nutrition makes a difference. Limit intake of caffeine and alcohol (alcohol actually disturbs regular sleep patterns), get adequate rest, exercise, and balance work and play.

**Share your feelings.** A conversation with a friend lets you know that you are not the only one having a bad day, caring for a sick child, or working in a busy office. Stay in touch with friends and family. Let them provide love, support, and guidance. Don't try to cope alone.

**Give in occasionally.** Be flexible. If you find you're meeting constant opposition in either your personal or professional life, rethink your position or strategy. Arguing only intensifies stressful feelings. If you know you are right, stand your ground, but do so calmly and rationally. Make allowances for others' opinions and be prepared to compromise. If you are willing to give in, others may meet you halfway.

Not only will you reduce your stress; you may find better solutions to your problems.

**Go easy with criticism.** You may expect too much of yourself and others. Try not to feel frustrated, let down, disappointed, or even "trapped" when another person does not measure up. The "other person" may be a wife, a husband, or child whom you are trying to change to suit yourself. Remember, everyone is unique, and has his or her own virtues, shortcomings, and right to develop as an individual.

## Where to Get Help

Help may be as close as a friend or spouse. But if you think that you or someone you know may be under more stress than just dealing with a passing difficulty, it may be helpful to talk with your doctor, spiritual advisor, or employee assistance professional. They may suggest you visit with a psychiatrist, psychologist, social worker, or other qualified counselor.

Ideas to consider when talking with a professional:

- List the things which cause stress and tension in your life.
- How does this stress and tension affect you, your family, and your job?
- Can you identify the stress and tensions in your life as short or long term?
- Do you have a support system of friends/family that will help you make positive changes?
- What are your biggest obstacles to reducing stress?
- What are you willing to change or give up for a less stressful and tension-filled life?
- What have you tried already that didn't work for you?
- If you do not have control of a situation, can you accept it and get on with your life?

# Chapter 34

# Post-Traumatic Stress Disorder (PTSD)

Post-traumatic stress disorder (PTSD) is an anxiety disorder that can develop after exposure to a terrifying event or ordeal in which grave physical harm occurred or was threatened. Traumatic events that can trigger PTSD include violent personal assaults such as rape or mugging, natural or human-caused disasters, accidents, or military combat. PTSD can be extremely disabling.

Military troops who served in the Vietnam and Gulf wars; rescue workers involved in the aftermath of disasters like the terrorist attacks on New York City and Washington, D.C.; survivors of the Oklahoma City bombing; survivors of accidents, rape, physical and sexual abuse, and other crimes; immigrants fleeing violence in their countries; survivors of the 1994 California earthquake, the 1997 North and South Dakota floods, and hurricanes Hugo and Andrew; and people who witness traumatic events are among those at risk for developing PTSD. Families of victims can also develop the disorder.

Fortunately, through research supported by the National Institute of Mental Health (NIMH) and the Department of Veterans Affairs (VA), effective treatments have been developed to help people with PTSD. Research is also helping scientists better understand the condition and how it affects the brain and the rest of the body.

Reprinted from "Facts about Post-traumatic Stress Disorder," National Institute of Mental Health, National Institutes of Health (NIH), updated October 5, 2001, http://www.nimh.nih.gov/anxiety/ptsdfacts.cfm. Also published as NIH Pub. No. OM-99 4157 (revised), 1999.

# What are the symptoms of PTSD?

Many people with PTSD repeatedly re-experience the ordeal in the form of flashback episodes, memories, nightmares, or frightening thoughts, especially when they are exposed to events or objects reminiscent of the trauma. Anniversaries of the event can also trigger symptoms. People with PTSD also experience emotional numbness and sleep disturbances, depression, anxiety, and irritability or outbursts of anger. Feelings of intense guilt are also common. Most people with PTSD try to avoid any reminders or thoughts of the ordeal. PTSD is diagnosed when symptoms last more than one month.

## How common is PTSD?

About 3.6 percent of U.S. adults ages 18 to 54 (5.2 million people) have PTSD during the course of a given year. About 30 percent of the men and women who have spent time in war zones experience PTSD. One million war veterans developed PTSD after serving in Vietnam. PTSD has also been detected among veterans of the 1991 Persian Gulf War, with some estimates running as high as 8 percent.

## When does PTSD first occur?

PTSD can develop at any age, including in childhood. Symptoms typically begin within three months of a traumatic event, although occasionally they do not begin until years later. Once PTSD occurs, the severity and duration of the illness varies. Some people recover within six months, while others suffer much longer.

## What treatments are available for PTSD?

Research has demonstrated the effectiveness of cognitive-behavioral therapy, group therapy, and exposure therapy, in which the patient gradually and repeatedly relives the frightening experience under controlled conditions to help him or her work through the trauma. Studies have also shown that medications help ease associated symptoms of depression and anxiety and help promote sleep. Scientists are attempting to determine which treatments work best for which type of trauma.

Some studies show that giving people an opportunity to talk about their experiences very soon after a catastrophic event may reduce some of the symptoms of PTSD. A study of 12,000 schoolchildren who lived through a hurricane in Hawaii found that those who got counseling early on were doing much better two years later than those who did not.

### Do other illnesses tend to accompany PTSD?

Co-occurring depression, alcohol or other substance abuse, or another anxiety disorder are not uncommon. The likelihood of treatment success is increased when these other conditions are appropriately identified and treated as well.

Headaches, gastrointestinal complaints, immune system problems, dizziness, chest pain, or discomfort in other parts of the body are common. Often, doctors treat the symptoms without being aware that they stem from PTSD. NIMH encourages primary care providers to ask patients about experiences with violence, recent losses, and traumatic events, especially if symptoms keep recurring. When PTSD is diagnosed, referral to a mental health professional who has had experience treating people with the disorder is recommended.

### Who is most likely to develop PTSD?

People who have suffered abuse as children or who have had other previous traumatic experiences are more likely to develop the disorder. Research is continuing to pinpoint other factors that may lead to PTSD.

It used to be believed that people who tend to be emotionally numb after a trauma were showing a healthy response, but now some researchers suspect that people who experience this emotional distancing may be more prone to PTSD.

### What are scientists learning from research?

NIMH and the VA sponsor a wide range of basic, clinical, and genetic studies of PTSD. In addition, NIMH has a special funding mechanism, called RAPID Grants, that allows researchers to immediately visit the scenes of disasters, such as plane crashes or floods and hurricanes, to study the acute effects of the event and the effectiveness of early intervention.

Studies in animals and humans have focused on pinpointing the specific brain areas and circuits involved in anxiety and fear, which are important for understanding anxiety disorders such as PTSD. Fear, an emotion that evolved to deal with danger, causes an automatic, rapid protective response in many systems of the body. It has been found that the body's fear response is coordinated by a small structure deep inside the brain, called the amygdala. The amygdala, although relatively small, is a very complicated structure, and recent research suggests that different anxiety disorders may be associated with abnormal activation of the amygdala.

The following are also recent research findings:

- In brain imaging studies, researchers have found that the hippocampus—a part of the brain critical to memory and emotion—appears to be different in cases of PTSD. Scientists are investigating whether this is related to short-term memory problems. Changes in the hippocampus are thought to be responsible for intrusive memories and flashbacks that occur in people with this disorder.

- People with PTSD tend to have abnormal levels of key hormones involved in response to stress. Some studies have shown that cortisol levels are lower than normal and epinephrine and norepinephrine are higher than normal.

- When people are in danger, they produce high levels of natural opiates, which can temporarily mask pain. Scientists have found that people with PTSD continue to produce those higher levels even after the danger has passed; this may lead to the blunted emotions associated with the condition.

- Research to understand the neurotransmitter systems involved in memories of emotionally charged events may lead to discovery of medications or psychosocial interventions that, if given early, could block the development of PTSD symptoms.

# Chapter 35

# *Depression*

Depression is a serious medical condition that affects the body, mood, and thoughts. It affects the way one eats and sleeps, one's self-concept, and the way one thinks about things. A depressive disorder is not the same as a passing blue mood. It is not a sign of personal weakness or a condition that can be willed or wished away. People with a depressive illness cannot merely "pull themselves together" and get better. Without treatment, symptoms can last for weeks, months, or years. Appropriate treatment, however, often involving medication and/or short-term psychotherapy, can help most people who suffer from depression.

> *"I can remember it started with a loss of interest in basically everything that I like doing. I just didn't feel like doing anything. I just felt like giving up. Sometimes I didn't even want to get out of bed."*

> —Rene Ruballo, police officer

Depression can strike anyone regardless of age, ethnic background, socioeconomic status, or gender; however, large-scale research studies have found that depression is about twice as common in women

Reprinted from "Men and Depression," National Institute of Mental Health, National Institutes of Health (NIH), 2003, http://menanddepression. nimh.nih.gov/infopage.asp?id=10, 2003. Also available in hard copy as NIH Pub. No. 03-4972, 2003.

as in men. In the United States, researchers estimate that in any given one-year period, depressive illnesses affect 12 percent of women (more than 12 million women) and nearly 7 percent of men (more than 6 million men). But important questions remain to be answered about the causes underlying this gender difference. For example, is depression truly less common among men, or are men just less likely than women to recognize, acknowledge, and seek help for depression?

In focus groups conducted by the National Institute of Mental Health (NIMH) to assess depression awareness, men described their own symptoms of depression without realizing that they were depressed. Notably, many were unaware that "physical" symptoms, such as headaches, digestive disorders, and chronic pain, can be associated with depression. In addition, they expressed concern about seeing a mental health professional or going to a mental health clinic, thinking that people would find out and that this might have a negative impact on their job security, promotion potential, or health insurance benefits. They feared that being labeled with a diagnosis of mental illness would cost them the respect of their family and friends, or their standing in the community.

Over the past 20 years, biomedical research including genetics and neuroimaging has helped to shed light on depression and other mental disorders—increasing our understanding of the brain, how its biochemistry can go awry, and how to alleviate the suffering that mental illnesses can cause. Brain-imaging technologies are now allowing scientists to see how effective treatment with medication or psychotherapy is reflected in changes in brain activity. As research continues to reveal that depressive disorders are real and treatable, and are no more a sign of weakness than cancer or any other serious illness, more and more men with depression may feel empowered to seek treatment and find improved quality of life.

## Types of Depression

Depression comes in different forms, just as is the case with other illnesses such as heart disease. This chapter briefly describes three of the most common types of depressive disorders. However, within these types there are variations in the number of symptoms, their severity, and persistence.

Major depression (or major depressive disorder) is manifested by a combination of symptoms (see symptom list below) that interferes with the ability to work, study, sleep, eat, and enjoy once-pleasurable activities. A major depressive episode may occur only once; but more commonly, several episodes may occur in a lifetime. Chronic major depression may require a person to continue treatment indefinitely.

A less severe type of depression, dysthymia (or dysthymic disorder), involves long-lasting symptoms that do not seriously disable, but keep one from functioning well or feeling good. Many people with dysthymia also experience major depressive episodes at some time in their lives.

Another type of depressive illness is bipolar disorder (or manic-depressive illness). Bipolar disorder is characterized by cycling mood changes: severe highs (mania) and lows (depression), often with periods of normal mood in between. Sometimes the mood switches are dramatic and rapid, but usually they are gradual. When in the depressed cycle, an individual can have any or all of the symptoms of depression. When in the manic cycle, the individual may be overactive, overtalkative, and have a great deal of energy. Mania often affects thinking, judgment, and social behavior in ways that cause serious problems and embarrassment. For example, the individual in a manic phase may feel elated, full of grand schemes that might range from unwise business decisions to romantic sprees and unsafe sex. Mania, left untreated, may worsen to a psychotic state.

## Symptoms of Depression and Mania

Not everyone who is depressed or manic experiences every symptom. Some people experience a few symptoms; some people suffer many. The severity of symptoms varies among individuals and also over time.

### *Depression*

- Persistent sad, anxious, or "empty" mood
- Feelings of hopelessness, pessimism
- Feelings of guilt, worthlessness, helplessness
- Loss of interest or pleasure in hobbies and activities that were once enjoyed, including sex
- Decreased energy, fatigue, being "slowed down"
- Difficulty concentrating, remembering, making decisions
- Trouble sleeping, early-morning awakening, or oversleeping
- Appetite and/or weight changes

- Thoughts of death or suicide, or suicide attempts

- Restlessness, irritability

- Persistent physical symptoms, such as headaches, digestive disorders, and chronic pain, which do not respond to routine treatment

*"You don't have any interest in thinking about the future, because you don't feel that there is going to be any future."*

—Shawn Colten, national diving champion

*"I wouldn't feel rested at all. I'd always feel tired. I could get from an hour's sleep to eight hours' sleep and I would always feel tired."*

—Rene Ruballo, police officer

### *Mania*

- Abnormal or excessive elation

- Unusual irritability

- Decreased need for sleep

- Grandiose notions

- Increased talking

- Racing thoughts

- Increased sexual desire

- Markedly increased energy

- Poor judgment

- Inappropriate social behavior

## Co-Occurrence of Depression with Other Illnesses

Depression can coexist with other illnesses. In such cases, it is important that the depression and each co-occurring illness be appropriately diagnosed and treated.

Research has shown that anxiety disorders, which include post-traumatic stress disorder (PTSD), obsessive-compulsive disorder, panic disorder, social phobia, and generalized anxiety disorder, commonly accompany depression. Depression is especially prevalent among people with PTSD, a debilitating condition that can occur after exposure to a terrifying event or ordeal in which grave physical harm occurred or was threatened. Traumatic events that can trigger PTSD include violent personal assaults such as rape or mugging, natural disasters, accidents, terrorism, and military combat. PTSD symptoms include: re-experiencing the traumatic event in the form of flashback episodes, memories, or nightmares; emotional numbness; sleep disturbances; irritability; outbursts of anger; intense guilt; and avoidance of any reminders or thoughts of the ordeal. In one NIMH-supported study, more than 40 percent of people with PTSD also had depression when evaluated at one month and four months following the traumatic event.

Substance use disorders (abuse or dependence) also frequently co-occur with depressive disorders. Research has revealed that people with alcoholism are almost twice as likely as those without alcoholism to also suffer from major depression. In addition, more than half of people with bipolar disorder type I (with severe mania) have a co-occurring substance use disorder.

Depression has been found to occur at a higher rate among people who have other serious illnesses such as heart disease, stroke, cancer, HIV, diabetes, and Parkinson's. Symptoms of depression are sometimes mistaken for inevitable accompaniments to these other illnesses. However, research has shown that the co-occurring depression can and should be treated, and that in many cases treating the depression can also improve the outcome of the other illnesses.

## *Causes of Depression*

Substantial evidence from neuroscience, genetics, and clinical investigation shows that depressive illnesses are disorders of the brain. However, the precise causes of these illnesses continue to be a matter of intense research.

Modern brain-imaging technologies are revealing that in depression, neural circuits responsible for the regulation of moods, thinking, sleep, appetite, and behavior fail to function properly, and that critical neurotransmitters—chemicals used by nerve cells to communicate—are out of balance. Genetics research indicates that risk for depression results from the influence of multiple genes acting together with environmental or other nongenetic factors. Studies of brain chemistry and the mechanisms of action of antidepressant medications continue to inform our understanding of the biochemical processes involved in depression.

Very often, a combination of genetic, cognitive, and environmental factors is involved in the onset of a depressive disorder. Trauma, loss of a loved one, a difficult relationship, a financial problem, or any stressful change in life patterns, whether the change is unwelcome or desired, can trigger a depressive episode in vulnerable individuals. Later episodes of depression may occur without an obvious cause.

In some families, depressive disorders seem to occur generation after generation; however, they can also occur in people who have no family history of these illnesses. Whether inherited or not, depressive disorders are associated with changes in brain structures or brain function, which can be seen using modern brain imaging technologies.

## Men and Depression

Researchers estimate that at least 6 million men in the United States suffer from a depressive disorder every year. Research and clinical evidence reveal that while both women and men can develop the standard symptoms of depression, they often experience depression differently and may have different ways of coping with the symptoms. Men may be more willing to acknowledge fatigue, irritability, loss of interest in work or hobbies, and sleep disturbances rather than feelings of sadness, worthlessness, and excessive guilt. Some researchers question whether the standard definition of depression and the diagnostic tests based upon it adequately capture the condition as it occurs in men.

> *"I'd drink and I'd just get numb. I'd get numb to try to numb my head. I mean, we're talking many, many beers to get to that state where you could shut your head off, but then you wake up the next day and it's still there. Because you have to deal with it, it doesn't just go away. It isn't a two-hour movie and then at the end it goes 'The End' and you press off. I mean it's a twenty-four hour a day movie and you're thinking there is no end. It's horrible."*

—Patrick McCathern, first sergeant, U.S. Air Force, retired

Men are more likely than women to report alcohol and drug abuse or dependence in their lifetime; however, there is debate among researchers as to whether substance use is a "symptom" of underlying depression in men or a co-occurring condition that more commonly develops in men. Nevertheless, substance use can mask depression, making it harder to recognize depression as a separate illness that needs treatment.

Instead of acknowledging their feelings, asking for help, or seeking appropriate treatment, men may turn to alcohol or drugs when they are depressed, or become frustrated, discouraged, angry, irritable, and, sometimes, violently abusive. Some men deal with depression by throwing themselves compulsively into their work, attempting to hide their depression from themselves, family, and friends; other men may respond to depression by engaging in reckless behavior, taking risks, and putting themselves in harm's way.

*"When I was feeling depressed I was very reckless with my life. I didn't care about how I drove, I didn't care about walking across the street carefully, I didn't care about dangerous parts of the city. I wouldn't be affected by any kinds of warnings on travel or places to go. I didn't care. I didn't care whether I lived or died and so I was going to do whatever I wanted whenever I wanted. And when you take those kinds of chances, you have a greater likelihood of dying."*

—Bill Maruyama, lawyer

Four times as many men as women die by suicide in the United States, even though women make more suicide attempts during their lives. In addition to the fact that the methods men use to attempt suicide are generally more lethal than those methods used by women, there may be other issues that protect women against suicide death. In light of research indicating that suicide is often associated with depression, the alarming suicide rate among men may reflect the fact that men are less likely to seek treatment for depression. Many men with depression do not obtain adequate diagnosis and treatment, which may be life saving.

More research is needed to understand all aspects of depression in men, including how men respond to stress and feelings associated with depression, how to make them more comfortable acknowledging these feelings and getting the help they need, and how to train physicians to better recognize and treat depression in men. Family members, friends, and employee assistance professionals in the workplace also can play important roles in recognizing depressive symptoms in men and helping them get treatment.

## Depression in Elderly Men

Men must cope with several kinds of stress as they age. If they have been the primary wage earners for their families and have identified heavily with their jobs, they may feel stress upon retirement—loss of an important role, loss of self-esteem—that can lead to depression. Similarly, the loss of friends and family and the onset of other health problems can trigger depression. Nevertheless, most elderly people feel satisfied with their lives, and it is not "normal" for older adults to feel depressed. Depression is an illness that can be effectively treated, thereby decreasing unnecessary suffering, improving the chances for recovery from other illnesses, and prolonging productive life.

However, health care professionals may miss depressive symptoms in older patients, who are often reluctant to discuss feelings of hope-lessness, sadness, loss of interest in normally pleasurable activities, or extremely prolonged grief after a loss, and who may complain pri-marily of physical symptoms. Also, it may be difficult to discern a co-occurring depressive disorder in patients who present with other illnesses, such as heart disease, stroke, or cancer, which in themselves may cause depressive symptoms, or which may be treated with medi-cations that have side effects resembling depression. If a depressive illness is diagnosed, treatment with appropriate medication and/or brief psychotherapy can help older adults manage both diseases, thus enhancing survival and quality of life.

*"As you get sick, as you become drawn in more and more by de-pression, you lose that perspective. Events become more irritat-ing, you get more frustrated about getting things done. You feel angrier, you feel sadder. Everything's magnified in an abnormal way."*

—Paul Gottlieb, publisher

The importance of identifying and treating depression in older adults is stressed by the statistics on suicide among the elderly. There is a common perception that suicide rates are highest among the young; however, it is the elderly, particularly older white males that have the highest rates. Over 70 percent of older suicide victims have been to their primary care physician within the month of their death, many with a depressive illness that was not detected. This has led to research efforts to determine how to best improve physicians' abili-ties to detect and treat depression in older adults.

Approximately 80 percent of older adults with depression improve when they receive treatment with antidepressant medication, psycho-therapy, or a combination of both. In addition, research has shown that a combination of psychotherapy and antidepressant medication is highly effective for reducing recurrences of depression among older adults. Psychotherapy alone has been shown to prolong periods of good health free from depression, and is particularly useful for older patients who cannot or will not take medication. Improved recognition and treatment of depression in late life will make those years more enjoyable and fulfilling for the depressed elderly person, the family, and caregivers.

## Depression in Boys and Adolescent Males

Only in the past two decades has depression in children been taken very seriously. An NIMH-sponsored study of nine- to 17-year-olds estimates that the prevalence of any depressive disorder is more than 6 percent in a six-month period, with 4.9 percent having major depression. Before puberty, boys and girls are equally likely to develop depressive disorders. After age 14, however, females are twice as likely as males to have major depression or dysthymia. The risk of developing bipolar disorder remains approximately equal for males and females throughout adolescence and adulthood.

Research has revealed that depression is occurring earlier in life today than in past decades. In addition, research has shown that early-onset depression often persists, recurs, and continues into adulthood, and that depression in youth may also predict more severe illness in adult life. Depression in young people frequently co-occurs with other mental disorders, most commonly anxiety, disruptive behavior, or substance abuse disorders, as well as with other serious illnesses such as diabetes. The depressed younger child may say he is sick, refuse to go to school, cling to a parent, or worry that the parent may die. The depressed older child may sulk, get into trouble at school, be negative, grouchy, and feel misunderstood.

Among both children and adolescents, depressive disorders confer an increased risk for illness and interpersonal and psychosocial difficulties that persist long after the depressive episode is resolved; in adolescents there is also an increased risk for substance abuse and suicidal behavior. Unfortunately, these disorders often go unrecognized by families and physicians alike. Signs of depressive disorders in young people are often viewed as normal mood swings typical of a particular developmental stage. In addition, health care professionals may be reluctant to prematurely "label" a young person with a mental illness diagnosis. However, early diagnosis and treatment of depressive disorders are critical to healthy emotional, social, and behavioral development.

Although the scientific literature on treatment of children and adolescents with depression is far less extensive than that for adults, a number of recent studies have confirmed the short-term efficacy and safety of treatments for depression in youth. Larger research studies on treatments are under way to determine which ones work best for which youngsters. Additional research is needed on how to best incorporate these treatments into primary care practice.

Bipolar disorder, although rare in young children, can appear in both children and adolescents. The unusual shifts in mood, energy, and functioning that are characteristic of bipolar disorder may begin with manic, depressive, or mixed manic and depressive symptoms. It is more likely to affect the children of parents who have the illness. Twenty to 40 percent of adolescents with major depression go on to reveal bipolar disorder within five years after the onset of depression.

Depression in children and adolescents is associated with an increased risk of suicidal behaviors. This risk may rise, particularly among adolescent males, if the depression is accompanied by conduct disorder and alcohol or other substance abuse. In 2000, suicide was the third leading cause of death among young males, age 10 to 24. NIMH-supported researchers found that among adolescents who develop major depressive disorder, as many as 7 percent may die by suicide in the young adult years. Therefore, it is important for doctors and parents to take seriously any remarks about suicide.

NIMH researchers are developing and testing various interventions to prevent suicide in children and adolescents. Early diagnosis and treatment, accurate evaluation of suicidal thinking, and limiting young people's access to lethal agents—including firearms and medications—may hold the greatest suicide prevention value.

## Suicide

*"You are pushed to the point of considering suicide, because living becomes very painful. You are looking for a way out, you're looking for a way to eliminate this terrible psychic pain. And I remember, I never really tried to commit suicide, but I came awful close, because I used to play matador with buses. You know, I would walk out into the traffic of New York City, with no reference to traffic lights, red or green, almost hoping that I would get knocked down."*

—Paul Gottlieb, publisher

Sometimes depression can cause people to feel like putting themselves in harm's way or killing themselves. Although the majority of people with depression do not die by suicide, having depression does increase suicide risk compared to people without depression.

If you are thinking about suicide, get help immediately:

- Call your doctor's office.

- Call 911 for emergency services.

- Go to the emergency room of the nearest hospital

- Ask a family member or friend to take you to the hospital or call your doctor.

- Call 1-800-SUICIDE (1-800-784-2433), the toll-free, 24-hour hotline of the National Hopeline Network sponsored by the Kristin Brooks Hope Center, to be connected to a trained counselor at a suicide crisis center nearest you.

## *Diagnostic Evaluation and Treatment*

*"Your tendency is just to wait it out, you know, let it get better. You don't want to go to the doctor. You don't want to admit to how bad you're really feeling."*

—Paul Gottlieb, publisher

The first step to getting appropriate treatment for depression is a physical examination by a physician. Certain medications as well as some medical conditions such as a viral infection, thyroid disorder, or low testosterone level can cause the same symptoms as depression, and the physician should rule out these possibilities through examination, interview, and lab tests. If no such cause of the depressive symptoms is found, a psychological evaluation for depression should be done by the physician or by referral to a mental health professional.

A good diagnostic evaluation will include a complete history of symptoms—i.e., when they started, how long they have lasted, how severe they are, whether the patient had them before and, if so, whether the symptoms were treated and what treatment was given. The doctor should ask about alcohol and drug use, and if the patient has thoughts about death or suicide. Further, a history should include questions about whether other family members have had a depressive illness and, if treated, what treatments they may have received and if they were effective. Last, a diagnostic evaluation should include a mental status examination to determine if speech, thought patterns, or memory has been affected, as sometimes happens with depressive disorders.

Treatment choice will depend on the patient's diagnosis, severity of symptoms, and preference. There are a variety of treatments, including medications and short-term psychotherapies (i.e., "talking" therapies), that have proven effective for depressive disorders. In general, severe depressive illnesses, particularly those that are recurrent, will require a combination of treatments for the best outcome.

## Medications

There are several types of medications used to treat depression. These include newer antidepressant medications—chiefly the selective serotonin reuptake inhibitors (SSRIs)—and older ones—the tricyclics and the monoamine oxidase inhibitors (MAOIs). The SSRIs, and other newer medications that affect neurotransmitters such as dopamine or norepinephrine, generally have fewer side effects than tricyclics. Sometimes the doctor will try a variety of antidepressants before finding the most effective medication or combination of medications for the patient. Sometimes the dosage must be increased to be effective. Although some improvements may be seen in the first couple of weeks, antidepressant medications must be taken regularly for three to four weeks (in some cases, as many as eight weeks) before the full therapeutic effect occurs.

Patients often are tempted to stop medication too soon. They may feel better and think they no longer need the medication, or they may think it isn't helping at all. It is important to keep taking medication until it has a chance to work, though side effects (see section on side effects) may appear before antidepressant activity does. Once the person is feeling better, it is important to continue the medication for at least four to nine months to prevent a relapse into depression. Some medications must be stopped gradually to give the body time to adjust, and many can produce withdrawal symptoms if discontinued abruptly. Therefore, medication should never be discontinued without talking to your doctor about it. For individuals with bipolar disorder and those with chronic or recurrent major depression, medication may have to be maintained indefinitely.

Research has shown that people with bipolar disorder are at risk of switching into mania, or of developing rapid cycling episodes, during treatment with antidepressant medication. Therefore, "mood-stabilizing" medications generally are required, alone or in combination with anti-depressants, to protect people with bipolar disorder from this switch. Lithium and valproate (Depakote®) are the most commonly used mood-stabilizing drugs today. However, the potential mood-stabilizing effects of newer medications continue to be evaluated through research.

Medications for depressive disorders are not habit-forming. Nevertheless, as is the case with any type of medication prescribed for more than a few days, these treatments have to be carefully monitored to see if the most effective dosage is being given. The doctor will check the dosage of each medicine and its effectiveness regularly.

For the small number of people for whom MAOIs are the best treatment, it is necessary to avoid certain foods that contain high levels of tyramine, including many cheeses, wines, and pickles, as well as medications such as decongestants. The interaction of tyramine with MAOIs can bring on a hypertensive crisis, a sharp increase in blood pressure that can lead to a stroke. The doctor should furnish a complete list of prohibited foods that the patient should carry at all times. Other forms of antidepressants require no food restrictions. Efforts are under way to develop a "skin patch" system for one of the newer MAOIs, selegiline; if successful, this may be a more convenient and safer medication option than the older MAOI tablets.

Medications of any kind—prescribed, over-the-counter, or borrowed—should never be mixed without consulting a doctor. Other health professionals, such as a dentist or other medical specialist, who may prescribe a drug should be told of the medications the patient is taking. Some medications, although safe when taken alone can, if taken with others, cause severe and dangerous side effects.

Alcohol, including wine, beer, and hard liquor, or street drugs may reduce the effectiveness of antidepressants and should be avoided. However, some people who have not had a problem with alcohol abuse or dependence may be permitted by their doctor to use a modest amount of alcohol while taking one of the newer antidepressants.

Anti-anxiety drugs or sedatives are not antidepressants. They are sometimes prescribed along with antidepressants, but they are not effective when taken alone for a depressive disorder. Stimulants, such as amphetamines, are also not effective antidepressants, but they are used occasionally under close supervision in medically ill depressed patients.

Lithium has for many years been the treatment of choice for bipolar disorder, as it can be effective in smoothing out the mood swings common to this illness. Its use must be carefully monitored, as the range between an effective dose and a toxic one is small. If a person has pre-existing thyroid, kidney, or heart disorders or epilepsy, lithium may not be recommended. Fortunately, other medications have been found to be of benefit in controlling mood swings. Among these are two mood-stabilizing anticonvulsants, valproate (Depakote®) and carbamazepine (Tegretol®). Both of these medications have gained wide acceptance in clinical practice, and valproate has been approved by the Food and Drug Administration for first-line treatment of acute mania. Other anticonvulsants that are being used now include lamotrigine (Lamictal®), topiramate (Topamax®), and gabapentin (Neurontin®); however, their role in the treatment of bipolar disorder is not yet proven and remains under study.

Most people who have bipolar disorder take more than one medication including, along with lithium and/or an anticonvulsant, a medication for accompanying agitation, anxiety, depression, or insomnia. Finding the best possible combination of these medications is of utmost importance to the patient and requires close monitoring by the physician.

Questions about any medication prescribed, or problems that may be related to it, should be discussed with your doctor.

### Side Effects

Before starting a new medication, ask the doctor to tell you about any side effects you may experience. Antidepressants may cause mild and usually temporary side effects (sometimes referred to as adverse effects) in some people. Typically these are annoying, but not serious. However, any unusual reactions or side effects, or those that interfere with functioning, should be reported to the doctor immediately.

The most common side effects of the newer antidepressants (SSRIs and others) are:

- *Headache*. This will usually go away.

- *Nausea*. This is also temporary, but even when it occurs, it is transient after each dose.

- *Nervousness and insomnia* (trouble falling asleep or waking often during the night). These may occur during the first few weeks; dosage reductions or time will usually resolve them.

- *Agitation* (feeling jittery). If this happens for the first time after the drug is taken and is more than transient, the doctor should be notified.

- *Sexual problems.* The doctor should be consulted if the problem is persistent or worrisome. Although depression itself can lower libido and impair sexual performance, it has been clearly established that SSRIs and other strongly serotonergic antidepressants (e.g., the tricyclic antidepressant clomipramine) provoke new, dose-dependent sexual dysfunction independent of their therapeutic activity in both men and women. These side effects can affect more than half of adults taking SSRIs. In men, common problems include reduced sexual drive, erectile dysfunction, and delayed ejaculation. In some cases of sexual dysfunction, the symptoms improve with the development of tolerance or lowering of the dose of medication; drug "holidays" in anticipation of sexual activity have proved to be successful for some patients taking shorter-acting SSRIs but are not feasible in the case of fluoxetine (Prozac®). Data describing differences among the SSRIs are limited, and there are no data showing a clinical benefit with respect to sexual dysfunction as a result of switching medications within this class. If an antidepressant must be changed, one from a different class should be substituted; bupropion (Wellbutrin®), mirtazapine (Remeron®), nefazodone (Serzone®), and venlafaxine (Effexor®) appear to be good choices on the basis of these side effects. Guided by a limited number of studies, some clinicians treating men with antidepressant-associated sexual dysfunction report improvement with the addition of bupropion (Wellbutrin®), buspirone (BuSpar®), or sildenafil (Viagra®) to ongoing treatment. Be sure to discuss the various options with your doctor, as there may be other interventions that can help.

Tricyclic antidepressants have different types of side effects:

- *Dry mouth.* It is helpful to drink sips of water, chew sugarless gum, and clean teeth daily.

- *Constipation.* Bran cereals, prunes, fruit, and vegetables should be in the diet.

- *Bladder problems.* Emptying the bladder may be troublesome, and the urine stream may not be as strong as usual; the doctor should be notified if there is marked difficulty or pain; may be particularly problematic in older men with enlarged prostate conditions.

- *Sexual problems.* Sexual functioning may change; men may experience some loss of interest in sex, difficulty in maintaining an erection or achieving orgasm. If worrisome, these side effects should be discussed with the doctor.

- *Blurred vision*. This will pass soon and will not usually necessitate new glasses.

- *Dizziness*. Rising from the bed or chair slowly is helpful.

- *Drowsiness as a daytime problem*. This usually passes soon. A person feeling drowsy or sedated should not drive or operate heavy equipment. The more sedating antidepressants are generally taken at bedtime to help sleep and minimize daytime drowsiness.

### Psychotherapies

Several forms of psychotherapy, including some short-term (10–20 weeks) therapies, can help people with depressive disorders. Two of the short-term psychotherapies that research has shown to be effective for depression are cognitive-behavioral therapy (CBT) and interpersonal therapy (IPT). Cognitive-behavioral therapists help patients change the negative thinking and behavior patterns that contribute to or result from depression. Through verbal exchange with the therapist, as well as "homework" assignments between therapy sessions, CBT helps patients gain insight into and resolve problems related to their depression. Interpersonal therapists help patients work through disturbed personal relationships that may be contributing to or worsening their depression. Psychotherapy is offered by a variety of licensed mental health providers, including psychiatrists, psychologists, social workers, and mental health counselors.

For many depressed patients, especially those with moderate to severe depression, a combination of antidepressant medication and psychotherapy is the preferred approach to treatment. Some psychiatrists offer both types of intervention. Alternatively, in many cases two mental health professionals collaborate in the treatment of a person with depression; for example, a psychiatrist or other physician, such as a family doctor, may prescribe medication while a nonmedical therapist provides ongoing psychotherapy.

> *"You start to have these little thoughts, 'Wait, maybe I can get through this. Maybe these things that are happening to me aren't so bad.' And you start thinking to yourself, 'Maybe I can deal with things for now.' And it's just little tiny thoughts until you realize that it's gone and then you go, 'Oh my God, thank you, I*

*don't feel sad anymore.' And then when it was finally gone, when I felt happy, I was back to the usual things that I was doing in my life. You get so happy because you think to yourself, 'I never thought it would leave.'"*

—Shawn Colten, national diving champion

## Electroconvulsive Therapy

Electroconvulsive therapy (ECT) is another treatment option that may be particularly useful for individuals whose depression is severe or life threatening, or who cannot take antidepressant medication. ECT often is effective in cases where antidepressant medications do not provide sufficient relief of symptoms. The exact mechanisms by which ECT exerts its therapeutic effect are not yet known.

In recent years, ECT has been much improved. A muscle relaxant is given before treatment, which is done under brief anesthesia. Electrodes are placed at precise locations on the head to deliver electrical impulses. The stimulation causes a brief (about 30 seconds) generalized seizure within the brain, which is necessary for therapeutic efficacy. The person receiving ECT does not consciously experience the electrical stimulus.

A typical course of ECT entails six to 12 treatments, administered at a rate of three times per week, on either an inpatient or outpatient basis. To sustain the response to ECT, continuation treatment, often in the form of antidepressant and/or mood stabilizer medication, must be instituted. Some individuals may require maintenance ECT, which is delivered on an outpatient basis at a rate of one treatment weekly to as infrequently as monthly. The most common side effects of ECT are confusion and memory loss for events surrounding the period of ECT treatment. The confusion and disorientation experienced upon awakening after ECT typically clear within an hour. More persistent memory problems are variable and can be minimized with the use of modern treatment techniques, such as application of both stimulus electrodes to the right side of the head (unilateral ECT).

## Herbal Therapy

In the past several years, there has been an increase in public interest in the use of herbs for the treatment of both depression and anxiety. The extract from St. John's wort (*Hypericum perforatum*), a wild-growing plant with yellow flowers, has been used extensively in Europe as a treatment for mild to moderate depression, and it now ranks among the top-selling botanical products in the United States. Because of the increase in Americans' use of St. John's wort and the need to answer important remaining questions about the herb's efficacy and long-term use for depression, the National Institutes of Health (NIH) conducted a four-year, $6 million clinical trial to determine whether a well-standardized extract of St. John's wort is effective in the treatment of adults suffering from major depression of moderate severity. The trial found that St. John's wort was no more effective for treating major depression of moderate severity than placebo. More research is needed to confirm the role of the herb in managing less severe forms of depression.

The Food and Drug Administration issued a Public Health Advisory on February 10, 2000, about the use of St. John's wort. It stated that the herb appears to affect an important metabolic pathway that is used by many drugs prescribed to treat conditions such as heart disease, depression, seizures, certain cancers, and rejection of organ transplants. Also, St. John's wort reduces blood levels of some HIV medications. If taken together, the combination could allow the AIDS virus to rebound, perhaps in a drug-resistant form. (See the alert on the NIMH Web site: http://www.nimh.nih.gov/events/stjohnwort.cfm). Health care providers should alert their patients about these potential drug interactions, and patients should always consult their health care provider before taking any herbal supplement.

## How to Help Yourself If You Are Depressed

*"It affects the way you think. It affects the way you feel. It just simply invades every pore of your skin. It's a blanket that covers everything. The act of pretending to be well was so exhausting. All I could do was shut down. At times you just say, 'It's enough already.'"*

—Steve Lappen, writer

Depressive disorders make one feel exhausted, worthless, helpless, and hopeless. Such negative thoughts and feelings make some people feel like giving up. It is important to realize that these negative views are part of the depression and typically do not accurately reflect the actual circumstances. Negative thinking fades as treatment begins to take effect. In the meantime:

- Mild exercise, going to a movie, a ballgame, or participating in religious, social, or other activities may help.

- Set realistic goals in light of the depression and assume a reasonable amount of responsibility.

- Break large tasks into small ones, set some priorities, and do what you can as you can.

- Try to be with other people and to confide in someone; it is usually better than being alone and secretive.

- Participate in activities that may make you feel better.

- Expect your mood to improve gradually, not immediately. Feeling better takes time. Often during treatment of depression, sleep and appetite will begin to improve before the depressed mood lifts.

- It is advisable to postpone important decisions until the depression has lifted. Before deciding to make a significant transition—change jobs, get married or divorced—discuss it with others who know you well and have a more objective view of your situation.

- People rarely "snap out of" a depression. But they can feel a little better day by day.

- Remember, positive thinking will replace the negative thinking that is part of the depression and will disappear as your depression responds to treatment.

- Let your family and friends help you.

## How Family and Friends Can Help

The most important thing anyone can do for a man who may have depression is to help him get to a doctor for a diagnostic evaluation and treatment. First, try to talk to him about depression—help him understand that depression is a common illness among men and is nothing to be ashamed about. Perhaps share this information with him. Then encourage him to see a doctor to determine the cause of his symptoms and obtain appropriate treatment.

Occasionally, you may need to make an appointment for the depressed person and accompany him to the doctor. Once he is in treatment, you may continue to help by encouraging him to stay with treatment until symptoms begin to lift (several weeks), or to seek different treatment if no improvement occurs. This may also mean monitoring whether he is taking prescribed medication and/or attending therapy sessions. Encourage him to be honest with the doctor about his use of alcohol and prescription or recreational drugs, and to follow the doctor's orders about the use of these substances while on antidepressant medication.

The second most important thing is to offer emotional support to the depressed person. This involves understanding, patience, affection, and encouragement. Engage him in conversation and listen carefully. Do not disparage the feelings he may express, but point out realities and offer hope. Do not ignore remarks about suicide. Report them to the depressed person's doctor. In an emergency, call 911. Invite him for walks, outings, to the movies, and other activities. Be gently insistent if your invitation is refused. Encourage participation in some activities that once gave pleasure, such as hobbies, sports, religious or cultural activities, but do not push him to undertake too much too soon. The depressed person needs diversion and company, but too many demands can increase feelings of failure.

Do not accuse the depressed person of faking illness or of laziness, or expect him "to snap out of it." Eventually, with treatment, most people do get better. Keep that in mind, and keep reassuring him that, with time and help, he will feel better.

## Where to Get Help

If unsure where to go for help, talk to someone you trust who has experience in mental health—for example, a doctor, nurse, social worker, or religious counselor. Ask their advice on where to seek treatment. If there is a university nearby, its departments of psychiatry or psychology may offer private and/or sliding-scale fee clinic treatment options. Otherwise, check the Yellow Pages under "mental health," "health," "social services," "suicide prevention," "crisis intervention services," "hotlines," "hospitals," or "physicians" for phone numbers and addresses. In times of crisis, the emergency room doctor at a hospital may be able to provide temporary help for a mental health problem, and will be able to tell you where and how to get further help.

Listed below are the types of people and places that will make a referral to, or provide, diagnostic and treatment services:

- Family doctors

- Mental health specialists, such as psychiatrists, psychologists, social workers, or mental health counselors

- Religious leaders/counselors

- Health maintenance organizations
- Community mental health centers
- Hospital psychiatry departments and outpatient clinics
- University- or medical school-affiliated programs
- State hospital outpatient clinics
- Social service agencies
- Private clinics and facilities
- Employee assistance programs
- Local medical and/or psychiatric societies

Within the federal government, the Substance Abuse and Mental Health Services Administration (SAMHSA) offers a "Services Locator" for mental health and substance abuse treatment programs and resources nationwide. Visit the website at http://www.mentalhealth. samhsa.gov/databases/ or call toll-free (800) 789-2647.

## Conclusion

Have you known a man who is grumpy, irritable, and has no sense of humor? Maybe he drinks too much or abuses drugs. Maybe he physically or verbally abuses his wife and his kids. Maybe he works all the time, or compulsively seeks thrills in high-risk behavior. Or maybe he seems isolated, withdrawn, and no longer interested in the people or activities he used to enjoy.

Perhaps this man is you. If so, it is important to understand that there is a disease of the brain called depression that may be underlying these feelings and behaviors. It's real: Scientists have developed sensitive imaging devices that enable us to see it in the brain. And it's treatable: More than 80 percent of those suffering from depression respond to existing treatments, and new ones are continually becoming available and helping more people. Talk to a health care provider about how you are feeling, and ask for help.

Or perhaps this man is someone you care about. Try to talk to him or to someone who has a chance of getting through to him. Help him to understand that depression is a common illness among men and is nothing to be ashamed about. Encourage him to see a doctor and get an evaluation for depression.

For most men with depression, life doesn't have to be so dark and hopeless. Life is hard enough as it is, and treating depression can free up vital resources to cope with life's challenges effectively. When a man is depressed, he's not the only one who suffers. His depression also darkens the lives of his family, his friends, virtually everyone close to him. Getting him into treatment can send ripples of healing and hope into all of those lives.

Depression is a real illness; it is treatable; and men can have it. It takes courage to ask for help, but help can make all the difference.

> *"And pretty soon you start having good thoughts about yourself and that you're not worthless and you kind of turn your head over your shoulder and look back at that, that rutted, muddy, dirt road that you just traveled and now you're on some smooth asphalt and go, 'Wow, what a trip. Still got a ways to go, but I wouldn't want to go down that road again.'"*

—Patrick McCathern, first sergeant, U.S. Air Force, retired

# Chapter 36

# *Domestic Violence*

## *Chapter Contents*

## Section 36.1

## *Questions and Answers about Domestic Violence*

Reprinted with permission from "Domestic Violence," American College of Emergency Physicians, http://www.acep.org/1,391,0.html, January 1998. © 1998 American College of Emergency Physicians. Reviewed by David A. Cooke, M.D., July 10, 2003.

- Domestic violence is a widespread problem that occurs among all ages, races, educational backgrounds, and socioeconomic groups.

- Emergency physicians are patient advocates who see the problem first-hand and can play an important role in breaking the cycle of domestic violence. Despite the magnitude of the problem, identifying domestic violence victims is still a complex issue.

- For help, talk to your physician before you end up in the emergency department, or call the National Domestic Violence Hotline at (800) 799-SAFE.

### *What is domestic violence, and who are its victims?*

Domestic violence, also known as partner abuse, spouse abuse, or battering, occurs when one person uses force to inflict injury, either emotional or physical, upon another person they have, or had, a relationship with. It occurs between spouses and partners, parents and children, children and grandparents, and brothers and sisters. Victims can be individuals of any age, race, or gender.

### *How extensive is the problem?*

Domestic violence is the single largest cause of injury to women between the ages of 15 and 44 in the United States, more than muggings, car accidents, and rapes combined. Each year between 2 and 4 million women are battered, and 2,000 of these battered women will die of their injuries. Violence against men by women is also a problem, according to the August issue of *Annals of Emergency Medicine*. In a study of an inner city hospital, men reported slightly more physical violence than women (20 percent of men and 19 percent of women), although women reported significantly more past and present nonphysical violence than men.

- A recent study by the U.S. Department of Justice shows that emergency departments treated more than 243,000 people in 1994 for injuries inflicted in the home by someone they knew intimately, four times higher than previous estimates of such crimes.

- Research studies show that approximately 900,000 parents are beaten or abused by their children each year. In 1988, researchers estimated that only one in four elder abuse incidents are reported, suggesting that 2 million incidents of elder abuse occurred that year.

- Approximately 2 million children in the United States are seriously abused by their parents, guardians, or others each year, and more than 1,000 children die as a result of their injuries. Recent studies suggest that approximately 20 percent of children will be sexually abused in some way before they become adults, usually by someone they know.

### Who are the most common victims of domestic violence?

There are no typical victims. Domestic abuse occurs among all ages, races, and socioeconomic classes. It occurs in families of all educational backgrounds, including physicians. Individuals may be living together or separated, divorced, or prohibited from contact by temporary or permanent restraining orders.

### What can emergency physicians do to stop domestic violence?

Despite the magnitude of the problem, identifying domestic violence victims is still a complex issue. It can be difficult to know whether someone fell or was pushed, and emergency physicians are working to improve identification of domestic violence when it occurs.

- The first thing a physician can do is recognize the signs of violence. These vary depending upon the type of abuse and the victim's position in the family.

- Medical findings such as these should prompt direct questioning about domestic violence:

    - Central pattern of injuries

    - Contusions or injuries in the head, neck, or chest

    - Injuries that suggest a defensive posture

    - Types or extent of injury that are inconsistent with the patient's explanation

    - Substantial delay between when the injury occurred and when the patient came for treatment

    - Injuries during pregnancy

    - Pattern of repeated visits to the emergency department

    - Evidence of alcohol or drug use

    - Arriving in the emergency department as a result of a suicide attempt or rape

- Physicians also can gain clues from observing a battered patient and his or her partner. For example, the patient may seem evasive, embarrassed, or inappropriately unconcerned with his or her injuries while the partner may be overly solicitous and answer questions for the patient. Or the partner of the victim may be openly hostile, defensive, or aggressive, setting up communication barriers between emergency personnel and the patient.

- Some physicians may not be familiar with the emotional, psychological, and social issues that can predispose someone to accept abuse. Emergency physicians in particular are trained to rapidly recognize and stabilize medical emergencies and therefore may place less emphasis on psychosocial factors. They also may be unfamiliar with the clinical presentations of domestic violence or may have prejudices or misunderstandings that prevent them from considering this possibility. For example, they may be concerned about intruding into the family unit or feel that victims could simply choose to leave abusive situations.

### When emergency physicians know or suspect abuse, are they required to report it to the police?

Battering is a crime, and few states specifically require reporting of domestic violence. A small number of states require mandatory arrest of batterers, and a few jurisdictions aggressively pursue cases of domestic violence and prosecute batterers even when victims refuse to press charges.

- Even when emergency physicians detect abuse, mandatory reporting to authorities—especially against a victim's will—may not be the best thing to do because it can put the victim at greater risk of injury and even death. Studies show that women who leave batterers are at a 75 percent greater risk of being killed by them.

- Virtually all jurisdictions impose civil or criminal penalties for failing to report suspected incidents of child abuse or neglect.

- It is extremely important for emergency physicians to know the laws of their states and how their local criminal justice systems deal with the issue so they can properly and adequately inform their patients.

## What kinds of help can emergency physicians offer to victims of domestic violence?

Because family violence often makes victims feel helpless and alone, emergency physicians can play an extremely important role in breaking the cycle of domestic violence.

- Even if a victim is not ready to leave the relationship or identify the batterer, physicians can recognize and confirm to her that this is a serious problem that must be solved, letting victims know that they are not alone, that they don't deserve to be beaten, and that help is available.

- Every emergency department should have written material with the names and telephone numbers of local shelters, advocacy groups, and legal assistance to give to patients if they feel it's safe to take it.

Section 36.2

# Hurting the One You Love: Intimate Partner Violence

Reprinted from "Intimate Partner Violence Fact Sheet," National Center for Injury Prevention and Control, Centers for Disease Control, reviewed February 28, 2003, http://www.cdc.gov/ncipc/factsheets/ipvfacts.htm.

Intimate partner violence—or IPV—is actual or threatened physical or sexual violence or psychological and emotional abuse directed toward a spouse, ex-spouse, current or former boyfriend or girlfriend, or current or former dating partner. Intimate partners may be heterosexual or of the same sex. Some of the common terms used to describe intimate partner violence are domestic abuse, spouse abuse, domestic violence, courtship violence, battering, marital rape, and date rape.

CDC uses the term "intimate partner violence" because it describes violence that occurs within all intimate relationships. Some of the other terms are overlapping and may be used to mean other forms of violence including abuse of elders, children, and siblings

## Occurrence

- Approximately 1.5 million women and 834,700 men are raped and/or physically assaulted by an intimate partner each year.

- Nearly two-thirds of women who reported being raped, physically assaulted, or stalked since age 18 were victimized by a current or former husband, cohabiting partner, boyfriend, or date.

- Among women who are physically assaulted or raped by an intimate partner, one in three is injured. Each year, more than 500,000 women injured as a result of IPV require medical treatment.

- As many as 324,000 women each year experience IPV during their pregnancy.

- Firearms were the major weapon type used in intimate partner homicides from 1981 to 1998.

## Consequences

- Intimate partner violence is associated with both short- and long-term problems, including physical injury and illness, psychological symptoms, economic costs, and death.

- As a consequence of severe intimate partner violence, female victims are more likely than male victims to need medical attention and take time off from work; they also spend more days in bed and suffer more from stress and depression.

- Each year, thousands of American children witness IPV within their families. Witnessing violence is a risk factor for long-term physical and mental health problems, including alcohol and substance abuse, being a victim of abuse, and perpetrating IPV.

- The estimated yearly direct medical cost of caring for battered women is about $1.8 billion.

## Groups at Risk

- More women than men experience intimate partner violence. According to the National Violence against Women Survey, one out of four U.S. women has been physically assaulted or raped by an intimate partner; one out of every 14 U.S. men reported such an experience.

- Women are more likely than men to be murdered in the context of intimate partner violence. Women ages 20 to 29 years are at greatest risk of being killed by an intimate partner.

- Nearly one-third of African American women experience IPV in their lifetimes compared with one-fourth of white women.

- According to the National Violence against Women Survey, American Indian/Alaska Native women and men were most likely to report IPV, and Asian/Pacific Islander women and men were least likely to report IPV. It is unclear whether this difference is due to variations in willingness to report information about violence or to variations in incidence of IPV.

## Risk Factors

- Alcohol use is frequently associated with violence between intimate partners. It is estimated that in 45 percent of cases of IPV, men had been drinking, and in about 20 percent of cases, women had been drinking.

- One study recently found that male partners' unemployment and drug or alcohol use were associated with increased risk for physical, sexual, and/or emotional abuse.

- Witnessing IPV as a child or adolescent, or experiencing violence from caregivers as a child, increases one's risk of both perpetrating IPV and becoming a victim of IPV.

- Men who are physically violent towards their partners are also likely to be sexually violent towards their partners and are likely to use violence towards children.

- Perpetrators of IPV may lack some social skills, such as lack of communication skills, particularly in the context of problematic situations with their intimate partners.

- Research has determined that violent husbands report more anger and hostility toward women when compared with nonviolent husbands.

- A high proportion of IPV perpetrators report more depression, lower self-esteem, and more aggression than nonviolent intimate partners. Evidence indicates that violent intimate partners may be more likely to have personality disorders such as schizoidal/borderline personality, antisocial or narcissistic behaviors, and dependency and attachment problems.

## Prevention: What You Can Do

At CDC, the National Center for Injury Prevention and Control (NCIPC) is actively working toward reducing the incidence of intimate partner violence through research on causes, risk factors, and intervention strategies.

What can you do if you are a victim? Contact your local battered women's shelter or the National Domestic Violence Hotline by telephone at (800) 799-SAFE (7233) or (800) 787-3224 (TDD) or on the Internet at http://www.ndvh.org/. The Hotline can provide you with helpful information and advice.

What can you do as a citizen? Learn more about intimate partner violence. Information is available in libraries, from local and national domestic violence organizations, and through the Internet. The NCIPC web page is a good place to start. The more you understand intimate partner violence, the easier it will be to recognize it and help friends who may be victims.

Other sources of information about intimate partner violence and prevention activities can be found on the Internet using the search words such as "domestic violence" and "spouse abuse."

# Chapter 37

# *When Men Are Raped*

Society is becoming increasingly aware of male rape. However, experts believe that current male rape statistics vastly underrepresent the actual number of males age 12 and over who are raped each year. Rape crisis counselors estimate that while only one in 50 raped women report the crime to the police, the rates of underreporting among men are even higher. Until the mid-1980s, most literature discussed this violent crime in the context of women only. The lack of tracking of sexual crimes against men and the lack of research about the effects of male rape are indicative of the attitude held by society at large—that while male rape occurs, it is not an acceptable topic for discussion.

Historically, the rape of males was more widely recognized in ancient times. Several of the legends in Greek mythology involved abductions and sexual assaults of males by other males or gods. The rape of a defeated male enemy was considered the special right of the victorious soldier in some societies and was a signal of the totality of the defeat. There was a widespread belief that a male who was sexually penetrated, even if it was by forced sexual assault, thus "lost his manhood," and could no longer be a warrior or ruler. Gang rape of a male was considered an ultimate form of punishment and, as such, was known to the Romans as punishment for adultery and the Persians and Iranians as punishment for violation of the sanctity of the harem.

Nicholas Groth, a clinical psychologist and author of *Men Who Rape: The Psychology of the Offender*, says all sexual assault is an act of aggression, regardless of the gender or age of the victim or the assailant. Neither sexual desire nor sexual deprivation is the primary motivating force behind sexual assault. It is not about sexual gratification, but rather a sexual aggressor using somebody else as a means of expressing his own power and control.

Much has been written about the psychological trauma associated with the rape of female victims. While less research has been conducted about male rape victims, case research suggests that males also commonly experience many of the reactions that females experience. These reactions include: depression, anger, guilt, self-blame, sexual dysfunctions, flashbacks, and suicidal feelings. Other problems facing males include an increased sense of vulnerability, damaged self-image, and emotional distancing. Male rape victims not only have to confront unsympathetic attitudes if they choose to press charges; they also often hear unsupportive statements from their friends, family, and acquaintances. People will tend to fault the male victim instead of the rapist. Stephen Donaldson, president of Stop Prisoner Rape (a national education and advocacy group), says that the suppression of knowledge of male rape is so powerful and pervasive that criminals such as burglars and robbers sometimes rape their male victims as a sideline solely to prevent them from going to the police.

There are many reasons that male victims do not come forward and report being raped, but perhaps the biggest reason for many males is the fear of being perceived as homosexual. However, male sexual assault has nothing to do with the sexual orientation of the attacker or the victim, just as a sexual assault does not make the victim survivor gay, bisexual, or heterosexual. It is a violent crime that affects heterosexual men as much as gay men. The phrase "homosexual rape," for instance, which is often used by uninformed persons to designate male-male rape, camouflages the fact that the majority of the rapists are not generally homosexual.

In a well-known study of offenders and victims conducted by Nicholas Groth and Ann Burgess, one-half of the offender population described their consenting sexual encounters to be with women only, while 38 percent had consenting sexual encounters with men and women. Additionally, one-half of the victim population was strictly heterosexual. Among the offenders studied, the gender of the victim did not appear to be of specific significance to half of the offenders. Instead, they appeared to be relatively indiscriminate with regard to their choice of a victim—that is, their victims included both males and females, as well as both adults and children. The choice of a victim seemed to be more a matter of accessibility than of sexual orientation, gender, or age.

Many people believe that the majority of male rape occurs in prison; however, there is existing research which shatters this myth. A study of incarcerated and nonincarcerated male rape victims in Tennessee concluded that the similarities between these two groups would suggest that the sexual assault of men may not be due to conditions unique to a prison and that all men are potential victims.

Research indicates that the most common sites for male rape involving postpuberty victims are outdoors in remote areas and in automobiles (the latter usually involving hitchhikers). Boys in their early and mid-teens are more likely to be victimized than older males (studies indicate a median victim age of 17). The form of assault usually involves penetration of the victim anally and/or orally, rather than stimulation of the victim's penis. Gang rape is more common in cases involving male victims than those involving female victims. Also, multiple sexual acts are more likely to be demanded, weapons are more likely to be displayed and used, and physical injury is more likely to occur, with the injuries that do occur being more serious than with injured female rape victims.

## Definition

Sexual assault and rape include any unwanted sexual acts. The assailant can be a stranger, an acquaintance, a family member, or someone the victim knows well and trusts. Rape and sexual assault are crimes of violence and are used to exert power and control over another person. The legal definitions of rape and sexual assault can vary from state to state. However, usually a sexual assault occurs when someone touches any part of another person's body in a sexual way, even through their clothes, without that person's consent. Rape of males is any kind of sexual assault that involves forced penetration of the anus or mouth by a penis, finger, or any other object. Both rape and sexual assault include situations when the victim cannot say "no" because he is disabled, unconscious, drunk, or high.

In some states, the word "rape" is used only to define a forced act of vaginal sexual intercourse, and an act of forced anal intercourse is termed "sodomy." In some states, the crime of sodomy also includes any oral sexual act. There are some states that now use gender-neutral terms to define acts of forced anal, vaginal, or oral intercourse. Also, some states no longer use the terms "rape" and "sodomy"; rather, all sex crimes are described as sexual assaults or criminal sexual conduct of various degrees depending on the use and amount of force or coercion on the part of the assailant.

## Victims' Response

It is not uncommon for a male rape victim to blame himself for the rape, believing that he in some way gave permission to the rapist. Male rape victims suffer a similar fear that female rape victims face—that people will believe the myth that they may have enjoyed being raped. Some men may believe they were not raped or that they gave consent because they became sexually aroused, had an erection, or ejaculated during the sexual assault. These are normal, involuntary physiological reactions. It does not mean that the victim wanted to be raped or sexually assaulted, or that the survivor enjoyed the traumatic experience. Sexual arousal does not necessarily mean there was consent.

According to Groth, some assailants may try to get their victim to ejaculate because for the rapist, it symbolizes their complete sexual control over their victim's body. Since ejaculation is not always within conscious control but rather an involuntary physiological reaction, rapists frequently succeed at getting their male victims to ejaculate. As Groth and Burgess have found in their research, this aspect of the attack is extremely stressful and confusing to the victim. In misidentifying ejaculation with orgasm, the victim may be bewildered by his physiological response during the sexual assault and, therefore, may be discouraged from reporting the assault for fear his sexuality may become suspect.

Another major concern facing male rape victims is society's belief that men should be able to protect themselves and, therefore, it is somehow their fault that they were raped. The experience of a rape may affect gay and heterosexual men differently. Most rape counselors point out that gay men have difficulties in their sexual and emotional relationships with other men and think that the assault occurred because they are gay, whereas straight men often begin to question their sexual identity and are more disturbed by the sexual aspect of the assault than the violence involved.

## Male Rape as an Act of Anti-gay Violence

Unfortunately, incidents of anti-gay violence also include forcible rape, either oral or anal. Attackers frequently use verbal harassment and name-calling during such a sexual assault. Given the context of coercion, however, such technically homosexual acts seem to imply no homosexuality on the part of the offenders. The victim serves, both physically and symbolically, as a "vehicle for the sexual status needs of the offenders in the course of recreational violence," according to Harry Joseph in *Hate Crimes*.

## If You Are a Victim

Rape and sexual assault include any unwanted sexual acts. Even if you agree to have sex with someone, you have the right to say "no" at any time, and to say "no" to any sexual acts. If you are sexually assaulted or raped, it is never your fault—you are not responsible for the actions of others.

Richie J. McMullen, author of *Male Rape: Breaking the Silence on the Last Taboo*, encourages seeking immediate medical attention whether or not the incident is reported to police. Even if you do not seem injured, it is important to get medical attention. Sometimes injuries that seem minor at first can get worse. Survivors can sometimes contract a sexually transmitted disease during the sexual assault, but not suffer immediate symptoms. Even if the symptoms of that disease take weeks or months to appear, it might be easily treated with an early diagnosis. [If you are concerned about HIV exposure, it is important to talk to a counselor about the possibility of exposure and the need for testing. For more information about HIV transmission and testing, contact the Centers for Disease Control National HIV/AIDS Hotline at (800) 342-AIDS, (800) 344-SIDA (Spanish), or (800) 243-7889 (TDD).]

Medical considerations making immediate medical attention imperative include:

- Rectal and anal tearing and abrasions which may require attention and put you at risk for bacterial infections

- Potential HIV exposure

- Exposure to other sexually transmitted diseases

If you plan to report the rape to the police, an immediate medical examination is necessary to collect potential evidence for the investigation and prosecution.

Some of the physical reactions a survivor may experience in response to the trauma of a sexual assault or rape include:

- Loss of appetite
- Nausea and/or stomach aches
- Headaches
- Loss of memory and/or concentration
- Changes in sleep patterns

Some of the psychological and emotional reactions a sexual assault survivor may experience include:

- Denial and/or guilt
- Shame or humiliation
- Fear and a feeling of loss of control
- Loss of self-respect
- Flashbacks to the attack
- Anger and anxiety
- Retaliation fantasies (sometimes shocking the survivor with their graphic violence)
- Nervous or compulsive behavior
- Depression and mood swings
- Withdrawal from relationships
- Changes in sexual activity

Survivors of rape, and often of attempted rape, usually manifest some elements of what has come to be called rape-related post-traumatic stress disorder (RR-PTSD), a form of post-traumatic stress disorder (PTSD). Apart from a small number of therapists and counselors specializing in sexual assault cases, few psychotherapists are familiar with the symptoms and treatment of RR-PTSD. For this reason, a rape survivor is usually well-advised to consult with a rape crisis center or someone knowledgeable in this area rather than relying on general counseling resources. The same applies to those close to a rape victim, such as a partner, spouse, or parent; these persons become secondary victims of the sexual assault and have special issues and concerns that they may need assistance in dealing with effectively.

Local rape crisis centers offer male sexual assault victims direct services or referrals for services, including counseling, crisis services, and support services. Victims may contact their local rape crisis center, no matter how long it has been since the rape occurred. Counselors on staff can either provide support or help direct the victim to trained professionals who can provide support. Most rape programs are staffed by women; however, some programs have male and female counselors. If you prefer one or the other, make that preference known when you initially contact the program. Whether or not they have male staff on call, almost all rape crisis centers can make referrals to male counselors sensitive to the needs of male sexual assault survivors. In addition, many communities across the country have support groups for victims of anti-gay violence.

Counseling can help you cope with the physical and emotional reactions to the sexual assault or rape, as well as provide you with necessary information about medical and criminal justice system procedures. Seeking counseling is an important way to regain a sense of control over your life after surviving a sexual assault. Contact your local rape crisis program even if services are not expressly advertised for male rape survivors. The number can be found in your local phone book listed under "Community Services Numbers," "Emergency Assistance Numbers," "Survival Numbers" or "Rape."

Sexual assault and rape are serious crimes. As a sexual assault survivor, you have the right to report the crime to the police. This decision is one only you can make. But because authorities are not always sensitive to male sexual assault victims, it is important to have a friend or advocate go with you to report the crime for support and assistance.

# Part Five

# Wellness and Appearance

# Chapter 38

# *Nutrition and Diet*

## *Chapter Contents*

491

# Section 38.1

# *Eating for Health*

Good health comes from eating a well-balanced diet. This means making sure you regularly eat foods that have a lot of vitamins and minerals in them, as well as foods that are not high in fat. You should drink milk every day to give your bones the calcium that makes them strong. Foods that are high in fiber are good for you, and you should try to eat several fruits and vegetables every day.

## *Do I need to make changes in my diet?*

If you answer yes to any of the following questions, you may need to talk about nutrition with your doctor:

- Has your doctor talked with you about a medical problem or a risk factor, such as high blood pressure or high cholesterol?

- Did your doctor tell you that this condition could be improved by a change in your diet?

- Do diabetes, cancer, heart disease, or osteoporosis run in your family?

- Are you overweight or have you gained weight over the years?

- Do you have questions about what kinds of foods you should eat or whether you should take vitamins?

- Do you think that you would benefit from seeing a nutritionist? (A nutritionist is a registered dietitian who specializes in nutrition counseling.)

## *Won't it be hard to change my diet?*

Not necessarily. But it will take time, so try not to get discouraged. The key is to keep trying to eat the right foods and stay in touch with your doctor and nutritionist, to let them know how you're doing. Here are a few suggestions to help you change your diet:

- Find the strong points and weak points in your current diet. Do you eat three to five servings of fruits and vegetables every day? Do you get enough calcium? Do you eat high-fiber foods regularly? If so, good! You're on the right track. Keep it up. If not, you can learn the changes you need to make.

- Make small, slow changes, instead of trying to make large, fast changes. This will make it easier for the changes to become a part of your every-day life.

- Every few days, keep track of your food intake by writing down what you ate and drank that day. Use this record to help you see if you need to eat more from any food groups, such as fruits, vegetables, or dairy products.

- Think about asking for help from a nutritionist, if you haven't already done so—especially if you have a medical problem that requires you to follow a special diet.

### Can I trust nutrition information I get from newspapers and magazines?

Nutrition tips from different sources can sometimes conflict with each other. You should always check with your doctor first. Also, keep in mind this advice:

- There is no "magic bullet" when it comes to nutrition. There isn't one diet that works for every person. You need to find a diet that works for you.

- Good nutrition doesn't come in a vitamin pill. You can take a vitamin pill to be sure you're getting enough vitamins and minerals, but your body benefits the most from eating healthy foods.

- Eating all different kinds of foods is best for your body. Learn to try new foods.

- Fad diets offer short-term changes, but good health comes from long-term effort and commitment.

- Stories from people who have used a diet program or product, especially in commercials and infomercials, are a way to sell more of the product. Remember, weight gain or other problems that come up after the program is over are never talked about in the ads.

## What changes can I make now in my diet?

Almost everyone can benefit from cutting back on fat in their diet. If your current diet is high in fat, try making these changes:

- Eat three to four servings of low-fat dairy products every day. You can use reduced-fat cheeses and nonfat yogurt. For example, if you make pizza at home, try using part-skim mozzarella cheese on top.

- Eat baked, grilled, and broiled foods rather than fried foods. Take the skin off before eating chicken. Eat fish at least once a week.

- Cut back on the extra fat that sneaks into your diet, such as butter or margarine on bread, sour cream on baked potatoes, and salad dressings on salad.

- Eat plenty of fruits and vegetables with your meals and as snacks.

- When eating away from home, watch out for "hidden" fats and larger portion sizes.

- Read the nutrition labels on foods before you buy them. If you need help reading the labels, ask your doctor or your nutritionist.

- Drink milk. Milk is important because it's a rich source of calcium. However, if you're still drinking whole milk, you're getting too much fat. Sometimes people try skim milk once and don't like the taste (or the way it looks in coffee). They go back to drinking whole milk. It might help to make a gradual change, starting with 2 percent milk. After three to six months, change to 1 percent milk. You might try mixing whole milk and 2 percent milk or 2 percent milk and 1 percent milk for a few weeks. Soon, you'll be able to enjoy drinking skim milk.

There are many health benefits to a low-fat, high-fiber diet, even if your weight never changes. So try to set goals you have a good chance of reaching, such as losing one pound a week or lowering your blood cholesterol level.

# Section 38.2

# *Effective Weight Loss*

Reprinted from "Losing Weight: More Than Counting Calories," Food and Drug Administration, This article originally appeared in *FDA Consumer* in January–February 2002, updated April 2002 and March 2003, http:// www.fda.gov/fdac/features/2002/102_fat.html.

Americans are getting fatter. We're putting on the pounds at an alarmingly rapid rate. And we're sacrificing our health for the sake of supersize portions, biggie drinks, and two-for-one value meals, obesity researchers say.

More than 60 percent of U.S. adults are either overweight or obese, according to the Centers for Disease Control and Prevention (CDC). While the number of overweight people has been slowly climbing since the 1980s, the number of obese adults has nearly doubled since then.

## No Laughing Matter

Excess weight and physical inactivity account for more than 300,000 premature deaths each year in the United States, second only to deaths related to smoking, says the CDC. People who are overweight or obese are more likely to develop heart disease, stroke, high blood pressure, diabetes, gallbladder disease, and joint pain caused by excess uric acid (gout). Excess weight can also cause interrupted breathing during sleep (sleep apnea) and wearing away of the joints (osteoarthritis).

Carrying extra weight means carrying an extra risk for certain types of cancer. "[Our] researchers have concluded that obesity increases the risk for many of the most common cancers worldwide, and perhaps cancer in general," says Melanie Polk, R.D., director of nutrition education at the American Institute for Cancer Research (AICR), a nonprofit research and education organization in Washington, D.C.

In their review of more than 100 studies and international reports on obesity and cancer risk, completed in October 2001, researchers at the AICR concluded that obesity is consistently linked to postmenopausal breast cancer, colon cancer, endometrial cancer, prostate cancer, and kidney cancer.

To address the public health epidemic of being overweight or obese, former Surgeon General David Satcher issued a "call to action" in December 2001. *The Surgeon General's Call to Action to Prevent and Decrease Overweight and Obesity* outlined strategies that communities can use in helping to address the problems. Those options included requiring physical education at all school grades, providing more healthy food options on school campuses, and providing safe and accessible recreational facilities for residents of all ages.

## *Are You Overweight?*

Overweight refers to an excess of body weight, but not necessarily body fat. Obesity means an excessively high proportion of body fat. Health professionals use a measurement called body mass index (BMI) to classify an adult's weight as healthy, overweight, or obese. BMI describes body weight relative to height and is correlated with total body fat content in most adults.

To get your approximate BMI, multiply your weight in pounds by 703, then divide the result by your height in inches, and divide that result by your height in inches a second time. (Or you can use the interactive BMI calculator at www.nhlbisupport.com/bmi/bmicalc. htm.)

A BMI from 18.5 up to 25 is considered in the healthy range, from 25 up to 30 is overweight, and 30 or higher is obese. Generally, the higher a person's BMI, the greater the risk for health problems, according to the National Heart, Lung and Blood Institute (NHLBI). However, there are some exceptions. For example, very muscular people, like bodybuilders, may have a BMI greater than 25 or even 30, but this reflects increased muscle rather than fat. "It is excess body fat that leads to the health problems such as type 2 diabetes, high blood pressure, and high cholesterol," says Eric Colman, M.D., of the Food and Drug Administration's Division of Metabolic and Endocrine Drug Products.

In addition to a high BMI, having excess abdominal body fat is a health risk. Men with a waist of more than 40 inches around and women with a waist of 35 inches or more are at risk for health problems.

Obesity, once thought by many to be a moral failing, is now often classified as a disease. The NHLBI calls it a complex chronic disease involving social, behavioral, cultural, physiological, metabolic, and genetic factors. Although experts may have different theories on how and why people become overweight, they generally agree that the key to losing weight is a simple message: Eat less and move more. Your body needs to burn more calories than you take in.

## Successful "Losers"

A popular weight-loss myth is that everyone who loses weight eventually gains it back, says Rena Wing, Ph.D., a professor of psychiatry at Brown Medical School in Providence, Rhode Island. Wing, the co-developer of a research study known as the National Weight Control Registry, has worked to deflate this myth.

Tucked away in the registry's database is information about the weight-control behaviors of more than 3,000 American adults who have lost an average of 60 pounds and have kept it off for an average of six years.

How do they do it?

These successful losers report four common behaviors, says Wing. They eat a low-fat, high-carbohydrate diet; they monitor themselves by weighing in frequently; they are very physically active; and they eat breakfast. Eating breakfast every day is contrary to the typical pattern for the average overweight person who is trying to diet, says Wing. "They get up in the morning and say 'I'm going to start my diet today,' and they eat little or no breakfast and a light lunch. Then they get hungry and consume most of their calories late in the day. Successful weight losers have managed to change this pattern."

Six years after their weight loss, most of the registry's successful losers still report eating a low-calorie, low-fat diet, with about 24 percent of calories from fat. (The *Dietary Guidelines for Americans* recommend no more than 30 percent of daily calories from fat.) They also exercise for about an hour or more a day, expending about 2,800 calories per week on a variety of activities. This is equivalent to walking 28 miles a week, or four miles a day, says Wing.

Wing also reports that more than 70 percent of the registry's weight losers became overweight before age 18.

Although Barbara Croft of Columbus, Ohio, was not an overweight child, she gained weight once she left home and started cooking for herself. Replacing the plain and simple meals she had as a child with pizza, sodas, and meat and vegetables laden with sauces, the 5' 5" Croft worked her way up to 350 pounds. "I always ate from all the food groups—I just ate huge portions and I ate in between meals," says Croft.

When she was diagnosed with type 2 diabetes in February 1999, Croft got scared. "I worried about the health consequences—about going blind. I already have a little numbness in my feet."

Croft went on a diet and lost 200 pounds in 19 months. She has kept it off for two and a half years. "This is the third time I've lost over 100 pounds," says the 52-year-old, 150-pound Croft, "but this is the longest I've been able to keep the weight off." In her two previous weight losses, Croft ate nutritious meals, but didn't exercise. This time, she started walking for exercise, but could only walk about a block at first. "My husband went with me because he was afraid I wouldn't make it," she says. Now, Croft walks on a treadmill for 50 minutes a day—25 minutes each morning and night.

She still eats balanced meals, but restricts her portions. And she always eats breakfast. "I have Egg Beaters, two pieces of low-calorie bread, fruit, decaf coffee, and 8 ounces of water." Croft dines out almost every night, typically eating half her dinner of grilled chicken or salmon and a vegetable or salad. She sends the other half back, so she isn't tempted to overeat.

"Losing the weight was easy—maintaining it is much harder," says Croft.

Croft had tried commercial weight-loss programs in the past, but this last time she did it on her own. "You have to find out what works for you," she says. "If I eat butter or cheese, that seems to do me in. Beef is also a problem."

Croft's diabetes is under control now without medication. And she says her knees don't hurt anymore, she can buy clothes in a regular store, and she started traveling again now that she can fit into an airplane seat.

## Setting a Goal

The first step to weight loss is setting a realistic goal. By using a BMI chart and consulting with your health-care provider, you can determine what is a healthy weight for you.

Studies show that you can improve your health with just a small amount of weight loss. "We know that physical activity in combination with reduced calorie consumption can lead to the 5 to 10 percent weight loss necessary to achieve remission of the obesity-associated complications," says William Dietz, M.D., Ph.D., director of the Division of Nutrition and Physical Activity at the CDC. "Even these moderate weight losses can improve blood pressure and help control diabetes and high cholesterol in obese or overweight adults."

To reach your goal safely, plan to lose weight gradually. A weight loss of one-half to two pounds a week is usually safe, according to the *Dietary Guidelines for Americans*. This can be achieved by decreasing the calories eaten or increasing the calories used by 250 to 1,000 calories per day, depending on current calorie intake. (Some people with serious health problems due to obesity may lose weight more rapidly under a doctor's supervision.) If you plan to lose more than 15 to 20 pounds, have any health problems, or take medication on a regular basis, a doctor should evaluate you before you begin a weight-loss program.

## Changing Eating Habits

Dieting may conjure up visions of eating little but lettuce and sprouts—but you can enjoy all foods as part of a healthy diet as long as you don't overdo it on fat (especially saturated fat), protein, sugars, and alcohol. To be successful at losing weight, you need to change your lifestyle—not just go on a diet, experts say.

Limit portion sizes, especially of foods high in calories, such as cookies, cakes, and other sweets; french fries; and fats, oils and spreads. Reducing dietary fat alone—without reducing calories—will not produce weight loss, according to the NHLBI's guidelines on treating overweight and obesity in adults.

Use the Food Guide Pyramid (http://www.nalusda.gov/fnic/Fpyr/pyramid.gif), developed by the U.S. Department of Agriculture (USDA) and the Department of Health and Human Services, to help you choose a healthful assortment of foods that includes vegetables, fruits, grains (especially whole grains), fat-free milk, and fish, lean meat, poultry, or beans. Choose foods naturally high in fiber, such as fruits, vegetables, legumes (such as beans and lentils), and whole grains. The high fiber content of many of these foods may help you to feel full with fewer calories.

All calorie sources are not created equal. Carbohydrate and protein have about 4 calories per gram, but fat has more than twice that amount (9 calories per gram). Just as for the general population, weight-conscious consumers should aim for a daily fat intake of no more than 30 percent of total calories.

Keep your intake of saturated fat at less than 10 percent of calories. Saturated fats increase the risk for heart disease by raising blood cholesterol. Foods high in saturated fats include high-fat dairy products (like cheese, whole milk, cream, butter, and regular ice cream), fatty fresh and processed meats, the skin and fat of poultry, lard, palm oil, and coconut oil.

If you drink alcoholic beverages, do so in moderation. Alcoholic beverages supply calories but few nutrients. A 12-ounce regular beer contains about 150 calories, a 5-ounce glass of wine about 100 calories, and 1.5 ounces of 80-proof distilled spirits about 100 calories.

Limit your use of beverages and foods that are high in added sugars—those added to foods in processing or preparation, not the naturally occurring sugars in foods such as fruit or milk. Foods containing added sugars provide calories, but may have few vitamins and minerals. In the United States, the major sources of added sugars include nondiet soft drinks, sweets and candies, cakes and cookies, and fruit drinks and fruitades.

## Using the Food Label

Under regulations from the Food and Drug Administration (FDA) and the United States Department of Agriculture (USDA), the food label, found on almost all processed foods, offers more complete, useful and accurate nutrition information than ever before. Even when restricting calories and portions, you can use the part of the food label called the Nutrition Facts panel to make sure you get all the essential nutrients for good health.

You'll find the serving size and the number of servings per package listed at the top of the Nutrition Facts panel. The serving size affects all the nutrient amounts listed on the panel. For example, if there is one cup in a serving and the package contains two servings, you need to double the calories and other nutrient numbers if you eat the whole package. Many items sold as single portions—like a 20-ounce soft drink, a 3-ounce bag of chips, and a large bagel—actually provide two or more servings.

"If you zero in on the 'amount per serving' section of the Nutrition Facts panel, you can tell at a glance how many calories a serving has and whether a food is high in total fat, saturated fat, cholesterol, and sodium," says Naomi Kulakow, coordinator of food labeling education in the FDA's Center for Food Safety and Applied Nutrition. "These are items you should think about limiting in your diet."

The Nutrition Facts panel also shows how much dietary fiber, vitamin A, vitamin C, calcium, and iron are contained in a serving. These are nutrients you need for good health.

Also listed on the Nutrition Facts panel are the amounts of carbohydrates, protein, and sugars contained in a serving. Use the panel to compare the amount of total sugars among similar products, and try to choose ones lower in sugars.

In addition to listing some nutrients by weight, the panel also gives this information as a percent daily value (%DV). The %DV shows how a serving of a food fits in with recommendations for a healthful diet and allows consumers to make comparisons between similar products.

For example, shoppers can use the %DV figures to find out which frozen dinner is lower in saturated fat—particularly when it involves a comparative nutritional claim, such as reduced fat. "You don't need to know the precise definition of 'low' or 'reduced,'" says Kulakow. "Just look at the percent daily value and see which is higher or lower in the nutrient you are interested in." Foods with 5 percent or less of the daily value are considered low in a nutrient, while those with 20 percent or more are high in the nutrient.

The %DVs are based on a 2,000-calorie daily diet. But even if you eat less than 2,000 calories, the %DV can be used to determine whether a food is high or low in a particular nutrient.

"People use the food label too often to just restrict calories and fat—not to get enough nutrients," says Kulakow. While restricting calories is important for weight loss, "most people have no idea how many calories they consume every day—especially if they eat out." The %DV gives you a frame of reference and can be used to make dietary trade-offs, says Kulakow. "For example, if you eat a favorite food that's high in fat at one meal, balance it with low-fat foods at other times of the day."

Kulakow advises caution when choosing foods that are labeled "fat-free" and "low-fat." Fat-free doesn't mean calorie-free. To make a food tastier, sometimes extra sugars are added, which adds calories. So dieters should always check the Nutrition Facts panel to get complete information, says Kulakow.

For further guidance on using the Nutrition Facts panel, visit FDA's Center for Food Safety and Applied Nutrition (http://www.cfsan.fda.gov/~dms/foodlab.html).

## Increasing Physical Activity

Most health experts recommend a combination of a reduced-calorie diet and increased physical activity for weight loss. Most adults should get at least 30 minutes and children should get 60 minutes of moderate physical activity on most, and preferably all, days of the week. But fewer than one in three U.S. adults gets the recommended amount of physical activity, according to *The Surgeon General's Call to Action to Prevent and Decrease Overweight and Obesity*.

In addition to helping to control weight, physical activity decreases the risk of dying from coronary heart disease and reduces the risk of developing diabetes, hypertension, and colon cancer. Researchers also have found that daily physical activity may help a person lose weight by partially lessening the slowdown in metabolism that occurs during weight loss.

Exercise does not have to be strenuous to be beneficial. And some studies show that short sessions of exercise several times a day are just as effective at burning calories and improving health as one long session.

To lose weight and to maintain a healthy weight after weight loss, many adults will likely need to do more than 30 minutes of moderate physical activity daily.

## Prescription Weight-Loss Drugs

For obese people who have difficulty losing weight through diet and exercise alone, there are a number of FDA-approved prescription drugs that may help. "On average, individuals who use weight-loss drugs lose about 5 percent to 10 percent of their original weight, though some will lose less and some more," says the FDA's Colman.

All of the prescription weight-loss drugs work by suppressing the appetite except for Xenical® (orlistat). Approved by the FDA in 1999, Xenical is the first in a new class of anti-obesity drugs known as lipase inhibitors. Lipase is the enzyme that breaks down dietary fat for use by the body. Xenical interferes with lipase function, decreasing dietary fat absorption by 30 percent. Because the undigested fats are not absorbed, fewer calories are available to the body. This may help in controlling weight. The main side effects of Xenical are cramping, diarrhea, flatulence, intestinal discomfort, and leakage of oily stool.

Meridia® (sibutramine), approved by the FDA in 1997, increases the levels of certain brain chemicals that help reduce appetite. Because it may increase blood pressure and heart rate, Meridia should not be used by people with uncontrolled high blood pressure, a history of heart disease, congestive heart failure, irregular heartbeat, or stroke. Other common side effects of Meridia include headache, dry mouth, constipation, and insomnia.

Other anti-obesity prescription drugs that were approved by the FDA many years ago based on very short-term, limited data include: Bontril® (phendimetrazine tartrate), Desoxyn® (methamphetamine) and Ionamin and Adipex-P® (phentermine). They are "speed"-like drugs that should not be used by people with heart disease, high blood pressure, an overactive thyroid gland, or glaucoma. These drugs are approved only for short-term use, such as a few weeks. They generally don't cause weight loss beyond several weeks, and they have significant potential for physical dependence or addiction.

"There is no magic pill for obesity," says David Orloff, M.D., director of the FDA's Division of Metabolic and Endocrine Drug Products. "The best effect you're going to get is with a concerted long-term regimen of diet and exercise. If you choose to take a drug along with this effort, it may provide additional help."

Until September 1997, two other drugs, fenfluramine (Pondimin® and others) and dexfenfluramine (Redux®), were available for treating obesity. But at the FDA's request, the manufacturers of these drugs voluntarily withdrew them from the market after newer findings suggested that they were the likely cause of heart valve problems. The FDA recommended that people taking the drugs stop and that they contact their doctor to discuss their treatment. (For the latest information on this topic, visit www.fda.gov/cder/news/feninfo. htm.)

Prescription weight-loss drugs are approved only for those with a BMI of 30 and above, or 27 and above if they have other risk factors, such as high blood pressure or diabetes.

People should contact a doctor before using any kind of drug, including a weight-loss drug.

## Over-the-Counter Drugs

Until recently, weight-control drugs containing the active ingredient phenylpropanolamine (also used as a nasal decongestant) were available over the counter (OTC). However, based on evidence linking this ingredient to an increased risk of hemorrhagic stroke (bleeding in the brain), the FDA asked drug manufacturers to discontinue marketing products containing phenylpropanolamine. In addition, the FDA issued a public health advisory in November 2000 warning consumers to stop using products containing this ingredient.

The FDA is proposing to classify phenylpropanolamine as "not generally recognized as safe," and is proceeding with regulatory actions that will likely remove this ingredient from the market. Although cough-cold products were reformulated with other nasal decongestant ingredients, there is no currently available active ingredient that is generally recognized as safe and effective for use in an OTC weight-control drug product.

## Beware of Unproven Claims

Some dietary supplement makers claim their products work for weight loss. These products are not reviewed by the FDA before they are marketed. "Under our existing laws, manufacturers have the responsibility for ensuring that their dietary supplement products are safe and effective," says Christine Lewis Taylor, Ph.D., R.D., director of the FDA's Office of Nutritional Products, Labeling, and Dietary Supplements.

Many weight-loss products claim to be "natural" or "herbal," but this does not necessarily mean that they're safe. These ingredients may interact with drugs or may be dangerous for people with certain medical conditions. If you are unsure about a product's claims or the safety of any weight-loss product, check with your doctor before using it.

## Avoid 'Fad' Diets

The cabbage soup diet, the low-carbohydrate and high-protein diet, and other so-called "fad" diets are fundamentally different from federal nutrition dietary guidelines and are not recommended for losing weight.

Fad diets usually overemphasize one particular food or type of food, contradicting the guidelines for good nutrition, which recommend eating a variety of foods from the Food Guide Pyramid. These diets may work at first because they cut calories, but they rarely have a permanent effect.

A high-protein diet is one fad diet that has remained popular over the years. "High-protein items may also be high in fat," says Robert Eckel, M.D., professor of medicine at the University of Colorado Health Sciences Center in Denver. High-fat diets can raise blood cholesterol levels, which increases a person's risk for heart disease and certain cancers.

High-protein diets force the kidneys to try to get rid of the excess waste products of protein and fat, called ketones. A buildup of ketones in the blood (called ketosis) can cause the body to produce high levels of uric acid, which is a risk factor for gout (a painful swelling of the joints) and kidney stones. Ketosis can be especially risky for people with diabetes because it can speed the progression of diabetic renal disease, says Eckel.

"It's important for the public to understand that no scientific evidence supports the claim that high-protein diets enable people to maintain their initial weight loss," says Eckel. "In general, quick weight-loss diets don't work for most people."

## Tips for Eating Out

- Choose foods that are steamed, broiled, baked, roasted, poached, or stir-fried.

- Share food, such as a main dish or dessert, with your dining partner.

- Take part of the food home with you, and refrigerate immediately. You may want to ask for a take-home container when the meal arrives. Spoon half the meal into it, so you're more likely to eat only what's left on your plate.

- Request your meal to be served without gravy, sauces, butter, or margarine.

- Ask for salad dressing on the side, and use only small amounts of full-fat dressings.

## Worth the Effort

"Losing weight requires major lifestyle changes, including diet and nutrition, exercise, behavior modification, and—when appropriate—intervention with drug therapy," says Judith S. Stern, Sc.D., professor of nutrition and internal medicine at the University of California, Davis, and vice president of the American Obesity Association. "But it is always worth making the effort to improve your health."

*—by Linda Bren*

## Section 38.3

# *Weight Loss Drugs and Safety*

Plenty of pills claim to be the "easy" way to weight loss. For many of them safety may be an issue.

Weight-loss pills and beverages that contain ephedra or ma huang, for instance, continue to be questioned for their potential side effects. These energy enhancers can increase blood pressure and heart rate and elevate body temperature, with more serious side effects including stroke and heart attack. Ephedra is categorized as a dietary supplement, so regulations to control its use are limited.

In addition to the safety concerns, fast weight loss often isn't long-lasting weight loss. If you're trying to lose weight, resist the temptation of a quick fix and turn to the tried and true: Make lasting changes in what and how much you eat and include more physical activity.

Chapter 39

# Tobacco

## Chapter Contents

# Section 39.1

# *Nicotine Addiction and Health*

Reprinted from "Cigarettes and Other Nicotine Products," National Institute on Drug Abuse, National Institutes of Health, 2003, http://www.nida.nih.gov/Infofax/tobacco.html.

Nicotine is one of the most heavily used addictive drugs in the United States. Cigarette smoking has been the most popular method of taking nicotine since the beginning of the twentieth century. In 1998, 60 million Americans were current cigarette smokers (28 percent of all Americans aged 12 and older), and 4.1 million were between the ages of 12 and 17 (18 percent of youth in this age bracket).

In 1989, the U.S. Surgeon General issued a report that concluded that cigarettes and other forms of tobacco, such as cigars, pipe tobacco, and chewing tobacco, are addictive and that nicotine is the drug in tobacco that causes addiction. In addition, the report determined that smoking was a major cause of stroke and the third leading cause of death in the United States.

## *Health Hazards*

Nicotine is highly addictive. It is both a stimulant and a sedative to the central nervous system. The ingestion of nicotine results in an almost immediate "kick" because it causes a discharge of epinephrine from the adrenal cortex. This stimulates the central nervous system and other endocrine glands, which causes a sudden release of glucose. Stimulation is then followed by depression and fatigue, leading the abuser to seek more nicotine. Nicotine is absorbed readily from tobacco smoke in the lungs, and it does not matter whether the tobacco smoke is from cigarettes, cigars, or pipes.

Nicotine also is absorbed readily when tobacco is chewed. With regular use of tobacco, levels of nicotine accumulate in the body during the day and persist overnight. Thus, daily smokers or chewers are exposed to the effects of nicotine for 24 hours each day. Nicotine taken in by cigarette or cigar smoking takes only seconds to reach the brain but has a direct effect on the body for up to 30 minutes.

Research has shown that stress and anxiety affect nicotine tolerance and dependence. The stress hormone corticosterone reduces the effects of nicotine; therefore, more nicotine must be consumed to achieve the same effect. This increases tolerance to nicotine and leads to increased dependence. Studies in animals have also shown that stress can directly cause relapse to nicotine self-administration after a period of abstinence.

Other studies have shown that animals cannot discriminate between the effects of nicotine and the effects of cocaine. Studies have also shown that nicotine self-administration sensitizes animals to self-administer cocaine more readily. Addiction to nicotine results in withdrawal symptoms when a person tries to stop smoking. For example, a study found that when chronic smokers were deprived of cigarettes for 24 hours, they had increased anger, hostility, and aggression and loss of social cooperation. Persons suffering from withdrawal also take longer to regain emotional equilibrium following stress. During periods of abstinence and/or craving, smokers have shown impairment across a wide range of psychomotor and cognitive functions, such as language comprehension.

Adolescent smokeless tobacco users are more likely than nonusers to become cigarette smokers. Behavioral research is beginning to explain how social influences, such as observing adults or other peers smoking, affect whether adolescents begin to smoke cigarettes. Research has shown that teens are generally resistant to many kinds of anti-smoking messages.

In addition to nicotine, cigarette smoke is primarily composed of a dozen gases (mainly carbon monoxide) and tar. The tar in a cigarette, which varies from about 15 milligrams for a regular cigarette to 7 milligrams in a low-tar cigarette, exposes the user to a high expectancy rate of lung cancer, emphysema, and bronchial disorders. The carbon monoxide in the smoke increases the chance of cardiovascular diseases.

The Environmental Protection Agency has concluded that second-hand smoke causes lung cancer in adults and greatly increases the risk of respiratory illnesses in children and sudden infant death.

## Promising Research

Research has shown that nicotine, like cocaine, heroin, and marijuana, increases the level of the neurotransmitter dopamine, which affects the brain pathways that control reward and pleasure. Scientists now have pinpointed a particular molecule (the beta 2 subunit of the nicotine cholinergic receptor) as a critical component in nicotine addiction. Mice that lack this molecule fail to self-administer nicotine, implying that without the b2 molecule, the mice do not experience the positive reinforcing properties of nicotine. This new finding identifies a potential site for targeting the development of anti-nicotine addiction medications.

Other new research found that individuals have greater resistance to nicotine addiction if they have a genetic variant that decreases the function of the enzyme CYP2A6. The decrease in CYP2A6 slows the breakdown of nicotine and protects individuals against nicotine addiction. Understanding the role of this enzyme in nicotine addiction gives a new target for developing more effective medications to help people stop smoking. Medications might be developed that can inhibit the function of CYP2A6, thus providing a new approach to preventing and treating nicotine addiction.

Another study found dramatic changes in the brain's pleasure circuits during withdrawal from chronic nicotine use. These changes are comparable in magnitude and duration to similar changes observed during the withdrawal from other abused drugs such as cocaine, opiates, amphetamines, and alcohol. Scientists found significant decreases in the sensitivity of the brains of laboratory rats to pleasurable stimulation after nicotine administration was abruptly stopped. These changes lasted several days and may correspond to the anxiety and depression experienced by humans for several days after quitting smoking "cold turkey." The results of this research may help in the development of better treatments for the withdrawal symptoms that may interfere with individual's attempts to quit smoking.

## Treatment

Research suggests that smoking cessation should be a gradual process because withdrawal symptoms are less severe in those who quit gradually than in those who quit all at once. Rates of relapse are highest in the first few weeks and months and diminish considerably after three months.

Studies have shown that pharmacological treatment combined with psychological treatment, including psychological support and skills training to overcome high-risk situations, results in some of the highest long-term abstinence rates.

Behavioral economic studies find that alternative rewards and reinforcers can reduce cigarette use. One study found that the greatest reductions in cigarette use were achieved when smoking cost was increased in combination with the presence of alternative recreational activities.

Nicotine chewing gum is one medication approved by the Food and Drug Administration (FDA) for the treatment of nicotine dependence. Nicotine in this form acts as a nicotine replacement to help smokers quit the smoking habit.

The success rates for smoking cessation treatment with nicotine chewing gum vary considerably across studies, but evidence suggests that it is a safe means of facilitating smoking cessation if chewed according to instructions and restricted to patients who are under medical supervision.

Another approach to smoking cessation is the nicotine transdermal patch, a skin patch that delivers a relatively constant amount of nicotine to the person wearing it. A research team at the National Institute on Drug Abuse's Division of Intramural Research studied the safety, mechanism of action, and abuse liability of the patch that was consequently approved by FDA. Both nicotine gum and the nicotine patch, as well as other nicotine replacements such as sprays and inhalers, are used to help people fully quit smoking by reducing withdrawal symptoms and preventing relapse while undergoing behavioral treatment.

Another tool in treating nicotine addiction is a medication that goes by the trademark Zyban®. This is not a nicotine replacement, as are the gum and patch. Rather, this works on other areas of the brain, and its effectiveness is in helping to make controllable nicotine craving or thoughts about cigarette use in people trying to quit.

In the future, a nicotine vaccine may be an effective method for preventing and treating tobacco addiction. The vaccine would prevent nicotine from reaching the brain so as to reduce its effects and help keep people from becoming addicted.

Scientists recently developed an experimental nicotine vaccine consisting of a nicotine derivative attached to a large protein. The scientists injected a single dose of nicotine into vaccinated rats and found that the amount of nicotine reaching the brain was reduced by 64 percent. Further, the researchers found that administering doses of nicotine antibodies similar to those that are ordinarily produced by the vaccine greatly reduced the rise in blood pressure produced by a nicotine injection. The antibodies also completely prevented the increased movements ordinarily seen when rats are injected with nicotine.

The next steps will be to conduct additional safety studies, followed by clinical trials with the vaccine in human volunteers. These clinical trials are currently scheduled to begin in early 2002.

Section 39.2

# *The Risks of Cigars*

Reprinted with permission from the Academy of General Dentistry, © 2001. For additional oral health topics, toll-free access to a directory of members in your ZIP code area, and other consumer services, see page 583 of this *Sourcebook* or contact the Academy of General Dentistry, 211 E. Chicago Avenue, Suite 900, Chicago, IL 60611, (312) 440-4300, or visit the website at http://www.agd.org.

Viewed as a glamorous luxury by men and women, cigars are promoted by everyone from sport superstars to top movie stars to upscale clothing stores and clubs. U.S. consumers lit up 4.4 billion cigars last year, and sales continue to rise. As cigar connoisseurs are leisurely puffing, they fail to realize that their habit not only hurts their health and smiles, but also is addictive and may be more dangerous than cigarettes, say dental experts meeting at the Academy of General Dentistry's forty-fifth annual meeting.

And cigar smoking is not just a habit of older men, but increasingly of women and teens. The Centers for Disease Control and Prevention (CDC) reports 26.7 percent of teens ages 14 to 19 have smoked a cigar in the past year.

"Cigars provide a false sense of security because many people think that they are a safe alternative to cigarettes," says E. "Mac" Edington, D.D.S., M.A.G.D., president of the Academy of General Dentistry. "Cigars can have up to 40 times the nicotine and tar found in cigarettes."

Dentists are patients' first line of defense against the adverse effects of tobacco use and nicotine addiction stemming from cigars, cigarettes, and smokeless tobacco. Dentists routinely screen for oral cancer and can help patients with tobacco cessation programs.

"Cigars are marketed as an upscale habit of the wealthy," says Robert Mecklenburg, D.D.S., M.P.H., dental coordinator, Smoking and Tobacco Control Program of the National Cancer Institute. "They are portrayed as being related to having money, sophistication, and an important social image of which people want to be a part. And kids are aware of what adults partake in."

"People think smoking occasional cigars is fine, but smoking cigars increases nicotine levels in the body," says Dr. Mecklenburg. "And an increase in nicotine means an increase in dependence. In addition, tobacco carcinogens places them at risk of mouth and throat cancer."

Other facts about cigar smoking:

- Cigar smokers often have badly stained teeth and chronic bad breath.

- Cigar smokers have four to 10 times the risk of dying from oral, laryngeal, and esophageal cancers as nonsmokers.

- The risk of lung cancer for cigar smokers is three times that of nonsmokers.

- Cancer death rates among men who smoke cigars are 34 percent higher than among their nonsmoking peers.

## Section 39.3

# *The Myth of Smokeless Tobacco*

Reprinted with permission from the Academy of General Dentistry, © 2001. For additional oral health topics, toll-free access to a directory of members in your ZIP code area, and other consumer services, see page 583 of this *Sourcebook* or contact the Academy of General Dentistry, 211 E. Chicago Avenue, Suite 900, Chicago, IL 60611, (312) 440-4300, or visit the website at http://www.agd.org.

Spit tobacco affects your dental health as well as the rest of your body. If you use smokeless tobacco and have thought about quitting, your dentist can help. In the meantime, here are a few facts that may help you decide to join the 200 million Americans who are tobacco-free.

### *What is spit tobacco?*

Spit tobacco includes snuff, a finely ground version of processed tobacco, and chewing tobacco in the form of shredded or pressed bricks and cakes, called plugs, or rope-like strands called twists. Users "pinch" or "dip" tobacco and place a wad in their cheek or between their lower lip and gums. In the United Kingdom, users often snort snuff.

### *Isn't it safer than smoking?*

Absolutely not. Some wrongly believe that spit tobacco is safer than smoking cigarettes. But spit tobacco is more addictive because it contains higher levels of addictive nicotine than cigarettes and can be harder to quit than cigarettes. One can of snuff delivers as much nicotine as 60 cigarettes.

About 8,000 people die every year from various types of tobacco use. About 70 percent of those deaths are from oral cancer. Other cancers caused by tobacco include cancer of the pancreas, nasal cavity, urinary tract, esophagus, pharynx, larynx, intestines, and stomach. Kids who use spit tobacco products are four to six times more likely to develop oral cancer than nonusers, and tobacco juice–related cancers can form within five years of regular use. Among high school seniors who have ever used spit tobacco, almost three-fourths began by the ninth grade.

### *How does snuff and chewing tobacco harm my dental health?*

It causes bad breath, discolors teeth, and promotes tooth decay that leads to tooth loss. Spit tobacco users have a decreased sense of smell and taste, and they are at greater risk of developing cavities. The grit in snuff eats away at gums, exposing tooth roots which are sensitive to hot and cold temperatures and can be painful. Sugar in spit tobacco causes decay. Spit tobacco users also have a hard time getting their teeth clean.

### *What about mouth sores?*

The most common sign of possible cancer in smokeless tobacco users is leukoplakia (loo-ko-play-key-ah), a white scaly patch or lesion inside the mouth or lips, common among many spit tobacco users. Red sores are also a warning sign of cancer. Often, signs of precancerous lesions are undetectable. Dentists can diagnose and treat such cases before the condition develops into oral cancer. If a white or red sore appears and doesn't heal, see your dentist immediately for a test to see if it's precancerous. Spit tobacco users also should see their dentist every three months, to make sure a problem doesn't develop.

Studies have found that 60 to 78 percent of spit tobacco users have oral lesions.

## What are double dippers?

Double dippers, who mix snuff and chewing tobacco, are more likely to develop precancerous lesions than those who use only one type of spit tobacco. Long-term snuff users have a 50 percent greater risk of developing oral cancer than nonusers, and spit tobacco users are more likely to become cigarette smokers.

## How do you kick the habit?

Your dentist can help you kick your spit tobacco habit. In addition to cleaning teeth and treating bad breath and puffy, swollen gums associated with tobacco use, your dentist may prescribe a variety of nicotine replacement therapies, such as the transdermal nicotine patch or chewing gum that helps to wean addicted snuff dippers or tobacco chewers. Nicotine patches are worn for 24 hours over several weeks, supplying a steady flow of nicotine. The four brands of patches are Habitrol®, Nicoderm®, Nicotrol®, and ProStep®. Over the course of treatment the amount of nicotine in the patch decreases. The nicotine patch has a 25 percent success rate. Or you may try nicotine gum therapy on your quit day. One piece of gum is slowly chewed every one to two hours. Each piece should be discarded after 20 to 30 minutes.

**Make goals.** Make the following goals to quit and never resume chewing or dipping:

- Pick a date and taper use as the date nears. Instead of using spit tobacco, carry substitutes like gum, hard candy, and sunflower seeds.

- Cut back on when and where you dip and chew. Let friends and family know that you're quitting and solicit their support. If they dip and chew, ask them not to do it around you.

- Make a list of three situations you're most likely to dip and chew, and make every effort to avoid using tobacco at those times.

- Switch to a lower-nicotine brand to help cut down your dose.

Chapter 40

# *Alcohol*

## *Chapter Contents*

# Section 40.1

# *Alcoholism and Alcohol Abuse*

Reprinted from "Alcoholism: Getting the Facts," National Institute on Alcohol Abuse and Alcoholism, National Institutes of Health (NIH). Originally published as NIH Pub. No. 96-3770, 1996, last reviewed May 28, 2001, http://www.niaaa.nih.gov/publications/booklet.htm.

For many people, the facts about alcoholism are not clear. What is alcoholism, exactly? How does it differ from alcohol abuse? When should a person seek help for a problem related to his or her drinking? The National Institute on Alcohol Abuse and Alcoholism (NIAAA) has prepared this information to help individuals and families answer these and other common questions about alcohol problems. This chapter explains both alcoholism and alcohol abuse, the symptoms of each, when and where to seek help, treatment choices, and additional helpful resources.

## *A Widespread Problem*

For most people who drink, alcohol is a pleasant accompaniment to social activities. Moderate alcohol use—up to two drinks per day for men and one drink per day for women and older people—is not harmful for most adults. (A standard drink is one 12-ounce bottle or can of either beer or wine cooler, one 5-ounce glass of wine, or 1.5 ounces of 80-proof distilled spirits.) Nonetheless, a large number of people get into serious trouble because of their drinking. Currently, nearly 14 million Americans—one in every 13 adults—abuse alcohol or are alcoholic. Several million more adults engage in risky drinking that could lead to alcohol problems. These patterns include binge drinking and heavy drinking on a regular basis. In addition, 53 percent of men and women in the United States report that one or more of their close relatives have a drinking problem.

The consequences of alcohol misuse are serious—in many cases, life threatening. Heavy drinking can increase the risk for certain cancers, especially those of the liver, esophagus, throat, and larynx (voice box). Heavy drinking can also cause liver cirrhosis, immune system problems, brain damage, and harm to the fetus during pregnancy. In addition, drinking increases the risk of death from automobile crashes as well as recreational and on-the-job injuries. Furthermore, both homicides and suicides are more likely to be committed by persons who have been drinking. In purely economic terms, alcohol-related problems cost society approximately $185 billion per year. In human terms, the costs cannot be calculated.

## What Is Alcoholism?

Alcoholism, also known as alcohol dependence, is a disease that includes four symptoms:

- *Craving*: A strong need, or compulsion, to drink.

- *Loss of control*: The inability to limit one's drinking on any given occasion.

- *Physical dependence*: Withdrawal symptoms, such as nausea, sweating, shakiness, and anxiety, occur when alcohol use is stopped after a period of heavy drinking.

- *Tolerance*: The need to drink greater amounts of alcohol in order to "get high."

People who are not alcoholic sometimes do not understand why an alcoholic can't just "use a little willpower" to stop drinking. However, alcoholism has little to do with willpower. Alcoholics are in the grip of a powerful "craving," or uncontrollable need, for alcohol that overrides their ability to stop drinking. This need can be as strong as the need for food or water.

Although some people are able to recover from alcoholism without help, the majority of alcoholics need assistance. With treatment and support, many individuals are able to stop drinking and rebuild their lives.

Many people wonder why some individuals can use alcohol without problems but others cannot. One important reason has to do with genetics. Scientists have found that having an alcoholic family member makes it more likely that if you choose to drink you too may develop alcoholism. Genes, however, are not the whole story. In fact, scientists now believe that certain factors in a person's environment influence whether a person with a genetic risk for alcoholism ever develops the disease. A person's risk for developing alcoholism can increase based on the person's environment, including where and how he or she lives;

family, friends, and culture; peer pressure; and even how easy it is to get alcohol.

## What Is Alcohol Abuse?

Alcohol abuse differs from alcoholism in that it does not include an extremely strong craving for alcohol, loss of control over drinking, or physical dependence. Alcohol abuse is defined as a pattern of drinking that results in one or more of the following situations within a 12-month period:

- Failure to fulfill major work, school, or home responsibilities

- Drinking in situations that are physically dangerous, such as while driving a car or operating machinery

- Having recurring alcohol-related legal problems, such as being arrested for driving under the influence of alcohol or for physically hurting someone while drunk

- Continued drinking despite having ongoing relationship problems that are caused or worsened by the drinking

Although alcohol abuse is basically different from alcoholism, many effects of alcohol abuse are also experienced by alcoholics.

## What Are the Signs of a Problem?

How can you tell whether you may have a drinking problem? Answering the following four questions can help you find out:

- Have you ever felt you should cut down on your drinking?

- Have people annoyed you by criticizing your drinking?

- Have you ever felt bad or guilty about your drinking?

- Have you ever had a drink first thing in the morning (as an "eye opener") to steady your nerves or get rid of a hangover?

One "yes" answer suggests a possible alcohol problem. If you answered "yes" to more than one question, it is highly likely that a problem exists. In either case, it is important that you see your doctor or other health care provider right away to discuss your answers to these questions. He or she can help you determine whether you have a drinking problem and, if so, recommend the best course of action.

Even if you answered "no" to all of the above questions, if you encounter drinking-related problems with your job, relationships, health, or the law, you should seek professional help. The effects of alcohol abuse can be extremely serious—even fatal—both to you and to others.

## The Decision to Get Help

Accepting the fact that help is needed for an alcohol problem may not be easy. But keep in mind that the sooner you get help, the better are your chances for a successful recovery.

Any concerns you may have about discussing drinking-related problems with your health care provider may stem from common misconceptions about alcoholism and alcoholic people. In our society, the myth prevails that an alcohol problem is a sign of moral weakness. As a result, you may feel that to seek help is to admit some type of shameful defect in yourself. In fact, alcoholism is a disease that is no more a sign of weakness than is asthma. Moreover, taking steps to identify a possible drinking problem has an enormous payoff—a chance for a healthier, more rewarding life.

When you visit your health care provider, he or she will ask you a number of questions about your alcohol use to determine whether you are having problems related to your drinking. Try to answer these questions as fully and honestly as you can. You also will be given a physical examination. If your health care provider concludes that you may be dependent on alcohol, he or she may recommend that you see a specialist in treating alcoholism. You should be involved in any referral decisions and have all treatment choices explained to you.

## Getting Well

### Alcoholism Treatment

The type of treatment you receive depends on the severity of your alcoholism and the resources that are available in your community. Treatment may include detoxification (the process of safely getting alcohol out of your system); taking doctor-prescribed medications, such as disulfiram (Antabuse®) or naltrexone (ReVia™), to help prevent a return (or relapse) to drinking once drinking has stopped; and individual and/or group counseling. There are promising types of counseling that teach alcoholics to identify situations and feelings that trigger the urge to drink and to find new ways to cope that do not include alcohol use. These treatments are often provided on an outpatient basis.

Because the support of family members is important to the recovery process, many programs also offer brief marital counseling and family therapy as part of the treatment process. Programs may also link individuals with vital community resources, such as legal assistance, job training, child care, and parenting classes.

### Alcoholics Anonymous

Virtually all alcoholism treatment programs also include Alcoholics Anonymous (AA) meetings. AA describes itself as a "worldwide fellowship of men and women who help each other to stay sober." Although AA is generally recognized as an effective mutual help program for recovering alcoholics, not everyone responds to AA's style or message, and other recovery approaches are available. Even people who are helped by AA usually find that AA works best in combination with other forms of treatment, including counseling and medical care.

## Can Alcoholism Be Cured?

Although alcoholism can be treated, a cure is not yet available. In other words, even if an alcoholic has been sober for a long time and has regained health, he or she remains susceptible to relapse and must continue to avoid all alcoholic beverages. "Cutting down" on drinking doesn't work; cutting out alcohol is necessary for a successful recovery.

However, even individuals who are determined to stay sober may suffer one or several "slips," or relapses, before achieving long-term sobriety. Relapses are very common and do not mean that a person has failed or cannot recover from alcoholism. Keep in mind, too, that every day that a recovering alcoholic has stayed sober prior to a relapse is extremely valuable time, both to the individual and to his or her family. If a relapse occurs, it is very important to try to stop drinking once again and to get whatever additional support you need to abstain from drinking.

## Help for Alcohol Abuse

If your health care provider determines that you are not alcohol-dependent but are nonetheless involved in a pattern of alcohol abuse, he or she can help you to:

- Examine the benefits of stopping an unhealthy drinking pattern.

- Set a drinking goal for yourself. Some people choose to abstain from alcohol. Others prefer to limit the amount they drink.

- Examine the situations that trigger your unhealthy drinking patterns, and develop new ways of handling those situations so that you can maintain your drinking goal.

Some individuals who have stopped drinking after experiencing alcohol-related problems choose to attend AA meetings for information and support, even though they have not been diagnosed as alcoholic.

## New Directions

With NIAAA's support, scientists at medical centers and universities throughout the country are studying alcoholism. The goal of this research is to develop better ways of treating and preventing alcohol problems. Today, NIAAA funds approximately 90 percent of all alcoholism research in the United States. Some of the more exciting investigations focus on the causes, consequences, treatment, and prevention of alcoholism.

### Genetics

Alcoholism is a complex disease. Therefore, there are likely to be many genes involved in increasing a person's risk for alcoholism. Scientists are searching for these genes, and have found areas on chromosomes where they are probably located. Powerful new techniques may permit researchers to identify and measure the specific contribution of each gene to the complex behaviors associated with heavy drinking. This research will provide the basis for new medications to treat alcohol-related problems.

### Treatment

NIAAA-supported researchers have made considerable progress in evaluating commonly used therapies and in developing new types of therapies to treat alcohol-related problems. One large-scale study sponsored by NIAAA found that each of three commonly used behavioral treatments for alcohol abuse and alcoholism—motivation enhancement therapy, cognitive-behavioral therapy, and 12-step facilitation therapy—significantly reduced drinking in the year following treatment. This study also found that approximately one-third of the study participants who were followed up either were still abstinent or were drinking without serious problems three years after the study ended. Other therapies that have been evaluated and found effective in reducing alcohol problems include brief intervention for alcohol abusers (individuals who are not dependent on alcohol) and behavioral marital therapy for married alcohol-dependent individuals.

## Medications Development

NIAAA has made developing medications to treat alcoholism a high priority. We believe that a range of new medications will be developed based on the results of genetic and neuroscience research. In fact, neuroscience research has already led to studies of one medication—naltrexone (ReVia™)—as an anti-craving medication. NIAAA-supported researchers found that this drug, in combination with behavioral therapy, was effective in treating alcoholism. Naltrexone, which targets the brain's reward circuits, is the first medication approved to help maintain sobriety after detoxification from alcohol since the approval of disulfiram (Antabuse®) in 1949. The use of acamprosate, an anti-craving medication that is widely used in Europe, is based on neuroscience research. Researchers believe that acamprosate works on different brain circuits to ease the physical discomfort that occurs when an alcoholic stops drinking. Acamprosate should be approved for use in the United States in the near future, and other medications are being studied as well.

## Combined Medications/Behavioral Therapies

NIAAA-supported researchers have found that available medications work best with behavioral therapy. Thus, NIAAA has initiated a large-scale clinical trial to determine which of the currently available medications and which behavioral therapies work best together. Naltrexone and acamprosate will each be tested separately with different behavioral therapies. These medications will also be used together to determine if there is some interaction between the two that makes the combination more effective than the use of either one alone.

In addition to these efforts, NIAAA is sponsoring promising research in other vital areas, such as fetal alcohol syndrome, alcohol's effects on the brain and other organs, aspects of drinkers' environments that may contribute to alcohol abuse and alcoholism, strategies to reduce alcohol-related problems, and new treatment techniques. Together, these investigations will help prevent alcohol problems; identify alcohol abuse and alcoholism at earlier stages; and make available new, more effective treatment approaches for individuals and families.

## Section 40.2

# *How to Cut Down on Drinking*

Reprinted from "How to Cut Down on Your Drinking," National Institute on Alcohol Abuse and Alcoholism, National Institutes of Health (NIH). Originally published as NIH Pub. No. 96-3770, 1996, last reviewed May 28, 2001, http://www.niaaa.nih.gov/publications/handout.htm.

If you are drinking too much, you can improve your life and health by cutting down. How do you know if you drink too much? Read these questions and answer "yes" or "no":

- Do you drink alone when you feel angry or sad?

- Does your drinking ever make you late for work?

- Does your drinking worry your family?

- Do you ever drink after telling yourself you won't?

- Do you ever forget what you did while you were drinking?

- Do you get headaches or have a hang-over after you have been drinking?

If you answered "yes" to any of these questions, you may have a drinking problem. Check with your doctor to be sure. Your doctor will be able to tell you whether you should cut down or abstain. If you are alcoholic or have other medical problems, you should not just cut down on your drinking—you should stop drinking completely. Your doctor will advise you about what is right for you.

If your doctor tells you to cut down on your drinking, these steps can help you:

## 1. Write Your Reasons for Cutting Down or Stopping.

Why do you want to drink less? There are many reasons why you may want to cut down or stop drinking. You may want to improve your health, sleep better, or get along better with your family or friends. Make a list of the reasons you want to drink less.

## 2. Set a Drinking Goal.

Choose a limit for how much you will drink. You may choose to cut down or not to drink at all. If you are cutting down, keep below these limits:

- Women: No more than one drink a day
- Men: No more than two drinks a day

A drink is:

- A 12-ounce bottle of beer *or*
- A 5-ounce glass of wine *or*
- A 1 1/2-ounce shot of liquor

These limits may be too high for some people who have certain medical problems or who are older. Talk with your doctor about the limit that is right for you.

Now, write your drinking goal on a piece of paper. Put it where you can see it, such as on your refrigerator or bathroom mirror. Your paper might look like this:

- I will start on this day _____.
- I will not drink more than _____ drinks in one day.
- I will not drink more than _____ drinks in one week.

  or

- I will stop drinking alcohol.

## 3. Keep a "Diary" of Your Drinking.

To help you reach your goal, keep a "diary" of your drinking. For example, write down every time you have a drink for one week. Try to keep your diary for three or four weeks. This will show you how much you drink and when. You may be surprised. How different is your goal from the amount you drink now?

Now you know why you want to drink less and you have a goal. There are many ways you can help yourself to cut down.

## Tips

**Watch it at home.** Keep a small amount or no alcohol at home. Don't keep temptations around.

**Drink slowly.** When you drink, sip your drink slowly. Take a break of one hour between drinks. Drink soda, water, or juice after a drink with alcohol. Do not drink on an empty stomach. Eat food when you are drinking.

**Take a break from alcohol.** Pick a day or two each week when you will not drink at all. Then, try to stop drinking for one week. Think about how you feel physically and emotionally on these days. When you succeed and feel better, you may find it easier to cut down for good.

**Learn how to say no.** You do not have to drink when other people drink. You do not have to take a drink that is given to you. Practice ways to say no politely. For example, you can tell people you feel better when you drink less. Stay away from people who give you a hard time about not drinking.

**Stay active.** What would you like to do instead of drinking? Use the time and money spent on drinking to do something fun with your family or friends. Go out to eat, see a movie, or play sports or a game.

**Get support.** Cutting down on your drinking may be difficult at times. Ask your family and friends for support to help you reach your goal. Talk to your doctor if you are having trouble cutting down. Get the help you need to reach your goal.

**Watch out for temptations.** Watch out for people, places, or times that make you drink, even if you do not want to. Stay away from people who drink a lot or bars where you used to go. Plan ahead of time what you will do to avoid drinking when you are tempted.

Do not drink when you are angry or upset or have a bad day. These are habits you need to break if you want to drink less.

**Do not give up.** Most people do not cut down or give up drinking all at once. Just like a diet, it is not easy to change. That is OK. If you do not reach your goal the first time, try again. Remember, get support from people who care about you and want to help. Do not give up.

Chapter 41

# *Recreational Drugs*

## *Chapter Contents*

# Section 41.1

# *Marijuana*

Reprinted from "Marijuana," National Institute on Drug Abuse, U.S. Department of Health and Human Services, updated October 2002, http://www.nida.nih.gov/Infofax/marijuana.html.

Marijuana is the most commonly used illicit drug in the United States. A dry, shredded green-brown mix of flowers, stems, seeds, and leaves of the hemp plant *Cannabis sativa*, it usually is smoked as a cigarette (joint, nail) or in a pipe (bong). It also is smoked in blunts, which are cigars that have been emptied of tobacco and refilled with marijuana, often in combination with another drug. Use also might include mixing marijuana in food or brewing it as a tea. As a more concentrated, resinous form, it is called hashish and, as a sticky black liquid, hash oil. Marijuana smoke has a pungent and distinctive, usually sweet-and-sour odor. There are countless street terms for marijuana including pot, herb, weed, grass, widow, ganja, and hash, as well as terms derived from trademarked varieties of cannabis, such as Bubble Gum®, Northern Lights®, Juicy Fruit®, Afghani #1®, and a number of Skunk® varieties.

The main active chemical in marijuana is THC (delta-9-tetrahydrocannabinol). The membranes of certain nerve cells in the brain contain protein receptors that bind to THC. Once securely in place, THC kicks off a series of cellular reactions that ultimately lead to the high that users experience when they smoke marijuana.

## *Extent of Use*

In 2001, over 12 million Americans age 12 and older used marijuana at least once in the month prior to being surveyed. That is more than three-quarters (76 percent) of the total number of Americans who used any illicit drug in the past month in 2001. Of the 76 percent, more than half (56 percent) consumed only marijuana; 20 percent used marijuana and another illicit drug; and the remaining 24 percent used an illicit drug or drugs other than marijuana.

Although marijuana is the most commonly used illicit drug in the United States, among students in the eighth, tenth, and twelfth grades nationwide its use remained stable from 1999 through 2001. Among eighth graders, however, past year use has decreased, from 18.3 percent in 1996 to 15.4 percent in 2001. Also in 2001, more than half (57.4 percent) of twelfth graders believed it was harmful to smoke marijuana regularly and 79.3 percent disapproved of regular marijuana use. Since 1975, 83 percent to 90 percent of every twelfth grade class surveyed has found it "fairly easy" or "very easy" to obtain marijuana.

Data for drug-related hospital emergency department visits in the continental United States recently showed a 15 percent increase in the number of visits to an emergency room that were induced by or related to the use of marijuana (referred to as mentions), from 96,426 in 2000 to 110,512 in 2001. The 12-to-34 age range was involved most frequently in these mentions. For emergency room patients in the 12-to-17 age range, the rate of marijuana mentions increased 23 percent between 1999 and 2001 (from 55 to 68 per 100,000 population) and 126 percent (from 30 to 68 per 100,000 population) since 1994.

## Effects on the Brain

Scientists have learned a great deal about how THC acts in the brain to produce its many effects. When someone smokes marijuana, THC rapidly passes from the lungs into the bloodstream, which carries the chemical to organs throughout the body, including the brain.

In the brain, THC connects to specific sites called cannabinoid receptors on nerve cells and influences the activity of those cells. Some brain areas have many cannabinoid receptors; others have few or none. Many cannabinoid receptors are found in the parts of the brain that influence pleasure, memory, thought, concentration, sensory and time perception, and coordinated movement.

The short-term effects of marijuana use can include problems with memory and learning; distorted perception; difficulty in thinking and problem solving; loss of coordination; and increased heart rate. Research findings for long-term marijuana use indicate some changes in the brain similar to those seen after long-term use of other major drugs of abuse. For example, cannabinoid (THC or synthetic forms of THC) withdrawal in chronically exposed animals leads to an increase in the activation of the stress-response system and changes in the activity of nerve cells containing dopamine. Dopamine neurons are involved in the regulation of motivation and reward, and are directly or indirectly affected by all drugs of abuse.

### Effects on the Heart

One study has indicated that a user's risk of heart attack more than quadruples in the first hour after smoking marijuana. The researchers suggest that such an effect might occur from marijuana's effects on blood pressure and heart rate and reduced oxygen-carrying capacity of blood.

### Effects on the Lungs

A study of 450 individuals found that people who smoke marijuana frequently but do not smoke tobacco have more health problems and miss more days of work than nonsmokers. Many of the extra sick days among the marijuana smokers in the study were for respiratory illnesses.

Even infrequent use can cause burning and stinging of the mouth and throat, often accompanied by a heavy cough. Someone who smokes marijuana regularly may have many of the same respiratory problems that tobacco smokers do, such as daily cough and phlegm production, more frequent acute chest illness, a heightened risk of lung infections, and a greater tendency to obstructed airways.

Cancer of the respiratory tract and lungs may also be promoted by marijuana smoke. A study comparing 173 cancer patients and 176 healthy individuals produced strong evidence that smoking marijuana increases the likelihood of developing cancer of the head or neck, and the more marijuana smoked the greater the increase. A statistical analysis of the data suggested that marijuana smoking doubled or tripled the risk of these cancers.

Marijuana use has the potential to promote cancer of the lungs and other parts of the respiratory tract because it contains irritants and carcinogens. In fact, marijuana smoke contains 50 to 70 percent more carcinogenic hydrocarbons than does tobacco smoke. It also produces high levels of an enzyme that converts certain hydrocarbons into their carcinogenic form—levels that may accelerate the changes that ultimately produce malignant cells. Marijuana users usually inhale more deeply and hold their breath longer than tobacco smokers do, which increases the lungs' exposure to carcinogenic smoke. These facts suggest that, puff for puff, smoking marijuana may increase the risk of cancer more than smoking tobacco.

## Other Health Effects

Some of marijuana's adverse health effects may occur because THC impairs the immune system's ability to fight off infectious diseases and cancer. In laboratory experiments that exposed animal and human cells to THC or other marijuana ingredients, the normal disease-preventing reactions of many of the key types of immune cells were inhibited. In other studies, mice exposed to THC or related substances were more likely than unexposed mice to develop bacterial infections and tumors.

## Effects of Heavy Marijuana Use on Learning and Social Behavior

Depression, anxiety, and personality disturbances are all associated with marijuana use. Research clearly demonstrates that marijuana use has potential to cause problems in daily life or make a person's existing problems worse. Because marijuana compromises the ability to learn and remember information, the more a person uses marijuana the more he or she is likely to fall behind in accumulating intellectual, job, or social skills. Moreover, research has shown that marijuana's adverse impact on memory and learning can last for days or weeks after the acute effects of the drug wear off.

Students who smoke marijuana get lower grades and are less likely to graduate from high school, compared to their nonsmoking peers. In one study, researchers compared marijuana-smoking and nonsmoking twelfth-graders' scores on standardized tests of verbal and mathematical skills. Although all of the students had scored equally well in fourth grade, the marijuana smokers' scores were significantly lower in twelfth grade.

A study of 129 college students found that, for heavy users of marijuana (those who smoked the drug at least 27 of the preceding 30 days), critical skills related to attention, memory, and learning were significantly impaired even after they had not used the drug for at least 24 hours. The heavy marijuana users in the study had more trouble sustaining and shifting their attention and in registering, organizing, and using information than did the study participants who had used marijuana no more than three of the previous 30 days. As a result, someone who smokes marijuana once daily may be functioning at a reduced intellectual level all of the time.

More recently, the same researchers showed that the ability of a group of long-term heavy marijuana users to recall words from a list remained impaired for a week after quitting, but returned to normal within four weeks. An implication of this finding is that some cognitive abilities may be restored in individuals who quit smoking marijuana, even after long-term heavy use.

Workers who smoke marijuana are more likely than their co-workers to have problems on the job. Several studies associate workers' marijuana smoking with increased absences, tardiness, accidents, workers' compensation claims, and job turnover. A study of municipal workers found that those who used marijuana on or off the job reported more "withdrawal behaviors"—such as leaving work without permission, daydreaming, spending work time on personal matters, and shirking tasks—that adversely affect productivity and morale.

## Effects on Pregnancy

Research has shown that babies born to women who used marijuana during their pregnancies display altered responses to visual stimuli, increased tremulousness, and a high-pitched cry, which may indicate problems with neurological development. During infancy and preschool years, marijuana-exposed children have been observed to have more behavioral problems and poorer performance on tasks of visual perception, language comprehension, sustained attention, and memory. In school, these children are more likely to exhibit deficits in decision-making skills, memory, and the ability to remain attentive.

## Addictive Potential

Long-term marijuana use can lead to addiction for some people; that is, they use the drug compulsively even though it often interferes with family, school, work, and recreational activities. Drug craving and withdrawal symptoms can make it hard for long-term marijuana smokers to stop using the drug. People trying to quit report irritability, sleeplessness, and anxiety. They also display increased aggression on psychological tests, peaking approximately one week after the last use of the drug.

## Genetic Vulnerability

Scientists have found that whether an individual has positive or negative sensations after smoking marijuana can be influenced by heredity. A 1997 study demonstrated that identical male twins were more likely than nonidentical male twins to report similar responses to marijuana use, indicating a genetic basis for their response to the drug. (Identical twins share all of their genes.)

It also was discovered that the twins' shared or family environment before age 18 had no detectable influence on their response to marijuana. Certain environmental factors, however, such as the availability of marijuana, expectations about how the drug would affect them, the influence of friends and social contacts, and other factors that differentiate experiences of identical twins were found to have an important effect.

## Treating Marijuana Problems

The latest treatment data indicate that, in 1999, marijuana was the primary drug of abuse in about 14 percent of all admissions to treatment facilities in the United States. Marijuana admissions were primarily male (77 percent), white (58 percent), and young (47 percent under 20 years old). Those in treatment for primary marijuana use had begun use at an early age; 57 percent had used it by age 14 and 92 percent had used it by 18.

One study of adult marijuana users found comparable benefits from a 14-session cognitive-behavioral group treatment and a two-session individual treatment that included motivational interviewing and advice on ways to reduce marijuana use. Participants were mostly men in their early thirties who had smoked marijuana daily for more than 10 years. By increasing patients' awareness of what triggers their marijuana use, both treatments sought to help patients devise avoidance strategies. Use, dependence symptoms, and psychosocial problems decreased for at least one year following both treatments; about 30 percent of users were abstinent during the last three-month follow-up period.

Another study suggests that giving patients vouchers that they can redeem for goods—such as movie passes, sporting equipment, or vocational training—may further improve outcomes.

Although no medications are currently available for treating marijuana abuse, recent discoveries about the workings of the THC receptors have raised the possibility of eventually developing a medication that will block the intoxicating effects of THC. Such a medication might be used to prevent relapse to marijuana abuse by lessening or eliminating its appeal.

# Section 41.2

# *Cocaine and Crack*

Reprinted from "Crack and Cocaine," National Institute on Drug Abuse, U.S. Department of Health and Human Services, 2003, http://www.nida.nih.gov/Infofax/cocaine.html.

Cocaine is a powerfully addictive drug of abuse. Once having tried cocaine, an individual cannot predict or control the extent to which he or she will continue to use the drug.

The major routes of administration of cocaine are sniffing or snorting, injecting, and smoking (including free-base and crack cocaine). Snorting is the process of inhaling cocaine powder through the nose where it is absorbed into the bloodstream through the nasal tissues. Injecting is the act of using a needle to release the drug directly into the bloodstream. Smoking involves inhaling cocaine vapor or smoke into the lungs where absorption into the bloodstream is as rapid as by injection.

"Crack" is the street name given to cocaine that has been processed from cocaine hydrochloride to a free base for smoking. Rather than requiring the more volatile method of processing cocaine using ether, crack cocaine is processed with ammonia or sodium bicarbonate (baking soda) and water and heated to remove the hydrochloride, thus producing a form of cocaine that can be smoked. The term "crack" refers to the crackling sound heard when the mixture is smoked (heated), presumably from the sodium bicarbonate.

There is great risk whether cocaine is ingested by inhalation (snorting), injection, or smoking. It appears that compulsive cocaine use may develop even more rapidly if the substance is smoked rather than snorted. Smoking allows extremely high doses of cocaine to reach the brain very quickly and brings an intense and immediate high. The injecting drug user is at risk for transmitting or acquiring HIV infection or AIDS if needles or other injection equipment are shared.

## Health Hazards

Cocaine is a strong central nervous system stimulant that interferes with the reabsorption process of dopamine, a chemical messenger associated with pleasure and movement. Dopamine is released as part of the brain's reward system and is involved in the high that characterizes cocaine consumption.

Physical effects of cocaine use include constricted peripheral blood vessels, dilated pupils, and increased temperature, heart rate, and blood pressure. The duration of cocaine's immediate euphoric effects, which include hyperstimulation, reduced fatigue, and mental clarity, depends on the route of administration. The faster the absorption, the more intense the high. On the other hand, the faster the absorption, the shorter the duration of action. The high from snorting may last 15 to 30 minutes, while that from smoking may last five to 10 minutes. Increased use can reduce the period of stimulation.

Some users of cocaine report feelings of restlessness, irritability, and anxiety. An appreciable tolerance to the high may be developed, and many addicts report that they seek but fail to achieve as much pleasure as they did from their first exposure. Scientific evidence suggests that the powerful neuropsychologic reinforcing property of cocaine is responsible for an individual's continued use, despite harmful physical and social consequences. In rare instances, sudden death can occur on the first use of cocaine or unexpectedly thereafter. However, there is no way to determine who is prone to sudden death.

High doses of cocaine and/or prolonged use can trigger paranoia. Smoking crack cocaine can produce a particularly aggressive paranoid behavior in users. When addicted individuals stop using cocaine, they often become depressed. This also may lead to further cocaine use to alleviate depression. Prolonged cocaine snorting can result in ulceration of the mucous membrane of the nose and can damage the nasal septum enough to cause it to collapse. Cocaine-related deaths are often a result of cardiac arrest or seizures followed by respiratory arrest.

## Added Danger: Cocaethylene

When people mix cocaine and alcohol consumption, they are compounding the danger each drug poses and unknowingly forming a complex chemical experiment within their bodies. NIDA-funded researchers have found that the human liver combines cocaine and alcohol and manufactures a third substance, cocaethylene, that intensifies cocaine's euphoric effects, while possibly increasing the risk of sudden death.

## Treatment

The widespread abuse of cocaine has stimulated extensive efforts to develop treatment programs for this type of drug abuse.

The National Institute on Drug Abuse's (NIDA) top research priority is to find a medication to block or greatly reduce the effects of cocaine, to be used as one part of a comprehensive treatment program. NIDA-funded researchers are also looking at medications that help alleviate the severe craving that people in treatment for cocaine addiction often experience. Several medications are currently being investigated to test their safety and efficacy in treating cocaine addiction.

In addition to treatment medications, behavioral interventions, particularly cognitive-behavioral therapy, can be effective in decreasing drug use by patients in treatment for cocaine abuse. Providing the optimal combination of treatment services for each individual is critical to successful treatment outcome.

## Extent of Use

### Monitoring the Future Study (MTF)

MTF is an annual survey on drug use and related attitudes of America's adolescents that began in 1975. The survey is conducted by the University of Michigan's Institute for Social Research and is funded by NIDA. The MTF assesses the extent of drug use among adolescents and young adults across the country. Copies of the latest survey are available from the National Clearinghouse for Alcohol and Drug Information at (800) 729-6686.

The proportion of high school seniors who have used cocaine at least once in their lifetimes has increased from a low of 5.9 percent in 1994 to 9.8 percent in 1999. However, this is lower than its peak of 17.3 percent in 1985. Current (past month) use of cocaine by seniors decreased from a high of 6.7 percent in 1985 to 2.6 percent in 1999. Also in 1999, 7.7 percent of tenth-graders had tried cocaine at least once, up from a low of 3.3 percent in 1992. The percentage of eighth-graders who had ever tried cocaine has increased from a low of 2.3 percent in 1991 to 4.7 percent in 1999.

Of college students one to four years beyond high school, in 1995, 3.6 percent had used cocaine within the past year, and 0.7 percent had used cocaine in the past month.

### Community Epidemiology Work Group (CEWG)

CEWG is a NIDA-sponsored network of researchers from 20 major U.S. metropolitan areas and selected foreign countries who meet semiannually to discuss the current epidemiology of drug abuse.

Although demographic data continue to show most cocaine users as older, inner-city crack addicts, isolated field reports indicate new groups of users: teenagers smoking crack with marijuana in some cities; Hispanic crack users in Texas; and in the Atlanta area, middle-class suburban users of cocaine hydrochloride and female crack users in their thirties with no prior drug history.

### National Household Survey on Drug Abuse (NHSDA)

NHSDA is an annual survey conducted by the Substance Abuse and Mental Health Services Administration. Copies of the latest survey are available from the National Clearinghouse for Alcohol and Drug Information at (800) 729-6686.

In 1998, about 1.7 million Americans were current (at least once per month) cocaine users. This is about 0.8 percent of the population age 12 and older; about 437,000 of these used crack. The rate of current cocaine use in 1998 was highest among Americans ages 18 to 25 (2.0 percent). The rate of use for this age group was significantly higher in 1998 than in 1997, when it was 1.2 percent.

## Section 41.3

# *Ecstasy and Club Drugs*

Reprinted from "Club Drugs," National Institute on Drug Abuse, U.S. Department of Health and Human Services, revised April, 2001, http://www.nida.nih.gov/Infofax/Clubdrugs.html.

MDMA (ecstasy), Rohypnol®, GHB, and ketamine are among the drugs used by teens and young adults who are part of a nightclub, bar, rave, or trance scene. Raves and trance events are generally night-long dances, often held in warehouses. Many who attend raves and trances do not use drugs, but those who do may be attracted to the generally low cost, seemingly increased stamina, and intoxicating highs that are said to deepen the rave or trance experience.

Current science, however, is showing change to critical parts of the brain from use of these drugs. Also, in high doses most of these drugs can cause a sharp increase in body temperature (malignant hyperthermia) leading to muscle breakdown and kidney and cardiovascular system failure.

## *MDMA (Ecstasy)*

MDMA is a synthetic, psychoactive drug with both stimulant (like amphetamines) and hallucinogenic (like LSD) properties. Street names for MDMA include ecstasy, Adam, XTC, hug, beans, and love drug. Its chemical structure (3-4 methylenedioxymethamphetamine, or MDMA) is similar to methamphetamine, methylenedioxyamphetamine (MDA), and mescaline; these are synthetic drugs known to cause brain damage. MDMA usually is taken in pill form, but some users snort it, inject it, or use it in suppository form.

Many problems MDMA users encounter are similar to those found with the use of amphetamines and cocaine. Psychological difficulties can include confusion, depression, sleep problems, severe anxiety, and paranoia. Physical problems can include muscle tension, involuntary teeth clenching, nausea, blurred vision, faintness, and chills or sweating. Use of the drug has also been associated with increases in heart rate and blood pressure, which are special risks for people with circulatory or heart disease. Recent research also links MDMA use to long-term damage to those parts of the brain critical to thought, memory, and pleasure.

MDMA use is increasing in most metropolitan areas of the United States. In Boston and New York City, it appears to be spreading beyond the club scene to the streets. Content of the MDMA pills also varies widely, and may include caffeine, dextromethorphan, heroin, and mescaline. In some areas of the country, the MDMA-like substance paramethoxyamphetamine (PMA) has been involved in the deaths of people who mistakenly thought they were taking true MDMA. The deaths were due to complications from hyperthermia.

In a five-year retrospective of emergency room mentions of club drugs, the Substance Abuse and Mental Health Services Administration reports that emergency room mentions involving MDMA increased from 250 in 1994 to 2,850 in 1999.

## Rohypnol, GHB, and Ketamine

GHB, Rohypnol®, and ketamine are predominantly central nervous system depressants. Because they are often colorless, tasteless, and odorless, they can be added to beverages and ingested unknowingly.

These drugs emerged a few years ago as "date rape" drugs. Because of concern about their abuse, Congress passed the Drug-Induced Rape Prevention and Punishment Act of 1996 in October 1996. This legislation increased federal penalties for use of any controlled substance to aid in sexual assault.

## GHB

Since about 1990, GHB (gamma hydroxybutyrate) has been abused in the U.S. for euphoric, sedative, and anabolic (bodybuilding) effects. It is a central nervous system depressant that was widely available over-the-counter in health food stores during the 1980s and until 1992. It was purchased largely by bodybuilders to aid fat reduction and muscle building. Street names include liquid ecstasy, soap, easy lay, and Georgia home boy. Even though GHB may be difficult to distinguish from water, it has appeared in law enforcement indicators, including seizures of large amounts in Minneapolis–St. Paul and Phoenix.

Coma and seizures can occur following abuse of GHB and, when combined with methamphetamine, there appears to be an increased risk of seizure. Combining use with other drugs such as alcohol can result in nausea and difficulty breathing. GHB may also produce withdrawal effects, including insomnia, anxiety, tremors, and sweating.

GHB and two of its precursors, gamma butyrolactone (GBL) and 1,4 butanediol (BD), have been involved in poisonings, overdoses, date rapes, and deaths. These products, obtainable over the Internet and sometimes still sold in health food stores, are also available at some gyms, raves, nightclubs, gay male parties, college campuses, and the street. They are commonly mixed with alcohol (which may cause unconsciousness), have a short duration of action, and are not easily detectable on routine hospital toxicology screens.

GHB emergency room mentions increased from 55 in 1994 to 2,973 in 1999. In 1999, GHB accounted for 32 percent of illicit drug-related poison center calls in Boston. In Chicago and San Francisco, GHB use is reportedly low compared with MDMA, although GHB overdoses seem frequent compared with overdoses related to other club drugs.

## Rohypnol

Rohypnol, a trade name for flunitrazepam, has been of particular concern for the last few years because of its abuse in date rape. It belongs to a class of drugs knows as benzodiazepines. When mixed with alcohol, Rohypnol can incapacitate victims and prevent them from resisting sexual assault. It can produce "anterograde amnesia," which means individuals may not remember events they experienced while under the effects of the drugs. Also, Rohypnol may be lethal when mixed with alcohol and/or other depressants.

Rohypnol is not approved for use in the United States, and its importation is banned. Illicit use of Rohypnol started appearing in the United States in the early 1990s, where it became known as rophies, roofies, roach, and rope. Emergency room mentions of Rohypnol were 13 in 1994 and increased to 624 in 1998; they decreased to 540 in 1999.

Abuse of two other similar drugs appears to be replacing Rohypnol abuse in Miami, Texas, and Boston. These are clonazepam, marketed in the U.S. as Klonopin® and in Mexico as Rivotril®, and alprazolam (marketed as Xanax®). Rohypnol, however, continues to be a problem among treatment admissions in Texas, particularly among young Hispanic males along the Mexican border.

## Ketamine

Ketamine is an anesthetic that has been approved for both human and animal use in medical settings since 1970; about 90 percent of the ketamine legally sold is intended for veterinary use. It can be injected or snorted. Ketamine is also known as special K or vitamin K.

Certain doses of ketamine can cause dreamlike states and hallucinations, and it has become common in club and rave scenes and has been used as a date rape drug.

At high doses, ketamine can cause delirium, amnesia, impaired motor function, high blood pressure, depression, and potentially fatal respiratory problems.

Emergency room mentions of ketamine rose from 19 in 1994 to 396 in 1999. Recent use has been reported more frequently among white youth in many cities, including Atlanta, Baltimore, Boston, Chicago, Minneapolis–St. Paul, Newark, New York City, Phoenix, San Diego, Texas, and Washington, D.C.

# Section 41.4

# *Methamphetamine*

Reprinted from " Methamphetamine," National Institute on Drug Abuse, U.S. Department of Health and Human Services, 2003, http://www.nida.nih.gov/Infofax/methamphetamine.html.

Methamphetamine is an addictive stimulant drug that strongly activates certain systems in the brain. Methamphetamine is closely related chemically to amphetamine, but the central nervous system effects of methamphetamine are greater. Both drugs have some medical uses, primarily in the treatment of obesity, but their therapeutic use is limited.

Methamphetamine is made in illegal laboratories and has a high potential for abuse and dependence. Street methamphetamine is referred to by many names, such as speed, meth, and chalk. Methamphetamine hydrochloride, clear chunky crystals resembling ice, which can be inhaled by smoking, is referred to as ice, crystal, and glass.

## Health Hazards

Methamphetamine releases high levels of the neurotransmitter dopamine, which stimulates brain cells, enhancing mood and body movement. It also appears to have a neurotoxic effect, damaging brain cells that contain dopamine and serotonin, another neurotransmitter. Over time, methamphetamine appears to cause reduced levels of dopamine, which can result in symptoms like those of Parkinson's disease, a severe movement disorder.

Methamphetamine is taken orally or intranasally (snorting the powder), by intravenous injection, and by smoking. Immediately after smoking or intravenous injection, the methamphetamine user experiences an intense sensation, called a "rush" or "flash," that lasts only a few minutes and is described as extremely pleasurable. Oral or intranasal use produces euphoria—a high, but not a rush. Users may become addicted quickly, and use it with increasing frequency and in increasing doses.

Animal research going back more than 20 years shows that high doses of methamphetamine damage neuron cell-endings. Dopamine- and serotonin-containing neurons do not die after methamphetamine use, but their nerve endings ("terminals") are cut back and regrowth appears to be limited.

The central nervous system (CNS) actions that result from taking even small amounts of methamphetamine include increased wakefulness, increased physical activity, decreased appetite, increased respiration, hyperthermia, and euphoria. Other CNS effects include irritability, insomnia, confusion, tremors, convulsions, anxiety, paranoia, and aggressiveness. Hyperthermia and convulsions can result in death.

Methamphetamine causes increased heart rate and blood pressure and can cause irreversible damage to blood vessels in the brain, producing strokes. Other effects of methamphetamine include respiratory problems, irregular heartbeat, and extreme anorexia. Its use can result in cardiovascular collapse and death.

A study in Seattle confirmed that methamphetamine use was widespread among the city's homosexual and bisexual populations. Of these groups, members using methamphetamine reported they practice sexual and needle-use behaviors that place them at risk of contracting and transmitting HIV and AIDS.

## Extent of Use

### *Monitoring the Future Study (MTF)*

MTF is an annual survey on drug use and related attitudes of America's adolescents that began in 1975. The survey is conducted by the University of Michigan's Institute for Social Research and is funded by National Institute on Drug Abuse (NIDA). Copies of the latest survey are available from the National Clearinghouse for Alcohol and Drug Information at (800) 729-6686. MTF assesses the extent of drug use among adolescents (eighth-, tenth-, and twelfth-graders) and young adults across the country.

Recent data from the survey:

- In 1997, 4.4 percent of high school seniors had used crystal methamphetamine at least once in their lifetimes—an increase from 2.7 percent in 1990.

- Data show that 2.3 percent of seniors reported past year use of crystal methamphetamine in 1997—an increase from 1.3 percent in 1990.

## *Community Epidemiology Work Group (CEWG)*

CEWG is a NIDA-sponsored network of researchers from 20 major U.S. metropolitan areas and selected foreign countries who meet semiannually to discuss the current epidemiology of drug abuse. CEWG's most recent reports are available on the CEWG website.

Methamphetamine is the dominant illicit drug problem in San Diego. San Francisco and Honolulu also have substantial methamphetamine-using populations. Patterns of increasing use have been seen in Denver, Los Angeles, Minneapolis, Phoenix, Seattle, and Tucson. New trafficking patterns have increased availability of the drug in Missouri, Nebraska, and Iowa.

## *National Household Survey on Drug Abuse (NHSDA)*

NHSDA is an annual survey conducted by the Substance Abuse and Mental Health Services Administration. Copies of the latest survey are available from the National Clearinghouse for Alcohol and Drug Information at (800) 729-6686.

According to the 1996 NHSDA, 4.9 million people (aged 12 and older) had tried methamphetamine at least once in their lifetimes (2.3 percent of population). This is not a statistically significant increase from 4.7 million people (2.2 percent) who reported using methamphetamine at least once in their lifetime in the 1995 NHSDA.

# Chapter 42

# *Exercise*

## Chapter Contents

# Section 42.1

# *The Basics of Healthy Exercise*

**Summary**: Emphasizes the importance of moderate physical activity and its health benefits.

What reduces the risk of heart disease, colon cancer, diabetes, reduces blood pressure, but lifts depression—and helps you sleep well? No, not a miracle drug, but something available to everyone—light exercise.

The new message from doctors is that we can gain real health benefits from exercise that's easy to do every day. It needn't be strenuous—a short, brisk walk will do. It doesn't have to take much time either—as little as 10 minutes counts towards the total of 30 minutes exercise we need to do each day. You can do this 30 minutes in one go, or break it up into shorter sessions of 10 or 15 minutes—this makes it easier to fit into your day. Exercise needn't be difficult—it just has to be regular. Here are some ideas to get you going.

Remember that some household chores count too. Washing the car, washing windows or floors, sweeping floors and outdoor areas, raking leaves, heavy digging, or weeding the garden are all vigorous enough to count as part of your daily 30 minutes.

## *Find Simple Ways to Get More Walking into Your Day.*

On your way to work, try getting off at an earlier bus stop, then take the stairs instead of the lift. Go for a walk in your lunch hour. If you get home from work and watch television before dinner, try a walk instead—a 10-minute walk can be more relaxing than 10 minutes in a chair. Walk to the shops instead of driving. Walk the dog to the nearest park and throw a ball around. Put the baby in a stroller and walk to visit a friend. Go for a walk around the nearest shopping center and remember to walk up the escalators instead of standing. Walk to a cafe to meet a friend for coffee.

## Get Active with the Family.

Find things to do together—regular physical activity is important for children and teenagers too. Make a list of parks, beaches, and bushland areas you've never visited before and take the family for a walk—encourage older relatives to come along too. Spend 10 minutes in the backyard or out on the street after work, throwing a ball or flying a kite with the children. Go swimming or cycling together. Shoot balls into a basketball hoop.

## Get Active with Friends.

Exercising with a friend can be more enjoyable because it gives you the chance to socialize as well. Find out what activities you can enjoy with other people in your area. Community health centers and local libraries are good places to find out about groups that do gentle exercise, tai chi, walking, dancing, or yoga. Form your own group—get friends together to play bocce, touch football, or a racquet sport.

What if you're afraid to walk in the street in your area? Walk with a group of friends. At weekends explore other areas where you feel safer. Hire an exercise video and work out at home. If you live in a block of units, always take the stairs instead of the lift.

## What If You Think You're Too Old?

You're not. Just start off slowly until you feel more confident. Encourage a friend to go for short walks with you and remind yourself that even though you're growing older, you can still improve with age. As well as all the other health benefits of exercise, regular activity can improve balance and muscle strength, reducing the risk of falls. Don't be put off if you have arthritis—regular light exercise can help control joint swelling and pain.

# Section 42.2

## *Choosing the Best Exercise for You*

**Summary**: What's the best exercise for you?

What's the best exercise for weight loss? Can you exercise if you have arthritis or have had a heart attack? What kind of activity can help prevent diseases like diabetes and high blood pressure? Here's what you need to know—and some realistic tips to get you started.

### How Much Activity Do You Need for Good Health?

Less than you think—you only have to take exercise regularly, not seriously. To help prevent problems like heart disease, diabetes, colon cancer, and high blood pressure, doctors now recommend 30 minutes of moderate activity on most days—preferably daily. You can break this 30 minutes into three 10-minute sessions, if it's easier to fit into your day. Besides walking, every-day activities like washing the car, sweeping the floor, or gardening can all count towards your 30 minutes. The important thing is to make activity a daily habit.

### What's the Best Exercise for Losing Weight?

If you're not already doing 30 minutes activity each day, this is a good way to start, but for successful weight loss you need to combine regular exercise with healthy, low-fat eating. It's also important to make healthy eating, and being more active, part of your life—once you stop being active and go back to eating fatty foods, you'll regain the weight you lost. If you're already active for 30 minutes a day, think of ways to increase this amount in ways you enjoy. The best type of exercise is one which uses the muscles in your legs and arms, together with your heart and lungs—this could be walking, swimming, cycling, dancing, aquarobics (gentle exercises in water), and low-impact aerobic classes—all good exercises for beginners. A good way to tell if you're exercising at the right level is the "talk test"—you should be able to talk while doing the activity (unless you're swimming). If not, you're working too hard. (If you're very overweight or unused to exercise, see your doctor before starting a new activity.)

## Can You Exercise after a Heart Attack or Heart Surgery?

Exercise is important for recovery from heart problems and will help prevent another attack or the need for more surgery, says the National Heart Foundation. But first, ask your doctor about how and when to start—some hospitals and community centers also have programs to help heart patients become active again. It's good to begin with gentle strolls for a few minutes and increase the amount of activity very gradually. Most people can return to activities like tennis, golf, or bowling after six to eight weeks.

Some people think physical activity can be dangerous, but over a lifetime it's more dangerous not to exercise than it is to be regularly active. This is also true if you have heart disease—just don't overdo it.

## Can You Exercise If You Have Arthritis?

Yes. Being active can help decrease pain and increase movement in the joints—tai chi, yoga, swimming, aquarobics, and walking can all help arthritis. The important thing is to find the right balance between rest and activity—rest can help ease an inflamed joint, but too much rest weakens muscles and increases stiffness. That's why it's best to exercise when you're least stiff and tired, have the least pain, and when your medication is working best. You'll exercise muscles and joints more effectively if they're warmed up—after a bath or a shower can be a good time.

For more information, see your doctor or ask him or her if you need to see a physiotherapist to help you with an exercise program. Ask the ethnic health worker at your community health center if there are any groups in your area for people with arthritis.

## Section 42.3

# *The Dangers of Steroid Abuse*

Reprinted from "Steroids (Anabolic-Androgenic)," National Institute on Drug Abuse, National Institutes of Health, revised January 2001, http://www.nida.nih.gov/Infofax/steroids.html.

Anabolic-androgenic steroids are man-made substances related to male sex hormones. "Anabolic" refers to muscle-building, and "androgenic" refers to increased masculine characteristics. "Steroids" refers to the class of drugs. These drugs are available legally only by prescription, to treat conditions that occur when the body produces abnormally low amounts of testosterone, such as delayed puberty and some types of impotence. They are also used to treat body wasting in patients with AIDS and other diseases that result in loss of lean muscle mass. Abuse of anabolic steroids, however, can lead to serious health problems, some irreversible.

Today, athletes and others abuse anabolic steroids to enhance performance and also to improve physical appearance. Anabolic steroids are taken orally or injected, typically in cycles of weeks or months (referred to as "cycling") rather than continuously. Cycling involves taking multiple doses of steroids over a specific period of time, stopping for a period, and starting again. In addition, users often combine several different types of steroids to maximize their effectiveness while minimizing negative effects (referred to as "stacking").

### Health Hazards

The major side effects from abusing anabolic steroids can include liver tumors and cancer, jaundice (yellowish pigmentation of skin, tissues, and body fluids), fluid retention, high blood pressure, increases in LDL (bad cholesterol), and decreases in HDL (good cholesterol). Other side effects include kidney tumors, severe acne, and trembling. In addition, there are some gender-specific side effects:

- For men—shrinking of the testicles, reduced sperm count, infertility, baldness, development of breasts, increased risk for prostate cancer.

- For women—growth of facial hair, male-pattern baldness, changes in or cessation of the menstrual cycle, enlargement of the clitoris, deepened voice.

- For adolescents—growth halted prematurely through premature skeletal maturation and accelerated puberty changes. This means that adolescents risk remaining short the remainder of their lives if they take anabolic steroids before the typical adolescent growth spurt.

In addition, people who inject anabolic steroids run the added risk of contracting or transmitting HIV/AIDS or hepatitis, which causes serious damage to the liver.

Scientific research also shows that aggression and other psychiatric side effects may result from abuse of anabolic steroids. Many users report feeling good about themselves while on anabolic steroids, but researchers report that extreme mood swings also can occur, including manic-like symptoms leading to violence. Depression often is seen when the drugs are stopped and may contribute to dependence on anabolic steroids. Researchers report also that users may suffer from paranoid jealousy, extreme irritability, delusions, and impaired judgment stemming from feelings of invincibility.

Research also indicates that some users might turn to other drugs to alleviate some of the negative effects of anabolic steroids. For example, a study of 227 men admitted in 1999 to a private treatment center for dependence on heroin or other opioids found that 9.3 percent had abused anabolic steroids before trying any other illicit drug. Of these 9.3 percent, 86 percent first used opioids to counteract insomnia and irritability resulting from the anabolic steroids.

## Extent of Use

The Monitoring the Future Study (MTF) survey is funded by National Institute on Drug Abuse, National Institutes of Health, and is conducted by the University of Michigan's Institute for Social Research. It assesses drug use among eighth, tenth, and twelfth graders nationwide, and has been conducted annually since 1975. Because of growing professional and public concern over anabolic steroids use by adolescents and young adults, questions regarding anabolic steroids use were added to the MTF in 1989 to give a better understanding of the extent of the problem. Between 1989 and 2000, lifetime prevalence of anabolic steroids use among twelfth graders fluctuated between a 3 percent high in 1989 and a 1.9 percent low in 1996.

In 1991, MTF was expanded to include assessment of eighth and tenth graders nationwide, in addition to twelfth graders. Use of steroids remained unchanged among eighth and twelfth graders from 1999 to 2000. Among tenth graders, however, the past year use of steroids increased from 1.7 percent in 1999 to 2.2 percent in 2000. In addition, the 2000 MTF noted a decrease among twelfth graders in the perceived risk of harm from using steroids.

Most anabolic steroids users are male, and among male students, past-year use of these substances was reported by 2.2 percent of eighth graders, 2.8 percent of tenth graders, and 2.5 percent of twelfth graders.

## Section 42.4

# *Sprains and Strains*

Reprinted from "Questions and Answers about Sprains and Strains," National Institute of Arthritis and Musculoskeletal and Skin Diseases, National Institutes of Health, November 1999. http://www.niams.nih.gov/hi/topics/strain_sprain/strain_sprain.htm. Reviewed by David A. Cooke, M.D., August 26, 2003.

This section contains general information about sprains and strains, which are both very common injuries. Individual parts describe what sprains and strains are, where they usually occur, what their signs and symptoms are, how they are treated, and how they can be prevented. If you have further questions, you may wish to discuss them with your doctor.

## What Is the Difference Between a Sprain and a Strain?

A sprain is an injury to a ligament—a stretching or a tearing. One or more ligaments can be injured during a sprain. The severity of the injury will depend on the extent of injury to a single ligament (whether the tear is partial or complete) and the number of ligaments involved.

A strain is an injury to either a muscle or a tendon. Depending on the severity of the injury, a strain may be a simple overstretch of the muscle or tendon, or it can result in a partial or complete tear.

## What Causes a Sprain?

A sprain can result from a fall, a sudden twist, or a blow to the body that forces a joint out of its normal position. This results in an overstretch or tear of the ligament supporting that joint. Typically, sprains occur when people fall and land on an outstretched arm, slide into base, land on the side of their foot, or twist a knee with the foot planted firmly on the ground.

## Where Do Sprains Usually Occur?

Although sprains can occur in both the upper and lower parts of the body, the most common site is the ankle. Ankle sprains are the most common injury in the United States and often occur during sports or recreational activities. Approximately one million ankle injuries occur each year, and 85 percent of them are sprains.

The talus bone and the ends of two of the lower leg bones (tibia and fibula) form the ankle joint (see Figure 42.1). This joint is supported by several lateral (outside) ligaments and medial (inside) ligaments. Most ankle sprains happen when the foot turns inward as a person runs, turns, falls, or lands on the ankle after a jump. This type of sprain is called an inversion injury. One or more of the lateral ligaments are injured, usually the anterior talofibular ligament. The calcaneofibular ligament is the second most frequently torn ligament.

The knee is another common site for a sprain. A blow to the knee or a fall is often the cause; sudden twisting can also result in a sprain (see Figure 42.2).

Sprains frequently occur at the wrist, typically when people fall and land on an outstretched hand.

## What Are the Signs and Symptoms of a Sprain?

The usual signs and symptoms include pain, swelling, bruising, and loss of the ability to move and use the joint (called functional ability). However, these signs and symptoms can vary in intensity, depending on the severity of the sprain. Sometimes people feel a pop or tear when the injury happens.

Doctors use many criteria to diagnose the severity of a sprain. In general, a grade I or mild sprain causes overstretching or slight tearing of the ligaments with no joint instability. A person with a mild sprain usually experiences minimal pain, swelling, and little or no loss of functional ability. Bruising is absent or slight, and the person is usually able to put weight on the affected joint. People with mild sprains usually do not need an x-ray, but one is sometimes performed if the diagnosis is unclear.

A grade II or moderate sprain causes partial tearing of the ligament and is characterized by bruising, moderate pain, and swelling. A person with a moderate sprain usually has some difficulty putting weight on the affected joint and experiences some loss of function. An x-ray may be needed to help the doctor determine if a fracture is causing the pain and swelling. Magnetic resonance imaging is occasionally used to help differentiate between a significant partial injury and a complete tear in a ligament.

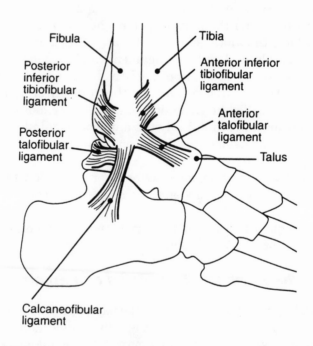

**Figure 42.1.** *View of the ankle joint from the side, showing the bones and ligaments.*

People who sustain a grade III or severe sprain completely tear or rupture a ligament. Pain, swelling, and bruising are usually severe, and the patient is unable to put weight on the joint. An x-ray is usually taken to rule out a broken bone.

When diagnosing any sprain, the doctor will ask the patient to explain how the injury happened. The doctor will examine the affected joint and check its stability and its ability to move and bear weight.

## When to See a Doctor for a Sprain

- You have severe pain and cannot put any weight on the injured joint.

- The area over the injured joint or next to it is very tender when you touch it.

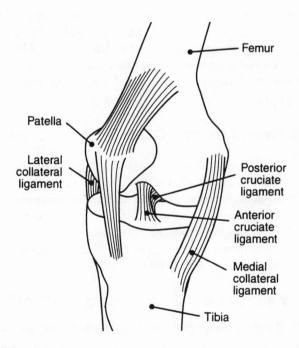

*Figure 42.2. View of the knee from the side, showing the bones and ligaments.*

- The injured area looks crooked or has lumps and bumps (other than swelling) that you do not see on the uninjured joint.

- You cannot move the injured joint.

- You cannot walk more than four steps without significant pain.

- Your limb buckles or gives way when you try to use the joint.

- You have numbness in any part of the injured area.

- You see redness or red streaks spreading out from the injury.

- You injure an area that has been injured several times before.

- You have pain, swelling, or redness over a bony part of your foot.

- You are in doubt about the seriousness of the injury or how to care for it.

## What Causes a Strain?

A strain is caused by twisting or pulling a muscle or tendon. Strains can be acute or chronic. An acute strain is caused by trauma or an injury such as a blow to the body; it can also be caused by improperly lifting heavy objects or overstressing the muscles. Chronic strains are usually the result of overuse—prolonged, repetitive movement of the muscles and tendons.

## Where Do Strains Usually Occur?

Two common sites for a strain are the back and the hamstring muscle (located in the back of the thigh). Contact sports such as soccer, football, hockey, boxing, and wrestling put people at risk for strains. Gymnastics, tennis, rowing, golf, and other sports that require extensive gripping can increase the risk of hand and forearm strains. Elbow strains sometimes occur in people who participate in racquet sports, throwing, and contact sports.

## What Are the Signs and Symptoms of a Strain?

Typically, people with a strain experience pain, muscle spasm, and muscle weakness. They can also have localized swelling, cramping, or inflammation and, with a minor or moderate strain, usually some loss of muscle function. Patients typically have pain in the injured area and general weakness of the muscle when they attempt to move it. Severe strains that partially or completely tear the muscle or tendon are often very painful and disabling.

## How Are Sprains and Strains Treated?

### Reduce Swelling and Pain

Treatment for sprains and strains is similar and can be thought of as having two stages. The goal during the first stage is to reduce swelling and pain. At this stage, doctors usually advise patients to follow a formula of rest, ice, compression, and elevation (RICE) for the first 24 to 48 hours after the injury. The doctor may also recommend an over-the-counter or prescription nonsteroidal anti-inflammatory drug, such as aspirin or ibuprofen, to help decrease pain and inflammation.

For people with a moderate or severe sprain, particularly of the ankle, a hard cast may be applied. Severe sprains and strains may require surgery to repair the torn ligaments, muscle, or tendons. Surgery is usually performed by an orthopedic surgeon.

It is important that moderate and severe sprains and strains be evaluated by a doctor to allow prompt, appropriate treatment to begin. Anyone who has any concerns about the seriousness of a sprain or strain should always contact a doctor for advice.

### RICE Therapy

**Rest.** Reduce regular exercise or activities of daily living as needed. Your doctor may advise you to put no weight on an injured area for 48 hours. If you cannot put weight on an ankle or knee, crutches may help. If you use a cane or one crutch for an ankle injury, use it on the uninjured side to help you lean away and relieve weight on the injured ankle.

**Ice.** Apply an ice pack to the injured area for 20 minutes at a time, four to eight times a day. A cold pack, ice bag, or plastic bag filled with crushed ice and wrapped in a towel can be used. To avoid cold injury and frostbite, do not apply the ice for more than 20 minutes.

**Compression.** Compression of an injured ankle, knee, or wrist may help reduce swelling. Examples of compression bandages are elastic wraps, special boots, air casts, and splints. Ask your doctor for advice on which one to use.

559

**Elevation.** If possible, keep the injured ankle, knee, elbow, or wrist elevated on a pillow, above the level of the heart, to help decrease swelling.

## Begin Rehabilitation

The second stage of treating a sprain or strain is rehabilitation, whose overall goal is to improve the condition of the injured part and restore its function. The health care provider will prescribe an exercise program designed to prevent stiffness, improve range of motion, and restore the joint's normal flexibility and strength. Some patients may need physical therapy during this stage.

When the acute pain and swelling have diminished, the health care provider or physical therapist will instruct the patient to do a series of exercises several times a day. These are very important because they help reduce swelling, prevent stiffness, and restore normal, pain-free range of motion. The health care provider can recommend many different types of exercises, depending on the injury. For example, people with an ankle sprain may be told to rest their heel on the floor and write the alphabet in the air with their big toe. A patient with an injured knee or foot will work on weight-bearing and balancing exercises. The duration of the program depends on the extent of the injury, but the regimen commonly lasts for several weeks.

Another goal of rehabilitation is to increase strength and regain flexibility. Depending on the patient's rate of recovery, this process begins about the second week after the injury. The health care provider or physical therapist will instruct the patient to do a series of exercises designed to meet these goals. During this phase of rehabilitation, patients progress to more demanding exercises as pain decreases and function improves.

The final goal is the return to full daily activities, including sports when appropriate. Patients must work closely with their health care provider or physical therapist to determine their readiness to return to full activity. Sometimes people are tempted to resume full activity or play sports despite pain or muscle soreness. Returning to full activity before regaining normal range of motion, flexibility, and strength increases the chance of reinjury and may lead to a chronic problem.

The amount of rehabilitation and the time needed for full recovery after a sprain or strain depend on the severity of the injury and individual rates of healing. For example, a moderate ankle sprain may require three to six weeks of rehabilitation before a person can return to full activity. With a severe sprain, it can take eight to 12 months before the ligament is fully healed. Extra care should be taken to avoid reinjury.

## Can Sprains and Strains Be Prevented?

There are many things people can do to help lower their risk of sprains and strains:

- Maintain a healthy, well-balanced diet to keep muscles strong.
- Maintain a healthy weight.
- Practice safety measures to help prevent falls (for example, keep stairways, walkways, yards, and driveways free of clutter, and salt or sand icy patches in the winter).
- Wear shoes that fit properly.
- Replace athletic shoes as soon as the tread wears out or the heel wears down on one side.
- Do stretching exercises daily.
- Be in proper physical condition to play a sport.
- Warm up and stretch before participating in any sports or exercise.
- Wear protective equipment when playing.
- Avoid exercising or playing sports when tired or in pain.
- Run on even surfaces.

Chapter 43

# Hair Loss

## Chapter Contents

# Section 43.1

# *Hair Loss and Its Causes*

Dating as far back as history will take us, baldness has been a part
of the aging process that many men fear the most. Before Rogaine®,
hair transplants and hair additions, men coped in various ways from
magic ointments to the styling of their hair. Julius Caesar grew his
hair long in the back and combed it all forward. Napoleon did the same
thing. Somehow we often disregard history and the fact that this has
been an age-old condition. We can't imagine or accept the fact that
there is not a cure.

Understanding the cause of male-pattern hair loss may better indicate exactly why it presently has no cure. Androgenetic alopecia—
the modern medical term for either male- or female-pattern hair
loss—can be broken down in two parts.

First, *androgenetic*, consisting of *androgen* (any of the various hormones that control the appearance and development of masculine
characteristics, such as testosterone). And *genetic*, the inheritance of
genes from either the mother's or the father's side of the family. Add
age, which when coupled with genetics, represents a time clock that
will signal the hair follicle to produce an enzyme named 5-alpha reductase. When the testosterone present in the follicle combines with
the enzyme 5-alpha reductase, it produces dihydrotestosterone (DHT).
Hair follicle receptors are sensitive to DHT and thereby start the process of male or female pattern hair loss.

Second, *alopecia* meaning hair loss, of which there are many types.

Put simply, scientists are working against aging, hormones, and
genetics. This is no easy task. Add the fact that male or female pattern hair loss is not life-threatening, and it is easy to see why many
physicians do not view hair loss as a priority in scientific research.

What is working for you in terms of research is that large pharmaceutical firms now know that a cure for hair loss could mean a for-
tune in revenue for their companies and stockholders. This is fuel
enough and the race has begun.

Although we may not see a cure in our lifetime, it is possible. Science is closer to understanding hair loss due to many recent advancements. To say the cure is around the corner would only be speculation, but hope certainly is alive.

Since there are other causes of hair loss, it is advisable to consult with a dermatologist who is competent and experienced with diagnosing hair loss. Confirming the type of hair loss you have will make it possible for you to know which treatment options may be best for you.

## Other Causes

- *Alopecia areata*: Generally thought to be an autoimmune disorder. Causes "patchy" hair loss, often in small circular areas in different areas of the scalp.

- *Alopecia totalis*: Total hair loss of the scalp (an advanced form of alopecia areata).

- *Alopecia universalis*: Hair loss of the entire body (also an advanced form of alopecia areata).

- *Traction alopecia*: Hair loss caused by physical stress and tension on the hair, such as prolonged use of hair weaving, corn rows, and so forth. Done too tightly on weak hair these can cause permanent hair loss.

- *Telogen effluvium*: Usually temporary hair loss. Causes: physical stress, emotional stress, thyroid abnormalities, medications, and hormonal causes normally associated with females.

- *Anagen effluvium*: Generally due to internally administered medications, such as chemotherapy agents, that poison the growing hair follicle.

All of these represent only a few of the different types of hair loss. Androgenetic alopecia represents close to 95 percent of all hair loss, however.

## Treatment Options Available for Androgenetic Alopecia

1. *Learning to live with hair loss*. Often the assistance of a professional counselor can be helpful in coping with hair loss.

2. *Hair styling* and cosmetic techniques, such as permanent waves and hair colors. The proper haircut alone can make a vast difference in diffusing hair loss.

3.  *Minoxidil*, the first FDA-approved topical treatment for male-
    or female-pattern hair loss. Although minoxidil is not effective
    in stimulating new hair growth in many males, it appears to
    be more effective in retarding hair loss in a substantial
    amount of both male and females. Currently, it is available
    over the counter in multiple brand-name (e.g., Rogaine™) and
    generic formulations.

4.  *Finasteride* (Propecia™), a second FDA-approved treatment
    for hair loss. Unlike minoxidil, this is only effective for male-
    pattern hair loss, and is taken orally. Like minoxidil,
    finasteride's effectiveness is limited, but it can prevent further
    hair loss.

5.  *Hair additions* have made many advances in both appearance
    and more secure attachment methods.

6.  *Hair replacement surgery* has also made many advances to-
    wards more natural-appearing results.

7.  A combination of #5—hair additions—with #6—hair replace-
    ment surgery.

# Section 43.2

# Hair Replacement: What Works, What Doesn't

Reprinted from "Hair Replacement: What Works, What Doesn't," *FDA Consumer,* March–April 1997, U.S. Food and Drug Administration. Also available at http://www.fda.gov/fdac/features/1997/397_hair.html. Reviewed and revised by David A. Cooke, M.D., on June 29, 2003.

When the advertising slogan "Be Like Mike" caught America's fancy, it wasn't because every man decided to go for the Michael Jordan look by reaching for a razor and shaving his head.

Sure, men like Jordan, Charles Barkley, and *Star Trek*'s Patrick Stewart are part of a small minority who are proud of their baldness. But combating and covering up hair loss hasn't turned into an estimated $1 billion-a-year industry because Americans like the idea of hair collecting in the shower drain.

"It probably represents aging," says Ken Washenik, M.D., director of dermatopharmacology at New York University Medical Center. "I think our concept of a bald person is of an older person. I think anything that reminds us in the mirror every day of the inevitability of aging is less than optimal."

When you talk about restoring hair, you're essentially looking at three different approaches. The first is to medicate, using a 2 percent solution of minoxidil found in Rogaine™ (and other brands since Pharmacia & Upjohn's patent expired in February 1996). Minoxidil was the first drug approved by the Food and Drug Administration (FDA) for regrowing hair. A second drug, finasteride, is marketed as Propecia™ by Merck as an oral tablet taken daily, but it is only effective for male-pattern hair loss.

That doesn't mean minoxidil or finasteride are by any means the panacea that men have been searching for since at least 1150 B.C., when Egyptians covered their baldness with a mixture of fats from ibex (a mountain goat), lion, crocodile, serpent, goose, and hippopotamus.

Surgical procedures, including hair transplantation and scalp reduction, are another modern-day approach. And, finally, there's the solution that Julius Caesar, according to legend, used in ancient days—cover it up. The most powerful man in the Roman Empire is said to have turned to the ceremonial wreath of laurel leaves to hide his ever-emerging scalp. The modern alternative is the hairpiece.

## Uncovering Baldness

When discussing baldness, which affects an estimated 40 million men and 20 million women in the United States, the topic is generally about a hereditary condition called androgenetic alopecia. Ninety-five percent of hair loss is of this variety.

Male-pattern baldness refers to the upward retreat of the hairline from the forehead, as well as an expanding area of fallout from the crown of the head. In the end, all that might be left is a horseshoe-shaped fringe around the sides and back of the head. Female-pattern baldness, which recently has received more attention since Pharmacia & Upjohn began packaging and marketing Rogaine separately for women, refers to a diffuse pattern of hair loss throughout the scalp.

Research continues in search of ways to treat androgenetic alopecia and allow hair to sprout in barren scalps. But, at this time, all you can do, if you're a man, is to look at your father's head and your mother's father's head to see how they fared, because chances are you'll wind up with a similar fate. In addition, female-pattern baldness can be passed down from mother to daughter.

"I think it's just the luck of the draw what your genetics are," says Allan Kayne, M.D., a dermatologist and assistant clinical professor of medicine at the University of Washington Medical Center in Seattle.

In male- and female-pattern baldness, the culprit is something called dihydrotestosterone, or DHT, which is derived from androgen, a male hormone. Circulating through the bloodstream, androgen is converted to DHT by the enzyme 5-alpha reductase. Those with greater enzyme activity have more DHT binding to hair-follicle receptors. If flooded by DHT, the follicles sprout thinner and thinner hairs until nothing regrows, and the follicles eventually wither away.

## Minoxidil

As Washenik explains, no one is quite certain how minoxidil, an oral medication originally approved to treat high blood pressure, works to grow hair.

To be effective, minoxidil must be used twice a day. It works better on those who are younger and whose hair loss is recent, according to clinical studies by Pharmacia & Upjohn.

Those studies show that 26 percent of men between 18 and 49 reported moderate to dense hair regrowth after four months of Rogaine treatment. An additional 33 percent had minimal hair regrowth. Almost 20 percent of women between 18 and 45 had moderate regrowth, while an additional 40 percent showed minimal regrowth.

A company spokesman said the research accounted for the fully pigmented hair fibers normally seen on the scalp and not vellus hair, which is more like peach fuzz. Many doctors, however, say the number of their patients who have as much success is much lower, and some find that only vellus hair appears.

"I have not been that impressed that it helps regrow hair," Kayne says. "I think that occurs in a very small minority."

One plus that Denise Cook, M.D., medical officer in FDA's division of dermatologic and dental drug products, points out is that patients report a decrease in shedding due to minoxidil use, though whether that perception is the result of fewer hairs being lost or more hairs being produced is unknown. Normally, you should lose only about 100 hairs a day.

One possible side effect of minoxidil is an itchy scalp. Another drawback is that it must be used for life or any regrown hair will fall out. Also, only those people losing hair on the crown, not in front, are candidates for regrowth.

### *Finasteride*

Finasteride, currently sold for hair loss as Propecia™, was developed as for treating urinary problems associated with age-related enlargement of the prostate gland. It is, in fact, marketed for this purpose as Proscar™, but at a different dose than Propecia.

Finasteride blocks the action of the 5-alpha reductase, the enzyme that converts androgens in the blood into DHT. This lowers levels of DHT in the scalp tissue and retards the hormone-related hair loss that occurs in male-pattern baldness. However, because of the way it works, finasteride is not effective for other forms of hair loss, and is completely ineffective in women, where hair loss is not due to DHT levels.

Like minoxidil, finasteride is modestly effective for male-pattern hair loss. It is usually necessary to use the medication for at least three months before any benefit can be seen. Whether it is any more effective than minoxidil for male-pattern hair loss remains a subject of debate.

Finasteride lowers blood levels of prostate specific antigen (PSA), a test that is sometimes used to screen for prostate cancer or to follow disease progress in patients who already have the disease. Therefore, it may affect the accuracy of this test. It can also have a negative effect on sexual interest and performance in some men.

As noted above, finasteride does not work for hair loss in women. Additionally, it can cause severe fetal malformations if taken by pregnant women. For this reason, pregnant women are advised even to avoid touching finasteride tablets if they are crushed or broken.

## Surgery

Twenty years ago, many people felt they risked looking like a Cabbage Patch doll if they chose surgery to eliminate baldness. Now, says Carlos Puig, D.O., director of Puig Medical Group, which is headquartered in Houston, better surgical techniques—used by increasingly skilled surgeons—are getting more eye-pleasing results.

"When I started in 1973 ... it was like the Stone Age," the cosmetic surgeon says, referring to the equipment and techniques in use. Now, he says, surgeons have learned to create a much more natural-looking hair line, using scalpels to cut either small slits or holes in the scalp to receive transplanted hair.

While there are numerous types of surgery, they can be sifted into two main categories: transplantation and scalp reduction.

Transplantation involves moving hair from densely covered sites on the sides or back of the head to bald areas of the scalp.

The key to success, explains Anthony Santangelo, president of the American Hair Loss Council, is to have good sites on the sides or back of the head from which to move hairs. Otherwise, patients can't expect ample coverage. Because their hair loss is diffuse, women generally lack good donor sites, making transplantation impractical for them.

The biggest improvement in transplants is with "micro" or "mini" grafts. "You're looking at one to two hairs shot into the head with a needle," Santangelo says. "It achieves a very, very fine, natural-looking hair line. The significant difference there is you need a lot of hair to do that."

Surgeons also use larger round plugs of seven to 10 hairs. Line grafts, the shifting of strips of nine to 12 hairs, are common, too.

One thing to keep in mind is that prosthetic hair fibers for transplantation are banned by FDA. Implanting them, according to Stephen Rhodes, acting chief of FDA's plastic and reconstructive surgery devices branch, caused a high incidence of adverse reactions, including infection.

If male-pattern baldness has left you with too much balding area to cover, you may benefit from scalp reduction: the surgical removal of large sections of a bald scalp. Extenders and expanders, elastic devices placed under the skin to stretch the hair-bearing scalp regions on the side of the head, have been used as a complement to reduction surgery.

Another surgical method is the flap technique, which rotates hair-bearing scalp areas from the sides or moves those areas from the back forward. The flap technique has the highest complication rate, though, Puig says. Bleeding, scarring, and infection can occur from surgery. But advances, such as knowing what size flap to use and how to enhance blood supply to the region, have cut down on the visibility of scars.

## Hairpieces

Finally, if you prefer to dodge the pain, time, and cost of surgery, there's always the old, reliable hairpiece.

Obviously, all toupees and wigs are not created equal. Just as the transplant is only as good as the surgeon, the hairpiece is only as good as the person creating it and the materials used.

There are a variety of ways of affixing the hairpiece, which consists of human or synthetic hair implanted one hair at a time into a nylon netting. No method is permanent.

The hair weave involves sewing a wig into existing hair.

Also there are more traditional methods: You can use bonding (a type of glue), metal clips, or simple tape to attach the hairpiece to the scalp. Unlike the weaves, these give you the option to take the hairpiece on or off with ease. Many companies advertise "hair systems" or "hair clubs," which, according to Santangelo, offer check-ups to clean, color, and tighten the hairpiece.

Lark Lambert, consumer complaint coordinator for FDA's Office of Cosmetics and Colors, notes that in addition to maintaining the cleanliness of hairpieces and wigs, it is important not to neglect the scalp under the wig. Keeping it clean and healthy avoids skin irritation and disease, he says. Also, as a precautionary safety measure, first-time users of hairpiece adhesives and solvents should test a patch of skin for 48 hours to determine possible skin sensitization to these products.

## Health-Related Hair Loss

While hair loss is more harmful to the psyche than anything else, some of the causes of baldness may represent serious health problems. That's why it's important to talk about hair loss with a physician.

One problem, says FDA's Cook, could be a condition called alopecia areata. It's an autoimmune disease of unknown cause in which inflammatory cells attack the bulbs of the follicles under the scalp, leaving hairless patches. In more serious cases, hair may fall out from the entire head—eyebrows and beard included—and the entire body. Many times, though, the hair returns spontaneously.

Childbirth, severe malnutrition, chemotherapy, thyroid problems, and a form of lupus can also cause hair loss.

Something as simple as pigtails or cornrows, if worn too long, can cause hair loss, too, because of the stress they cause to the hair shaft.

The medical opinion concerning the role of emotional stress in balding is mixed. If stress does play a role, however, it's only at times of extreme emotional trauma, according to Kayne at the University of Washington Medical Center.

## Mythical Treatments

The mythology of hair loss is a book unto itself. Wearing hats won't cause it, doctors say. Nor will standing on your head to increase blood flow cure it. Massaging your scalp and brushing your hair won't save you. Toweling off your head lightly rather than vigorously will only postpone the inevitable for a few days.

Perhaps the biggest myth is that cleaning your scalp of sebum (the semifluid secretion of glands attached to the follicle) will unclog those follicles and allow hair to grow. Surgeons will tell you that when they're performing transplants, there's no trapped hair to be found.

In 1989, FDA banned all nonprescription hair creams, lotions, or other external products claiming to grow hair or prevent baldness. And it has taken action against companies that continue to sell such products. In 1996, the agency sent a warning letter to Daniel Rogers Laboratories Inc., of Paramus, N.J., the manufacturer of "Natural Hairs," for claiming its product could promote hair growth and prevent hair loss. Two years earlier, after an FDA investigation, a U.S. district court judge enjoined the marketing of "Solution 109 Herbal Shampoo" because of claims that the product warded off hair loss.

Advertisements for "hair farming" products and others that hint they can regrow hair are still plentiful. But if you're desperate, keep one thing in mind:

"There will be never be a secret [ingredient] that works for hair loss," NYU's Washenik says. And, if they were to find it, he says: "It will be on the cover of the *New York Times*. It will be on the nightly news. ... When this happens, it's going to be wildness. You're not going to need an expert to tell you the name of the drug."

## *The Thick and Thin of Hair Cosmetics*

While minoxidil-based products and finasteride are giving consumers hopes of regrowing hair, another part of the hair-care industry has been jumping into the fray.

Drugstore chains, beauty shops, and salons are offering a number of products claiming to make hair appear thicker or fuller. While they won't solve baldness, such products can help women in particular by giving the appearance of more hair—if, and only if, the products are used regularly.

"The reality is," says Anthony Santangelo, president of the American Hair Loss Council, "[the products] just build hair for the day."

A quick walk down the store aisle shows a multitude of shampoos, conditioners, gels, mousses, and volumizers competing for your dollars. Many labeling claims target people with thinning hair, while others hint they can regrow hair, creating controversy about whether such a claim constitutes going too far. Any product claiming to regrow hair would have to file a new drug application. The Food and Drug Administration has approved only two products, the drugs minoxidil and finasteride, for regrowing hair.

"It's marketing; it's puffery," Santangelo says. "They'll take it as close as they possibly can without crossing the line, and they'll run with it."

Many of these products seem to thicken hair by coating it with chemicals called polymers. Hair has a negative charge, and the polymers' positive charge causes the polymers to adhere to the hair shaft, says Charles Fox, a Fair Lawn, N.J., consultant to the cosmetics industry. That results in better hair manageability and shine, he says. The hair also retains moisture, causing the shaft to swell and its diameter to expand slightly.

Also, says Stanley Milstein, Ph.D., special assistant to the director of FDA's Office of Cosmetics and Colors, some products coat the hair with various oils, waxes, and silicone, claiming to restore moisture balance as they thicken hair.

Clarence Robbins, vice president of advanced technology for Colgate-Palmolive Co. and author of Chemical and Physical Behavior of Human Hair, says that if the products work, it's because they keep hair shafts from sliding past each other (think of the fly-away hair you get after blow-drying on a winter day.) In that way, hair volume appears greater.

If you're one to use bleach (peroxide) occasionally, he says, the bleach can achieve that sliding effect. Perms also make your hair wavier and fuller looking.

Many promoters of these products say their pro-vitamin $B_5$ (panthenol) formulas can lead to fuller hair. Experts say don't bet on it, and according to the agency, the claim has never been proved.

By the way, there are products that simply color your scalp to create the appearance of hair. "But get any closer than 20 feet from an individual, they're gonna see your head's been spray-painted or covered with powder," Santangelo says.

# Part Six

# Additional
# Help and Information

# Chapter 44

# *Glossary of Terms Related to Men's Health*

**Acute bacterial prostatitis**: The least common form of prostatitis, caused by bacteria traveling up the urethra and the backward flow of infected urine into the prostatic ducts. [1]

**Alpha blockers:** Also known as alpha-adrenergic blockers. Drugs used to treat high blood pressure and other conditions like an enlarged prostate. [1]

**Analgesic:** A drug intended to alleviate pain. [1]

**Androgens:** A family of hormones that promote the development and maintenance of male sex characteristics. [3]

---

This glossary was compiled from three sources. Terms marked with [1] are reprinted with permission from American Urological Association Education and Research, Inc. For current information on urological health topics, visit http://www.UrologyHealth.org. © 2003 by American Urological Association Education and Research, Inc. All rights reserved. Terms marked with [2] are provided by KidsHealth, one of the largest resources online for medically reviewed health information written for parents, kids, and teens. For more articles like this one, visit www.KidsHealth.org or www.TeensHealth.org. © 2001 The Nemours Center for Children's Health Media, a division of The Nemours Foundation. Terms marked with [3] are taken from "What You Need To Know About™ Prostate Cancer," National Cancer Institute, http://www.nci.nih.gov/templates/page_print.aspx?viewid=b94a9092-bbc1-4ba2-8c75-6793238d92a4, updated September 16, 2002. Also available in hard copy as NIH Pub. No. 00-1576 via https://cissecure.nci.nih.gov/ncipubs/.

**Autoimmune disease:** Any disorder in which the body is attacked by its own immune system. [1]

**Azoospermia:** Absence of sperm in the ejaculate fluid. [1]

**Bacterial prostatitis:** Swelling of the prostate caused by bacteria. [1]

**Benign prostatic hyperplasia:** BPH. A benign (noncancerous) condition in which an overgrowth of prostate tissue pushes against the urethra and the bladder, blocking the flow of urine. Also called benign prostatic hypertrophy. [3]

**Bladder:** The balloon-shaped organ inside the pelvis that holds urine. [1]

**Catheter:** A tube that is inserted through the urethra to the bladder to drain urine. [1]

**Chronic bacterial prostatitis:** An uncommon form of prostatitis caused by bacteria traveling up the urethra and the backward flow of infected urine into the prostatic ducts causing recurrent infections. [1]

**Chronic prostatitis:** Inflammation of the prostate gland, developing slowly and lasting a long time. [1]

**Corpora cavernosa:** Two cylinder-shaped bodies that lie side by side in the penis and that, when filled with blood, enlarge to cause the penis to swell and become erect. [1]

**Corpus spongiosum:** A column of erectile tissue in the center of the penis and surrounding the urethra. When filled with blood, it enlarges and causes the penis to swell and become erect. [1]

**Cystoscopy:** Also known as cystourethroscopy. Examination with a narrow, tube-like instrument passed through the urethra to look inside the bladder. [1]

**Digital rectal examination:** Also known as DRE. Insertion of a gloved, lubricated finger into the rectum to feel the prostate and check for any abnormalities. [1]

**Dry orgasm:** Sexual climax without the release of semen from the penis. [3]

**Ejaculation:** The ejection of semen through the penis during sexual activity. [2]

**Epididymis:** A coiled tube attached to the back and upper side of the testicle that stores sperm and is connected to the vas deferens. [1]

**Erectile dysfunction:** Also known as ED or impotence. The inability to get or maintain an erection for satisfactory sexual intercourse. [1]

**Erection:** Enlargement and hardening of the penis caused by increased blood flow into the penis and decreased blood flow out of it as a result of sexual excitement. [1]

**Fertile:** Able to produce offspring. [1]

**Fibrous cavernositis:** Also known as Peyronie disease. Fibrous scarring causing the erect penis to be bent to such a degree that it interferes with sexual intercourse. [1]

**Genitals:** Organs of the reproductive system. [2]

**Genitourinary system:** The parts of the body that play a role in reproduction, getting rid of waste products in the form of urine, or both. [3]

**Gland:** A mass of cells or an organ that removes substances from the bloodstream and excretes them or secretes them back into the blood with a specific physiological purpose. [1]

**Groin:** The area where the upper thigh meets the lower abdomen. [1]

**Hydrocele:** A painless swelling of the scrotum caused by collection of fluid around the testicle. [1]

**Impotence:** The inability to get or maintain an erection of the penis for sexual activity. Also called erectile dysfunction. [1]

**Insemination:** Insertion of sperm into the woman's uterus. [1]

**Oligospermia:** Low number of sperm in the ejaculate. [1]

**Orchiectomy:** Surgery to remove one or both testicles. [3]

**Orgasm:** The climax of sexual excitement, consisting of intense muscle tightening around the genital area experienced as a pleasurable wave of tingling sensations through parts of the body. [1]

**Penile shaft:** The cylindrical body of the penis. [1]

**Penis:** Male reproductive organ that transfers sperm to the female. [2]

**Perineum:** The area between the anus and the scrotum in males and the area between the anus and the vagina in females. [1]

**Peyronie disease:** A plaque (hardened area) that forms on the penis, preventing that area from stretching. During erection, the penis bends in the direction of the plaque, or the plaque may lead to indentation and shortening of the penis. [1]

**Prostate gland:** Structure surrounding the ejaculatory ducts that produces some of the components of sperm. [2]

**Prostatectomy:** An operation to remove part or all of the prostate. Radical (or total) prostatectomy is the removal of the entire prostate and some of the tissue around it. [3]

**Prostatism:** A disorder of the prostate gland, especially enlargement that blocks or inhibits urine flow. [1]

**Prostatitis:** Inflammation of the prostate gland. Chronic prostatitis means the prostate gets inflamed over and over again. The most common form of prostatitis is not associated with any known infecting organism. [1]

**Prostatodynia:** Pain in the prostate. [1]

**PSA test:** Also referred to as prostate-specific antigen test. A blood test used to help detect prostate cancer. [1]

**Retrograde ejaculation:** Caused by the failure of the bladder neck to close during ejaculation, allowing the ejaculate to be propelled into the bladder instead of out the penis. [1]

**Scrotum:** Pouch-like structure containing the testes. [2]

**Semen:** The thick whitish fluid, produced by glands of the male reproductive system, that carries the sperm (reproductive cells) through the penis during ejaculation. [1]

**Seminal fluid:** Whitish fluid that mixes with sperm to form semen. [2]

**Seminal vesicles:** Sac-like structures attached to the vas deferens that provide fluids to lubricate the duct system and nourish the sperm. [2]

**Seminiferous tubules:** Tiny coiled tubes in the testes that produce sperm. [2]

**Sperm:** Also referred to as spermatozoa. Male germ cells that are produced by the testicles and that are capable of fertilizing the female partner's eggs. Cells resemble tadpoles if seen by the naked eye. [1]

**Testicle:** Also known as testis. Either of the paired, egg-shaped glands contained in a pouch (scrotum) below the penis. They produce sperm and the male hormone testosterone. [1]

**Testicular cancer:** Cancer of the testis. [1]

**Testosterone:** Major male sex hormone. [2]

**Transurethral resection of the prostate:** Surgical procedure to remove tissue from the prostate using an instrument inserted through the urethra. Also called TURP. [3]

**Urethra:** In males, this narrow tube carries urine from the bladder to the outside of the body and also serves as the channel through which semen is ejaculated. In females, this narrow tube carries urine from the bladder to the outside of the body. [1]

**Urinary tract:** The system that takes wastes from the blood and carries them out of the body in the form of urine. The urinary tract includes the kidneys, ureters, bladder, and urethra. [1]

**Urologist:** A doctor who specializes in diseases of the male and female urinary systems and the male reproductive system. [1]

**Varicoceles:** Dilated varicose veins in the scrotum that drain the testis and can impair the process of formation of sperm. [1]

**Vas deferens:** Muscular tube that passes upward alongside the testes and transports the sperm. [2]

**Vasectomy:** A surgical operation in which the vas deferens from each testicle is cut and tied to prevent the transfer of sperm during ejaculation. [1]

**Zygote:** The fertilized egg; a combination of egg and sperm. [2]

# Chapter 45

# *Directory of Organizational Resources in Men's Health*

Information in this chapter was compiled from many sources deemed accurate; inclusion does not constitute endorsement. All contact information verified in August 2003.

**Academy of General Dentistry**
211 E. Chicago Avenue
Suite 900
Chicago, IL 60611
Toll-free: (877) 2X-A-YEAR [(877)-292-9327]
Phone: (312) 440-4300
Website: http://www.agd.org
E-mail: agdtech@agd.org

The Academy of General Dentistry website serves as a consumer resource for current dental health information. Consumers can search more than 300 oral health topics:

- *SmileLine Online*, http://forums.agd.org/agdsmileline. Consumers can receive free dental advice by posting questions on the SmileLine Online, a message board on the Academy's website. Questions are answered within hours by an Academy member.

- *Find a Dentist*, http://www.agd.org/consumer/consumer/ index.html. Find a Dentist provides a listing of member dentists nationwide. When consumers provide a ZIP code, they will receive a randomly selected list of up to six dentists.

- *(877) 2X-A-YEAR* [(877) 292-9327]. The Academy sponsors a year-round, toll-free service to help consumers find a general dentist in their area and remind them to visit the dentist twice a year.

- *Free oral and overall health brochure*. Call (877) 292-9327.

- *Dentalnotes*. A quarterly public interest newsletter, *Dentalnotes* can be found in Academy members' offices nationwide. *Dentalnotes* provides dental tips for maintaining good oral health. To subscribe to this publication, log onto https:// www.agdwebapps.org/products.html.

- Online oral health topics, http://www.agd.org/consumers/ resources.html. This is a free resource containing information on everything from the history of dentistry to children's dental health information.

### Al-Anon Family Group Headquarters, Inc.
1600 Corporate Landing Parkway
Virginia Beach, VA 23454-5617
Toll-free: (888) 4AL-ANON
Phone: (757) 563-1600
Fax: (757) 563-1655
Website: http://www.al-anon.alateen.org
E-mail: WSO@al-anon.org

Al-Anon Family Group Headquarters, Inc. makes referrals to local Al-Anon groups, which are support groups for spouses and other significant adults in an alcoholic person's life. It also makes referrals to Alateen groups, which offer support to children of alcoholics. Free informational materials and locations of Al-Anon or Alateen meetings worldwide can be obtained by calling the toll-free number (888) 425-2666 from the United States or Canada, Monday through Friday, 8 a.m.–6 p.m. (Eastern Time).

### Alcoholics Anonymous (AA) World Services, Inc.
475 Riverside Drive
11th Floor
New York, NY 10115
Phone: (212) 870–3400
Fax: (212) 870–3003
Website: http://www.aa.org
E-mail: via AA's Website

Alcoholics Anonymous (AA) World Services, Inc. makes referrals to local AA groups and provides informational materials on the AA program. Many cities and towns also have a local AA office listed in the telephone book. All communication should be directed to AA's mailing address: AA World Services, Inc., Grand Central Station, P.O. Box 459, New York, NY 10163.

### American Academy of Family Physicians
11400 Tomahawk Creek Parkway
Leawood, KS 66211-2672
Toll-free: (800) 274-2237
Phone: (913) 906-6000
Website: http://familydoctor.org
E-mail: mail@familydoctor.org

The AAFP is an association of family doctors and other health care providers and students with an interest in family practice. Through their consumer oriented website, familydoctor.org, they provide information on a wide variety of health-related topics. A physician locator service is also available.

### American Diabetes Association (ADA)
National Office
1701 North Beauregard Street
Alexandria, VA 22311
Phone: (800) DIABETES [(800) 342-2383]
Website: http://www.diabetes.org
E-mail: AskADA@diabetes.org

The American Diabetes Association works toward preventing diabetes and finding a cure. It offers information through a variety of publications, provides funding for research, and serves in an advocacy role for people who's lives have been affected by diabetes.

### American Liver Foundation
75 Maiden Lane
Suite 603
New York, NY 10038
Toll-free: (800) GO-LIVER (465-4837) or (888) 443-7872
Phone: (212) 668-1000
Fax: (212) 483-8179
Website: http://www.liverfoundation.org
E-mail: info@liverfoundation.org

The American Liver Foundation seeks to help prevent, treat, and cure liver diseases, including hepatitis. Its educational programs work to increase awareness among the general public and to assist health care providers in making diagnostic and treatment decisions. The foundation also supports liver and biliary tract research.

### American Psychological Association
Office of Public Affairs
750 First St., N.E.
Washington, DC 20002-4242
Toll-free: (800) 374-2721
Phone: (202) 336-5700
TDD/TTY: (202) 336-6123
Website: http://www.apa.org

The American Psychological Association (APA) represents more than 150,000 psychologists worldwide. The association's mission includes promoting psychological research and developing professional standards. Their website offers information about a wide variety of topics, including attention deficit hyperactivity disorder, aging, anger, depression, divorce, sexuality, and stress, and numerous publications.

### American Urological Association
1000 Corporate Boulevard
Linthicum, MD 21090
Toll-free: (866) RING-AUA [(866) 746-4282]
Website: http://www.auanet.org
E-mail: aua@auanet.org

The AUA represents more than 13,000 health care providers who work in the field of urology and helps them stay abreast of current research. Patient information for people with urological conditions is available on the association's website.

### Arthritis Foundation
1330 West Peachtree Street
Atlanta, GA 30309
Phone: Call your local chapter (listed in the telephone directory) or toll-free (800) 283-7800
Website: http://www.arthritis.org

The foundation is a major voluntary organization devoted to supporting research on arthritis and other rheumatic diseases. The foundation publishes a free pamphlet on osteoarthritis and a magazine for members on arthritis and related conditions. It also provides up-to-date information on treatments, nutrition, alternative therapies, and self-management strategies. Chapters nationwide offer exercise programs, classes, support groups, physician referral services, and free literature.

## Centers for Disease Control and Prevention (CDC)
1600 Clifton Road
Atlanta, GA 30333
Toll-free: (800) 311-3435
Phone: (404) 639-3311
Fax: (404) 639-3312
Website: http://www.cdc.gov

The CDC is the lead federal agency for protecting the health and safety of Americans at home and abroad, providing credible information to enhance health decisions, and promoting health through strong partnerships. CDC serves as the national focus for developing and applying disease prevention and control, environmental health, and health promotion and education activities designed to improve the health of the people of the United States. CDC is an agency of the Department of Health and Human Services.

## Centers for Disease Control National AIDS Hotline
Phone: (800) 342-AIDS
Spanish: (800) 344-SIDA
TTY: (800) 243-7889

The CDC National AIDS Hotline, including its Spanish Service and TTY Service, is operated under contract with Centers for Disease Control and Prevention (CDC). The hotline handles about one million calls per year — about 2,740 calls per day — from people with questions about prevention, risk, testing, treatment, and other HIV/AIDS-related concerns. Information specialists are available 24 hours a day, seven days a week, to answer questions, provide referrals, and send free publications through e-mail and postal mail.

## Depression and Bipolar Support Alliance (formerly the National Depressive and Manic-Depressive Association)
730 N. Franklin Street, Suite 501
Chicago, IL 60601-7204
Toll-free (800) 826-3632
Phone: (312) 642-0049

## Depression and Bipolar Support Alliance, continued
Fax: (312) 642-7243
Website: http://www.dbsalliance.org

Depression and Bipolar Support Alliance is a patient-directed organization whose mission is to improve the lives of people living with
mood disorders.

## National Alliance for the Mentally Ill
Colonial Place Three
2107 Wilson Blvd., 3rd Floor
Arlington, VA 22201
Toll-free: (800) 950-NAMI (6264)
Phone: (703) 524-7600
Fax: (703) 524-9094
Website: http://www.nami.org

NAMI is a support and advocacy organization of consumers, families, and
friends of people with severe mental illness; over 1,200 state and local
affiliates. Local affiliates often give guidance in finding treatment.

## National Council on Alcoholism and Drug Dependence, Inc. (NCADD)
20 Exchange Place, Suite 2902
New York, NY 10005
HOPE LINE: (800) NCA-CALL (24-hour affiliate referral)
Phone: (212) 269-7797
Fax: (212) 269-7510
Website: http://www.ncadd.org
E-mail: national@ncadd.org

NCADD offers educational materials and information on alcoholism.
The council provides phone numbers of local NCADD Affiliates (who
can provide information on local treatment resources) via the toll-free,
24-hour HOPE LINE.

## National Foundation for Depressive Illness, Inc.
P.O. Box 2257
New York, NY 10116
Toll-free (800) 239-1265
Phone: (212) 268-4260
Website: http://www.depression.org

The foundation informs the public about depressive illness and its treatability and promotes programs of research, education, and treatment.

### National Herpes Resource Center and Hotline
American Social Health Association
P.O. Box 13827
Research Triangle Park, NC 27709-9940
Phone: (919) 361-8488 (9 a.m. to 7 p.m. Eastern Time, Monday through Friday)
Fax: (919) 361-8425
Website: http://www.ashastd.org/hrc/index.html

The Herpes Resource Center (HRC) provides facts about herpes and works to increase public awareness of related issues. The center offers information resources and referrals.

### National Institute of Allergy and Infectious Diseases (NIAID)
National Institutes of Health
31 Center Drive, MSC 2520
Bethesda, MD 20892-2520
Website: http://www.niaid.nih.gov

The National Institute of Allergy and Infectious Diseases (NIAID) is a component of the National Institutes of Health (NIH). NIAID conducts and supports research that strives to understand, treat, and ultimately prevent the myriad infectious, immunologic, and allergic diseases that threaten hundreds of millions of people worldwide. The institute's mission is driven by a strong commitment to basic research and the understanding that the fields of immunology, microbiology, and infectious disease are related and complementary. NIAID research centers on immune-mediated diseases (and immune tolerance), HIV/AIDS, emerging infectious diseases, and vaccines.

### National Institute of Mental Health (NIMH)
Office of Communications
Information Resources and Inquiries Branch
6001 Executive Boulevard, Room 8184, MSC 9663
Bethesda, MD 20892-9663
Toll-free: (866) 227-NIMH (6464)
Phone: (301) 443-4513

### National Institute of Mental Health (NIMH), continued
TTY: (301) 443-8431
Fax: (301) 443-4279
Fax4U: (301) 443-5158
Website: http://www.nimh.nih.gov
E-mail: nimhinfo@nih.gov

NIMH is a federal government agency whose mission is to reduce the burden of mental illness and behavioral disorders through research on mind, brain, and behavior. The National Institute of Mental Health is a part of the National Institutes of Health, U.S. Department of Health and Human Services.

### National Institute of Arthritis and Musculoskeletal and Skin Diseases (NIAMS)
National Institutes of Health
1 AMS Circle
Bethesda, MD 20892-3675
Toll-free: (877) 22-NIAMS
Phone: (301) 495-4484
TTY: (301) 565-2966
Fax: (301) 718-6366
Website www.niams.nih.gov
E-mail: niamsinfo@mail.nih.gov

NIAMS provides information about various forms of arthritis and rheumatic diseases. It distributes patient and professional education materials and also refers people to other sources of information.

### National Institute on Alcohol Abuse and Alcoholism (NIAAA)
Scientific Communications Branch
6000 Executive Boulevard
Willco Building, Suite 409
Bethesda, MD 20892-7003
Phone: (301) 443-3860
Fax: (301) 480-1726
Website: http://www.niaaa.nih.gov
E-mail: niaaaweb-r@exchange.nih.gov

NIAAA makes available free informational materials on all aspects of alcoholism, including the effects of drinking during pregnancy, alcohol use and the elderly, and help for cutting down on drinking.

## National Library of Medicine
MEDLINEplus
8600 Rockville Pike
Bethesda, MD 20894
Phone: (800) 338-7657
Website: http://medlineplus.gov
E-mail: custserv@nlm.nih.gov

MEDLINEplus is a gold mine of good health information from the world's largest medical library, the National Library of Medicine. Health professionals and consumers alike can depend on it for information that is authoritative and up-to-date. MEDLINEplus provides extensive information from the National Institutes of Health and other trusted sources on over 600 diseases and conditions. There are also lists of hospitals and physicians, a medical encyclopedia and a medical dictionary, health information in Spanish, extensive information on prescription and nonprescription drugs, health information from the media, and links to thousands of clinical trials.

## National Mental Health Association
2001 N. Beauregard Street, 12th Floor
Alexandria, VA 22311
Toll-free: (800) 969-NMHA (6642)
Toll-free TTY: (800) 433-5959
Phone: (703) 684-7722
Fax: (703) 684-5968
Website: http://www.nmha.org

This association works with more than 340 affiliates nationwide to promote mental health through advocacy, education, research, and services.

## Sexual Function Health Council
American Foundation for Urologic Disease
1128 North Charles Street
Baltimore, MD 21201
Toll-free: (800) 433-4215
Phone: (410) 468-1800
Website: http://www.impotence.org
E-mail: impotence@afud.org

The Sexual Function Health Council seeks to assist people in obtaining confidential and accurate information about erectile dysfunction.

Facts about treatment options are available on the council's website. E-mail and telephone contacts can be used to obtain answers to specific questions.

### Sexuality Information and Education Council of the United States (SIECUS)
130 W. 42nd Street, Suite 350
New York, NY 10036-7802
Phone: (212) 819-9770
Fax: (212) 819-9776
Website: http://www.siecus.org
E-mail: siecus@siecus.org

SIECUS provides information to the general public and to health care professionals about human sexuality. The organization's programs include projects to promote sexuality education, to help parents discuss related issues with their children, and to provide accurate information about AIDS and other sexually transmitted diseases.

### Substance Abuse and Mental Health Services Administration (SAMHSA)
National Mental Health Information Center
P.O. Box 42557
Washington, DC 20015
Toll-free: (800) 789-2647
Toll-free TTY: (866) 889-2647
Phone: (301) 443-1805
TTY: (301) 443-9006
Fax: (301) 984-8796
Website: http://www.mentalhealth.samhsa.gov
E-mail: info@mentalhealth.org

SAMHSA's National Mental Health Information Center provides the public with information on mental health services and referrals to federal, state, or local resources for more information and help. SAMHSA is an agency of the U.S. Department of Health and Human Services.

# *Index*

# Index

Page numbers followed by 'n' indicate a footnote. Page numbers in *italics* indicate a table or illustration.

## A

AICD *see* automated implantable cardiac defibrillator

AIDS *see* acquired immune deficiency syndrome

air pollution, chronic obstructive pulmonary disease 130

Al-Anon Family Group Headquarters, Inc., contact information 584

albumin 176

albuterol 132

alcoholic liver disease 185–86, 189

Alcoholics Anonymous (AA) World Services, Inc., contact information 584–85

alcoholism, overview 518–25

"Alcoholism: Getting the Facts" (NIH) 518n

alcohol use
  antidepressant medications 461
  cancer 52
  cocaine 537
  depression 453
  drinking diary 525–28
  hypertension 234
  stroke 101
  suicide 171–72

aldosterone 44

alendronate 275

*Alopecia areata* 565

*Alopecia totalis* 565

*Alopecia universalis* 565

alpha1 antitrypsin deficiency, liver disease 186

alpha1 antitrypsin deficiency related emphysema (AAT emphysema) 136–37

alpha-beta blockers 236

alpha blockers
  defined 577
  hypertension 235–36

alpha-fetoprotein (AFP) 91

alpha interferon 191–92, 203

Alport syndrome 180

alprazolam 542

alveoli, described 130–31

ambiguous genitalia, described 288

American Academy of Family Physicians (AAFP)
  contact information 585

American Academy of Family Physicians (AAFP), continued
  publications
    testicular cancer 89n
    tinea infections 239n

American Association of Retired Persons (AARP)
  driver safety program information 110
  driving decisions publication 111
  sexuality study 338

American Automobile Association (AAA), driver safety program information 110, 111

American College of Emergency Physicians, domestic violence publication 472n

American Diabetes Association (ADA), contact information 585

American Dietetic Association, weight loss medications publication 506n

American Heart Association, publications
  stroke 97n
  tobacco use 27n

American Liver Foundation, contact information 585

American Lung Association, chronic obstructive pulmonary disease publication 129n

"American Lung Association Fact Sheet: Chronic Obstructive Pulmonary Disease (COPD)" (American Lung Association) 129n

American Psychological Association (APA)
  contact information 586
  sexual orientation publication 289n

American Social Health Association (ASHA), contact information 370

American Urological Association (AUA), contact information 586

"Am I at Risk for Type 2 Diabetes?" (National Diabetes Information Clearinghouse) 145n

aminoglutethimide 86, 89

amitriptyline 279

amoxicillin 381

amprenavir 202

cimetidine 343
ciprofloxacin 373
circumcision 288, 295–97
cirrhosis 185–90
"Cirrhosis of the Liver" (National Digestive Diseases Information Clearinghouse) 185n
clinical trials
  cancer 57
  colorectal cancer 78
  lung cancer 69
  testicular cancer 94
clonazepam 542
clotting factor VIII 261, 263–65
club drugs 540–43
"Club Drugs" (DHHS) 540n
CMV *see* cytomegalovirus
cocaethylene 537
cocaine, overview 539
cognitive behavioral therapy
  alcoholism 524
  depression 464
  marijuana use 535
colchicine 322
Colman, Eric 496, 502
colon, described 72–73
colonoscopy, colorectal cancer 75, 76
colorectal cancer
  diagnosis 76
  overview 72–79
  symptoms 75
  treatment 77–78
colposcopy 384
coming out, described 292
Community Epidemiology Work Group (CEWG) 538–39, 545
computed tomography (CAT scan; CT scan)
  cancer 55
  liver disease 188
  lung cancer 67
  testicular cancer 94
"Conditions Men Get, Too" (FDA) 273n
condoms
  described *216*, 217–19
  HIV infection prevention 204
  overview 406–14
  STD prevention 401–2

congenital adrenal hyperplasia (CAH) 431
congestive heart failure
  diagnosis 40
  overview 36–45
  treatment 40–44
continuous positive airway pressure (CPAP) 270
contraception *see* family planning
Cook, Denise 569, 572
Cooke, David A. 6n, 8n, 36n, 251n, 364n, 481n, 548n, 550n, 554n, 567n
COPD *see* chronic obstructive pulmonary disease
coronary angiography *see* angiography
coronary angioplasty *see* angioplasty
coronary artery bypass graft, coronary heart disease 22
coronary heart disease (CHD)
  overview 14–22
  tobacco use 27–28
corpora cavernosa
  defined 578
  depicted *343*
  described 342, 578
corpus spongiosum
  defined 578
  depicted *343*
corticosteroids 133, 189
counseling
  cancer treatment 355–56
  depression 464–65
CPAP *see* continuous positive airway pressure
crab lice *see* pubic lice
"Crack and Cocaine" (DHHS) 536n
crack cocaine, described 536
creatine kinase 245
Crixivan (indinavir) 202
Cromie, William J. 8n, 11
cryoprecipitate 263
cryosurgery 354
cryptorchidism (undescended testicle)
  described 287
  testicular cancer 90
CT scan *see* computed tomography
curvature of spine *see* scoliosis
CVS *see* chorionic villus sampling
cyclosporine 189

# Health Reference Series
## COMPLETE CATALOG

## Adolescent Health Sourcebook

*Basic Consumer Health Information about Common Medical, Mental, and Emotional Concerns in Adolescents, Including Facts about Acne, Body Piercing, Mononucleosis, Nutrition, Eating Disorders, Stress, Depression, Behavior Problems, Peer Pressure, Violence, Gangs, Drug Use, Puberty, Sexuality, Pregnancy, Learning Disabilities, and More*

*Along with a Glossary of Terms and Other Resources for Further Help and Information*

Edited by Chad T. Kimball. 658 pages. 2002. 0-7808-0248-9. $78.

"It is written in clear, nontechnical language aimed at general readers. . . . Recommended for public libraries, community colleges, and other agencies serving health care consumers."
*— American Reference Books Annual, 2003*

"Recommended for school and public libraries. Parents and professionals dealing with teens will appreciate the easy-to-follow format and the clearly written text. This could become a 'must have' for every high school teacher." *— E-Streams, Jan '03*

"A good starting point for information related to common medical, mental, and emotional concerns of adolescents." *— School Library Journal, Nov '02*

"This book provides accurate information in an easy to access format. It addresses topics that parents and caregivers might not be aware of and provides practical, useable information." *— Doody's Health Sciences Book Review Journal, Sep-Oct '02*

"Recommended reference source."
*— Booklist, American Library Association, Sep '02*

## AIDS Sourcebook, 3rd Edition

*Basic Consumer Health Information about Acquired Immune Deficiency Syndrome (AIDS) and Human Immunodeficiency Virus (HIV) Infection, Including Facts about Transmission, Prevention, Diagnosis, Treatment, Opportunistic Infections, and Other Complications, with a Section for Women and Children, Including Details about Associated Gynecological Concerns, Pregnancy, and Pediatric Care*

*Along with Updated Statistical Information, Reports on Current Research Initiatives, a Glossary, and Directories of Internet, Hotline, and Other Resources*

Edited by Dawn D. Matthews. 664 pages. 2003. 0-7808-0631-X. $78.

*ALSO AVAILABLE: AIDS Sourcebook, 1st Edition.* Edited by Karen Bellenir and Peter D. Dresser. 831 pages. 1995. 0-7808-0031-1. $78.

*AIDS Sourcebook, 2nd Edition.* Edited by Karen Bellenir. 751 pages. 1999. 0-7808-0225-X. $78.

"Highly recommended."
*—American Reference Books Annual, 2000*

"Excellent sourcebook. This continues to be a highly recommended book. There is no other book that provides as much information as this book provides."
*— AIDS Book Review Journal, Dec-Jan 2000*

"Recommended reference source."
*—Booklist, American Library Association, Dec '99*

"A solid text for college-level health libraries."
*—The Bookwatch, Aug '99*

Cited in *Reference Sources for Small and Medium-Sized Libraries, American Library Association, 1999*

## Alcoholism Sourcebook

*Basic Consumer Health Information about the Physical and Mental Consequences of Alcohol Abuse, Including Liver Disease, Pancreatitis, Wernicke-Korsakoff Syndrome (Alcoholic Dementia), Fetal Alcohol Syndrome, Heart Disease, Kidney Disorders, Gastrointestinal Problems, and Immune System Compromise and Featuring Facts about Addiction, Detoxification, Alcohol Withdrawal, Recovery, and the Maintenance of Sobriety*

*Along with a Glossary and Directories of Resources for Further Help and Information*

Edited by Karen Bellenir. 613 pages. 2000. 0-7808-0325-6. $78.

"This title is one of the few reference works on alcoholism for general readers. For some readers this will be a welcome complement to the many self-help books on the market. Recommended for collections serving general readers and consumer health collections."
*— E-Streams, Mar '01*

"This book is an excellent choice for public and academic libraries."
*— American Reference Books Annual, 2001*

"Recommended reference source."
*—Booklist, American Library Association, Dec '00*

"Presents a wealth of information on alcohol use and abuse and its effects on the body and mind, treatment, and prevention." *— SciTech Book News, Dec '00*

"Important new health guide which packs in the latest consumer information about the problems of alcoholism." *— Reviewer's Bookwatch, Nov '00*

*SEE ALSO Drug Abuse Sourcebook, Substance Abuse Sourcebook*

# Allergies Sourcebook, 2nd Edition

*Basic Consumer Health Information about Allergic Disorders, Triggers, Reactions, and Related Symptoms, Including Anaphylaxis, Rhinitis, Sinusitis, Asthma, Dermatitis, Conjunctivitis, and Multiple Chemical Sensitivity*

*Along with Tips on Diagnosis, Prevention, and Treatment, Statistical Data, a Glossary, and a Directory of Sources for Further Help and Information*

Edited by Annemarie S. Muth. 598 pages. 2002. 0-7808-0376-0. $78.

**ALSO AVAILABLE:** *Allergies Sourcebook, 1st Edition.* Edited by Allan R. Cook. 611 pages. 1997. 0-7808-0036-2. $78.

"This book brings a great deal of useful material together. . . . This is an excellent addition to public and consumer health library collections."
— *American Reference Books Annual, 2003*

"This second edition would be useful to laypersons with little or advanced knowledge of the subject matter. This book would also serve as a resource for nursing and other health care professions students. It would be useful in public, academic, and hospital libraries with consumer health collections." — *E-Streams, Jul '02*

∎

# Alternative Medicine Sourcebook, 2nd Edition

*Basic Consumer Health Information about Alternative and Complementary Medical Practices, Including Acupuncture, Chiropractic, Herbal Medicine, Homeopathy, Naturopathic Medicine, Mind-Body Interventions, Ayurveda, and Other Non-Western Medical Traditions*

*Along with Facts about such Specific Therapies as Massage Therapy, Aromatherapy, Qigong, Hypnosis, Prayer, Dance, and Art Therapies, a Glossary, and Resources for Further Information*

Edited by Dawn D. Matthews. 618 pages. 2002. 0-7808-0605-0. $78.

**ALSO AVAILABLE:** *Alternative Medicine Sourcebook, 1st Edition.* Edited by Allan R. Cook. 737 pages. 1999. 0-7808-0200-4. $78.

"Recommended for public, high school, and academic libraries that have consumer health collections. Hospital libraries that also serve the public will find this to be a useful resource." — *E-Streams, Feb '03*

"Recommended reference source."
— *Booklist, American Library Association, Jan '03*

"An important alternate health reference."
— *MBR Bookwatch, Oct '02*

"A great addition to the reference collection of every type of library." — *American Reference Books Annual, 2000*

# Alzheimer's Disease Sourcebook, 3rd Edition

*Basic Consumer Health Information about Alzheimer's Disease, Other Dementias, and Related Disorders, Including Multi-Infarct Dementia, AIDS Dementia Complex, Dementia with Lewy Bodies, Huntington's Disease, Wernicke-Korsakoff Syndrome (Alcohol-Reated Dementia), Delirium, and Confusional States*

*Along with Information for People Newly Diagnosed with Alzheimer's Disease and Caregivers, Reports Detailing Current Research Efforts in Prevention, Diagnosis, and Treatment, Facts about Long-Term Care Issues, and Listings of Sources for Additional Information*

Edited by Karen Bellenir. 645 pages. 2003. 0-7808-0666-2. $78.

**ALSO AVAILABLE:** *Alzheimer's, Stroke & 29 Other Neurological Disorders Sourcebook, 1st Edition.* Edited by Frank E. Bair. 579 pages. 1993. 1-55888-748-2. $78.

**ALSO AVAILABLE:** *Alzheimer's Disease Sourcebook, 2nd Edition.* Edited by Karen Bellenir. 524 pages. 1999. 0-7808-0223-3. $78.

"Provides a wealth of useful information not otherwise available in one place. This resource is recommended for all types of libraries."
— *American Reference Books Annual, 2000*

"Recommended reference source."
— *Booklist, American Library Association, Oct '99*

**SEE ALSO** Brain Disorders Sourcebook

∎

# Arthritis Sourcebook

*Basic Consumer Health Information about Specific Forms of Arthritis and Related Disorders, Including Rheumatoid Arthritis, Osteoarthritis, Gout, Polymyalgia Rheumatica, Psoriatic Arthritis, Spondyloarthropathies, Juvenile Rheumatoid Arthritis, and Juvenile Ankylosing Spondylitis*

*Along with Information about Medical, Surgical, and Alternative Treatment Options, and Including Strategies for Coping with Pain, Fatigue, and Stress*

Edited by Allan R. Cook. 550 pages. 1998. 0-7808-0201-2. $78.

". . . accessible to the layperson."
— *Reference and Research Book News, Feb '99*

∎

# Asthma Sourcebook

*Basic Consumer Health Information about Asthma, Including Symptoms, Traditional and Nontraditional Remedies, Treatment Advances, Quality-of-Life Aids, Medical Research Updates, and the Role of Allergies, Exercise, Age, the Environment, and Genetics in the Development of Asthma*

*Along with Statistical Data, a Glossary, and Directories of Support Groups, and Other Resources for Further Information*

Edited by Annemarie S. Muth. 628 pages. 2000. 0-7808-0381-7. $78.

"A worthwhile reference acquisition for public libraries and academic medical libraries whose readers desire a quick introduction to the wide range of asthma information." — *Choice, Association of College & Research Libraries, Jun '01*

"Recommended reference source."
— *Booklist, American Library Association, Feb '01*

"Highly recommended." — *The Bookwatch, Jan '01*

"There is much good information for patients and their families who deal with asthma daily."
— *American Medical Writers Association Journal, Winter '01*

"This informative text is recommended for consumer health collections in public, secondary school, and community college libraries and the libraries of universities with a large undergraduate population."
— *American Reference Books Annual, 2001*

## Attention Deficit Disorder Sourcebook

*Basic Consumer Health Information about Attention Deficit/Hyperactivity Disorder in Children and Adults, Including Facts about Causes, Symptoms, Diagnostic Criteria, and Treatment Options Such as Medications, Behavior Therapy, Coaching, and Homeopathy*

*Along with Reports on Current Research Initiatives, Legal Issues, and Government Regulations, and Featuring a Glossary of Related Terms, Internet Resources, and a List of Additional Reading Material*

Edited by Dawn D. Matthews. 470 pages. 2002. 0-7808-0624-7. $78.

"Recommended reference source."
— *Booklist, American Library Association, Jan '03*

"This book is recommended for all school libraries and the reference or consumer health sections of public libraries." — *American Reference Books Annual, 2003*

## Back & Neck Disorders Sourcebook

*Basic Information about Disorders and Injuries of the Spinal Cord and Vertebrae, Including Facts on Chiropractic Treatment, Surgical Interventions, Paralysis, and Rehabilitation*

*Along with Advice for Preventing Back Trouble*

Edited by Karen Bellenir. 548 pages. 1997. 0-7808-0202-0. $78.

"The strength of this work is its basic, easy-to-read format. Recommended."
— *Reference and User Services Quarterly, American Library Association, Winter '97*

## Blood & Circulatory Disorders Sourcebook

*Basic Information about Blood and Its Components, Anemias, Leukemias, Bleeding Disorders, and Circulatory Disorders, Including Aplastic Anemia, Thalassemia, Sickle-Cell Disease, Hemochromatosis, Hemophilia, Von Willebrand Disease, and Vascular Diseases*

*Along with a Special Section on Blood Transfusions and Blood Supply Safety, a Glossary, and Source Listings for Further Help and Information*

Edited by Karen Bellenir and Linda M. Shin. 554 pages. 1998. 0-7808-0203-9. $78.

"Recommended reference source."
— *Booklist, American Library Association, Feb '99*

"An important reference sourcebook written in simple language for everyday, non-technical users. "
— *Reviewer's Bookwatch, Jan '99*

## Brain Disorders Sourcebook

*Basic Consumer Health Information about Strokes, Epilepsy, Amyotrophic Lateral Sclerosis (ALS/Lou Gehrig's Disease), Parkinson's Disease, Brain Tumors, Cerebral Palsy, Headache, Tourette Syndrome, and More*

*Along with Statistical Data, Treatment and Rehabilitation Options, Coping Strategies, Reports on Current Research Initiatives, a Glossary, and Resource Listings for Additional Help and Information*

Edited by Karen Bellenir. 481 pages. 1999. 0-7808-0229-2. $78.

"Belongs on the shelves of any library with a consumer health collection." — *E-Streams, Mar '00*

"Recommended reference source."
— *Booklist, American Library Association, Oct '99*

*SEE ALSO Alzheimer's Disease Sourcebook*

## Breast Cancer Sourcebook

*Basic Consumer Health Information about Breast Cancer, Including Diagnostic Methods, Treatment Options, Alternative Therapies, Self-Help Information, Related Health Concerns, Statistical and Demographic Data, and Facts for Men with Breast Cancer*

*Along with Reports on Current Research Initiatives, a Glossary of Related Medical Terms, and a Directory of Sources for Further Help and Information*

Edited by Edward J. Prucha and Karen Bellenir. 580 pages. 2001. 0-7808-0244-6. $78.

"It would be a useful reference book in a library or on loan to women in a support group."
— *Cancer Forum, Mar '03*

"Recommended reference source."
— *Booklist, American Library Association, Jan '02*

"This reference source is highly recommended. It is quite informative, comprehensive and detailed in nature, and yet it offers practical advice in easy-to-read language. It could be thought of as the 'bible' of breast cancer for the consumer."                *— E-Streams, Jan '02*

"The broad range of topics covered in lay language make the *Breast Cancer Sourcebook* an excellent addition to public and consumer health library collections."
*— American Reference Books Annual 2002*

"From the pros and cons of different screening methods and results to treatment options, *Breast Cancer Sourcebook* provides the latest information on the subject."
*— Library Bookwatch, Dec '01*

"This thoroughgoing, very readable reference covers all aspects of breast health and cancer.... Readers will find much to consider here. Recommended for all public and patient health collections."
*— Library Journal, Sep '01*

**SEE ALSO** *Cancer Sourcebook for Women, Women's Health Concerns Sourcebook*

■

# Breastfeeding Sourcebook

*Basic Consumer Health Information about the Benefits of Breastmilk, Preparing to Breastfeed, Breastfeeding as a Baby Grows, Nutrition, and More, Including Information on Special Situations and Concerns Such as Mastitis, Illness, Medications, Allergies, Multiple Births, Prematurity, Special Needs, and Adoption*

*Along with a Glossary and Resources for Additional Help and Information*

Edited by Jenni Lynn Colson. 388 pages. 2002. 0-7808-0332-9. $78.

**SEE ALSO** *Pregnancy & Birth Sourcebook*

"Particularly useful is the information about professional lactation services and chapters on breastfeeding when returning to work.... *Breastfeeding Sourcebook* will be useful for public libraries, consumer health libraries, and technical schools offering nurse assistant training, especially in areas where Internet access is problematic."
*— American Reference Books Annual, 2003*

■

# Burns Sourcebook

*Basic Consumer Health Information about Various Types of Burns and Scalds, Including Flame, Heat, Cold, Electrical, Chemical, and Sun Burns*

*Along with Information on Short-Term and Long-Term Treatments, Tissue Reconstruction, Plastic Surgery, Prevention Suggestions, and First Aid*

Edited by Allan R. Cook. 604 pages. 1999. 0-7808-0204-7. $78.

"This is an exceptional addition to the series and is highly recommended for all consumer health collections, hospital libraries, and academic medical centers."
*— E-Streams, Mar '00*

"This key reference guide is an invaluable addition to all health care and public libraries in confronting this ongoing health issue."
*— American Reference Books Annual, 2000*

"Recommended reference source."
*— Booklist, American Library Association, Dec '99*

**SEE ALSO** *Skin Disorders Sourcebook*

■

# Cancer Sourcebook, 4th Edition

*Basic Consumer Health Information about Major Forms and Stages of Cancer, Featuring Facts about Head and Neck Cancers, Lung Cancers, Gastrointestinal Cancers, Genitourinary Cancers, Lymphomas, Blood Cell Cancers, Endocrine Cancers, Skin Cancers, Bone Cancers, Sarcomas, and Others, and Including Information about Cancer Treatments and Therapies, Identifying and Reducing Cancer Risks, and Strategies for Coping with Cancer and the Side Effects of Treatment*

*Along with a Cancer Glossary, Statistical and Demographic Data, and a Directory of Sources for Additional Help and Information*

Edited by Karen Bellenir. 1,119 pages. 2003. 0-7808-0633-6. $78.

**ALSO AVAILABLE:** *Cancer Sourcebook, 1st Edition.* Edited by Frank E. Bair. 932 pages. 1990. 1-55888-888-8. $78.

*New Cancer Sourcebook, 2nd Edition.* Edited by Allan R. Cook. 1,313 pages. 1996. 0-7808-0041-9. $78.

*Cancer Sourcebook, 3rd Edition.* Edited by Edward J. Prucha. 1,069 pages. 2000. 0-7808-0227-6. $78.

"This title is recommended for health sciences and public libraries with consumer health collections."
*— E-Streams, Feb '01*

"... can be effectively used by cancer patients and their families who are looking for answers in a language they can understand. Public and hospital libraries should have it on their shelves."
*— American Reference Books Annual, 2001*

"Recommended reference source."
*— Booklist, American Library Association, Dec '00*

Cited in *Reference Sources for Small and Medium-Sized Libraries, American Library Association, 1999*

"The amount of factual and useful information is extensive. The writing is very clear, geared to general readers. Recommended for all levels."          *— Choice, Association of College & Research Libraries, Jan '97*

**SEE ALSO** *Breast Cancer Sourcebook, Cancer Sourcebook for Women, Pediatric Cancer Sourcebook, Prostate Cancer Sourcebook*

# Cancer Sourcebook for Women, 2nd Edition

Basic Consumer Health Information about Gynecologic Cancers and Related Concerns, Including Cervical Cancer, Endometrial Cancer, Gestational Trophoblastic Tumor, Ovarian Cancer, Uterine Cancer, Vaginal Cancer, Vulvar Cancer, Breast Cancer, and Common Non-Cancerous Uterine Conditions, with Facts about Cancer Risk Factors, Screening and Prevention, Treatment Options, and Reports on Current Research Initiatives

Along with a Glossary of Cancer Terms and a Directory of Resources for Additional Help and Information

Edited by Karen Bellenir. 604 pages. 2002. 0-7808-0226-8. $78.

***ALSO AVAILABLE:*** *Cancer Sourcebook for Women, 1st Edition.* Edited by Allan R. Cook and Peter D. Dresser. 524 pages. 1996. 0-7808-0076-1. $78.

"An excellent addition to collections in public, consumer health, and women's health libraries."
— *American Reference Books Annual, 2003*

"Overall, the information is excellent, and complex topics are clearly explained. As a reference book for the consumer it is a valuable resource to assist them to make informed decisions about cancer and its treatments."
— *Cancer Forum, Nov '02*

"Highly recommended for academic and medical reference collections." — *Library Bookwatch, Sep '02*

"This is a highly recommended book for any public or consumer library, being reader friendly and containing accurate and helpful information."
— *E-Streams, Aug '02*

"Recommended reference source."
— *Booklist, American Library Association, Jul '02*

***SEE ALSO*** *Breast Cancer Sourcebook, Women's Health Concerns Sourcebook*

---

# Cardiovascular Diseases & Disorders Sourcebook, 1st Edition

***SEE*** *Heart Diseases & Disorders Sourcebook, 2nd Edition*

---

# Caregiving Sourcebook

Basic Consumer Health Information for Caregivers, Including a Profile of Caregivers, Caregiving Responsibilities and Concerns, Tips for Specific Conditions, Care Environments, and the Effects of Caregiving

Along with Facts about Legal Issues, Financial Information, and Future Planning, a Glossary, and a Listing of Additional Resources

Edited by Joyce Brennfleck Shannon. 600 pages. 2001. 0-7808-0331-0. $78.

"Essential for most collections."
— *Library Journal, Apr 1, 2002*

"An ideal addition to the reference collection of any public library. Health sciences information professionals may also want to acquire the *Caregiving Sourcebook* for their hospital or academic library for use as a ready reference tool by health care workers interested in aging and caregiving." — *E-Streams, Jan '02*

"Recommended reference source."
— *Booklist, American Library Association, Oct '01*

---

# Childhood Diseases & Disorders Sourcebook

Basic Consumer Health Information about Medical Problems Often Encountered in Pre-Adolescent Children, Including Respiratory Tract Ailments, Ear Infections, Sore Throats, Disorders of the Skin and Scalp, Digestive and Genitourinary Diseases, Infectious Diseases, Inflammatory Disorders, Chronic Physical and Developmental Disorders, Allergies, and More

Along with Information about Diagnostic Tests, Common Childhood Surgeries, and Frequently Used Medications, with a Glossary of Important Terms and Resource Directory

Edited by Chad T. Kimball. 662 pages. 2003. 0-7808-0458-9. $78.

---

# Colds, Flu & Other Common Ailments Sourcebook

Basic Consumer Health Information about Common Ailments and Injuries, Including Colds, Coughs, the Flu, Sinus Problems, Headaches, Fever, Nausea and Vomiting, Menstrual Cramps, Diarrhea, Constipation, Hemorrhoids, Back Pain, Dandruff, Dry and Itchy Skin, Cuts, Scrapes, Sprains, Bruises, and More

Along with Information about Prevention, Self-Care, Choosing a Doctor, Over-the-Counter Medications, Folk Remedies, and Alternative Therapies, and Including a Glossary of Important Terms and a Directory of Resources for Further Help and Information

Edited by Chad T. Kimball. 638 pages. 2001. 0-7808-0435-X. $78.

"A good starting point for research on common illnesses. It will be a useful addition to public and consumer health library collections."
— *American Reference Books Annual 2002*

"Will prove valuable to any library seeking to maintain a current, comprehensive reference collection of health resources. . . . Excellent reference."
— *The Bookwatch, Aug '01*

"Recommended reference source."
— *Booklist, American Library Association, July '01*

# Communication Disorders Sourcebook

*Basic Information about Deafness and Hearing Loss, Speech and Language Disorders, Voice Disorders, Balance and Vestibular Disorders, and Disorders of Smell, Taste, and Touch*

Edited by Linda M. Ross. 533 pages. 1996. 0-7808-0077-X. $78.

"This is skillfully edited and is a welcome resource for the layperson. It should be found in every public and medical library." — *Booklist Health Sciences Supplement, American Library Association, Oct '97*

■

# Congenital Disorders Sourcebook

*Basic Information about Disorders Acquired during Gestation, Including Spina Bifida, Hydrocephalus, Cerebral Palsy, Heart Defects, Craniofacial Abnormalities, Fetal Alcohol Syndrome, and More*

*Along with Current Treatment Options and Statistical Data*

Edited by Karen Bellenir. 607 pages. 1997. 0-7808-0205-5. $78.

"Recommended reference source." — *Booklist, American Library Association, Oct '97*

*SEE ALSO Pregnancy & Birth Sourcebook*

■

# Consumer Issues in Health Care Sourcebook

*Basic Information about Health Care Fundamentals and Related Consumer Issues, Including Exams and Screening Tests, Physician Specialties, Choosing a Doctor, Using Prescription and Over-the-Counter Medications Safely, Avoiding Health Scams, Managing Common Health Risks in the Home, Care Options for Chronically or Terminally Ill Patients, and a List of Resources for Obtaining Help and Further Information*

Edited by Karen Bellenir. 618 pages. 1998. 0-7808-0221-7. $78.

"Both public and academic libraries will want to have a copy in their collection for readers who are interested in self-education on health issues." — *American Reference Books Annual, 2000*

"The editor has researched the literature from government agencies and others, saving readers the time and effort of having to do the research themselves. Recommended for public libraries." — *Reference and User Services Quarterly, American Library Association, Spring '99*

"Recommended reference source." — *Booklist, American Library Association, Dec '98*

# Contagious & Non-Contagious Infectious Diseases Sourcebook

*Basic Information about Contagious Diseases like Measles, Polio, Hepatitis B, and Infectious Mononucleosis, and Non-Contagious Infectious Diseases like Tetanus and Toxic Shock Syndrome, and Diseases Occurring as Secondary Infections Such as Shingles and Reye Syndrome*

*Along with Vaccination, Prevention, and Treatment Information, and a Section Describing Emerging Infectious Disease Threats*

Edited by Karen Bellenir and Peter D. Dresser. 566 pages. 1996. 0-7808-0075-3. $78.

■

# Death & Dying Sourcebook

*Basic Consumer Health Information for the Layperson about End-of-Life Care and Related Ethical and Legal Issues, Including Chief Causes of Death, Autopsies, Pain Management for the Terminally Ill, Life Support Systems, Insurance, Euthanasia, Assisted Suicide, Hospice Programs, Living Wills, Funeral Planning, Counseling, Mourning, Organ Donation, and Physician Training*

*Along with Statistical Data, a Glossary, and Listings of Sources for Further Help and Information*

Edited by Annemarie S. Muth. 641 pages. 1999. 0-7808-0230-6. $78.

"Public libraries, medical libraries, and academic libraries will all find this sourcebook a useful addition to their collections." — *American Reference Books Annual, 2001*

"An extremely useful resource for those concerned with death and dying in the United States." — *Respiratory Care, Nov '00*

"Recommended reference source." — *Booklist, American Library Association, Aug '00*

"This book is a definite must for all those involved in end-of-life care." — *Doody's Review Service, 2000*

■

# Dental Care & Oral Health Sourcebook, 2nd Edition

*Basic Consumer Health Information about Dental Care, Including Oral Hygiene, Dental Visits, Pain Management, Cavities, Crowns, Bridges, Dental Implants, and Fillings, and Other Oral Health Concerns, Such as Gum Disease, Bad Breath, Dry Mouth, Genetic and Developmental Abnormalities, Oral Cancers, Orthodontics, and Temporomandibular Disorders*

*Along with Updates on Current Research in Oral Health, a Glossary, a Directory of Dental and Oral Health Organizations, and Resources for People with Dental and Oral Health Disorders*

Edited by Amy L. Sutton. 609 pages. 2003. 0-7808-0634-4. $78.

# Depression Sourcebook

Basic Consumer Health Information about Unipolar Depression, Bipolar Disorder, Postpartum Depression, Seasonal Affective Disorder, and Other Types of Depression in Children, Adolescents, Women, Men, the Elderly, and Other Selected Populations

Along with Facts about Causes, Risk Factors, Diagnostic Criteria, Treatment Options, Coping Strategies, Suicide Prevention, a Glossary, and a Directory of Sources for Additional Help and Information

Edited by Karen Belleni. 602 pages. 2002. 0-7808-0611-5. $78.

# Diabetes Sourcebook, 3rd Edition

Basic Consumer Health Information about Type 1 Diabetes (Insulin-Dependent or Juvenile-Onset Diabetes), Type 2 Diabetes (Noninsulin-Dependent or Adult-Onset Diabetes), Gestational Diabetes, Impaired Glucose Tolerance (IGT), and Related Complications, Such as Amputation, Eye Disease, Gum Disease, Nerve Damage, and End-Stage Renal Disease, Including Facts about Insulin, Oral Diabetes Medications, Blood Sugar Testing, and the Role of Exercise and Nutrition in the Control of Diabetes

Along with a Glossary and Resources for Further Help and Information

Edited by Dawn D. Matthews. 622 pages. 2003. 0-7808-0629-8. $78.

ALSO AVAILABLE: Diabetes Sourcebook, 1st Edition. Edited by Karen Bellenir and Peter D. Dresser. 827 pages. 1994. 1-55888-751-2. $78.

Diabetes Sourcebook, 2nd Edition. Edited by Karen Bellenir. 688 pages. 1998. 0-7808-0224-1. $78.

# Diet & Nutrition Sourcebook, 2nd Edition

Basic Consumer Health Information about Dietary Guidelines, Recommended Daily Intake Values, Vitamins, Minerals, Fiber, Fat, Weight Control, Dietary Supplements, and Food Additives

Along with Special Sections on Nutrition Needs throughout Life and Nutrition for People with Such Specific Medical Concerns as Allergies, High Blood Cholesterol, Hypertension, Diabetes, Celiac Disease, Seizure Disorders, Phenylketonuria (PKU), Cancer, and Eating Disorders, and Including Reports on Current Nutrition Research and Source Listings for Additional Help and Information

Edited by Karen Bellenir. 650 pages. 1999. 0-7808-0228-4. $78.

ALSO AVAILABLE: Diet & Nutrition Sourcebook, 1st Edition. Edited by Dan R. Harris. 662 pages. 1996. 0-7808-0084-2. $78.

SEE ALSO Digestive Diseases & Disorders Sourcebook, Eating Disorders Sourcebook, Gastrointestinal Diseases & Disorders Sourcebook, Vegetarian Sourcebook

# Digestive Diseases & Disorders Sourcebook

Basic Consumer Health Information about Diseases and Disorders that Impact the Upper and Lower Digestive System, Including Celiac Disease, Constipation,

Crohn's Disease, Cyclic Vomiting Syndrome, Diarrhea, Diverticulosis and Diverticulitis, Gallstones, Heartburn, Hemorrhoids, Hernias, Indigestion (Dyspepsia), Irritable Bowel Syndrome, Lactose Intolerance, Ulcers, and More

Along with Information about Medications and Other Treatments, Tips for Maintaining a Healthy Digestive Tract, a Glossary, and Directory of Digestive Diseases Organizations

Edited by Karen Bellenir. 335 pages. 2000. 0-7808-0327-2. $78.

"This title would be an excellent addition to all public or patient-research libraries."
—American Reference Books Annual, 2001

"This title is recommended for public, hospital, and health sciences libraries with consumer health collections." —E-Streams, Jul-Aug '00

"Recommended reference source."
—Booklist, American Library Association, May '00

SEE ALSO Diet & Nutrition Sourcebook, Eating Disorders Sourcebook, Gastrointestinal Diseases & Disorders Sourcebook

■

# Disabilities Sourcebook

Basic Consumer Health Information about Physical and Psychiatric Disabilities, Including Descriptions of Major Causes of Disability, Assistive and Adaptive Aids, Workplace Issues, and Accessibility Concerns

Along with Information about the Americans with Disabilities Act, a Glossary, and Resources for Additional Help and Information

Edited by Dawn D. Matthews. 616 pages. 2000. 0-7808-0389-2. $78.

"It is a must for libraries with a consumer health section." —American Reference Books Annual 2002

"A much needed addition to the Omnigraphics Health Reference Series. A current reference work to provide people with disabilities, their families, caregivers or those who work with them, a broad range of information in one volume, has not been available until now. . . . It is recommended for all public and academic library reference collections." —E-Streams, May '01

"An excellent source book in easy-to-read format covering many current topics; highly recommended for all libraries." —Choice, Association of College and Research Libraries, Jan '01

"Recommended reference source."
—Booklist, American Library Association, Jul '00

■

# Domestic Violence & Child Abuse Sourcebook

Basic Consumer Health Information about Spousal/Partner, Child, Sibling, Parent, and Elder Abuse, Covering Physical, Emotional, and Sexual Abuse, Teen Dating Violence, and Stalking; Includes Information

about Hotlines, Safe Houses, Safety Plans, and Other Resources for Support and Assistance, Community Initiatives, and Reports on Current Directions in Research and Treatment

Along with a Glossary, Sources for Further Reading, and Governmental and Non-Governmental Organizations Contact Information

Edited by Helene Henderson. 1,064 pages. 2001. 0-7808-0235-7. $78.

"Interested lay persons should find the book extremely beneficial. . . . A copy of Domestic Violence and Child Abuse Sourcebook should be in every public library in the United States."
—Social Science & Medicine, No. 56, 2003

"This is important information. The Web has many resources but this sourcebook fills an important societal need. I am not aware of any other resources of this type." —Doody's Review Service, Sep '01

"Recommended for all libraries, scholars, and practitioners." —Choice, Association of College & Research Libraries, Jul '01

"Recommended reference source."
—Booklist, American Library Association, Apr '01

"Important pick for college-level health reference libraries." —The Bookwatch, Mar '01

"Because this problem is so widespread and because this book includes a lot of issues within one volume, this work is recommended for all public libraries."
—American Reference Books Annual, 2001

■

# Drug Abuse Sourcebook

Basic Consumer Health Information about Illicit Substances of Abuse and the Diversion of Prescription Medications, Including Depressants, Hallucinogens, Inhalants, Marijuana, Narcotics, Stimulants, and Anabolic Steroids

Along with Facts about Related Health Risks, Treatment Issues, and Substance Abuse Prevention Programs, a Glossary of Terms, Statistical Data, and Directories of Hotline Services, Self-Help Groups, and Organizations Able to Provide Further Information

Edited by Karen Bellenir. 629 pages. 2000. 0-7808-0242-X. $78.

"Containing a wealth of information . . . . This resource belongs in libraries that serve a lower-division undergraduate or community college clientele as well as the general public." —Choice, Association of College and Research Libraries, Jun '01

"Recommended reference source."
—Booklist, American Library Association, Feb '01

"Highly recommended." —The Bookwatch, Jan '01

"Even though there is a plethora of books on drug abuse, this volume is recommended for school, public, and college libraries."
—American Reference Books Annual, 2001

SEE ALSO Alcoholism Sourcebook, Substance Abuse Sourcebook

628

# Ear, Nose & Throat Disorders Sourcebook

*Basic Information about Disorders of the Ears, Nose, Sinus Cavities, Pharynx, and Larynx, Including Ear Infections, Tinnitus, Vestibular Disorders, Allergic and Non-Allergic Rhinitis, Sore Throats, Tonsillitis, and Cancers That Affect the Ears, Nose, Sinuses, and Throat*

*Along with Reports on Current Research Initiatives, a Glossary of Related Medical Terms, and a Directory of Sources for Further Help and Information*

Edited by Karen Bellenir and Linda M. Shin. 576 pages. 1998. 0-7808-0206-3. $78.

"Overall, this sourcebook is helpful for the consumer seeking information on ENT issues. It is recommended for public libraries."
— *American Reference Books Annual, 1999*

"Recommended reference source."
— *Booklist, American Library Association, Dec '98*

■

# Eating Disorders Sourcebook

*Basic Consumer Health Information about Eating Disorders, Including Information about Anorexia Nervosa, Bulimia Nervosa, Binge Eating, Body Dysmorphic Disorder, Pica, Laxative Abuse, and Night Eating Syndrome*

*Along with Information about Causes, Adverse Effects, and Treatment and Prevention Issues, and Featuring a Section on Concerns Specific to Children and Adolescents, a Glossary, and Resources for Further Help and Information*

Edited by Dawn D. Matthews. 322 pages. 2001. 0-7808-0335-3. $78.

"Recommended for health science libraries that are open to the public, as well as hospital libraries. This book is a good resource for the consumer who is concerned about eating disorders." — *E-Streams, Mar '02*

"This volume is another convenient collection of excerpted articles. Recommended for school and public library patrons; lower-division undergraduates; and two-year technical program students." — *Choice, Association of College & Research Libraries, Jan '02*

"Recommended reference source." — *Booklist, American Library Association, Oct '01*

SEE ALSO *Diet & Nutrition Sourcebook, Digestive Diseases & Disorders Sourcebook, Gastrointestinal Diseases & Disorders Sourcebook*

■

# Emergency Medical Services Sourcebook

*Basic Consumer Health Information about Preventing, Preparing for, and Managing Emergency Situations, When and Who to Call for Help, What to Expect in the Emergency Room, the Emergency Medical Team, Patient Issues, and Current Topics in Emergency Medicine*

*Along with Statistical Data, a Glossary, and Sources of Additional Help and Information*

Edited by Jenni Lynn Colson. 494 pages. 2002. 0-7808-0420-1. $78.

"Handy and convenient for home, public, school, and college libraries. Recommended."
— *Choice, Association of College and Research Libraries, Apr '03*

"This reference can provide the consumer with answers to most questions about emergency care in the United States, or it will direct them to a resource where the answer can be found."
— *American Reference Books Annual, 2003*

"Recommended reference source."
— *Booklist, American Library Association, Feb '03*

■

# Endocrine & Metabolic Disorders Sourcebook

*Basic Information for the Layperson about Pancreatic and Insulin-Related Disorders Such as Pancreatitis, Diabetes, and Hypoglycemia; Adrenal Gland Disorders Such as Cushing's Syndrome, Addison's Disease, and Congenital Adrenal Hyperplasia; Pituitary Gland Disorders Such as Growth Hormone Deficiency, Acromegaly, and Pituitary Tumors; Thyroid Disorders Such as Hypothyroidism, Graves' Disease, Hashimoto's Disease, and Goiter; Hyperparathyroidism; and Other Diseases and Syndromes of Hormone Imbalance or Metabolic Dysfunction*

*Along with Reports on Current Research Initiatives*

Edited by Linda M. Shin. 574 pages. 1998. 0-7808-0207-1. $78.

"Omnigraphics has produced another needed resource for health information consumers."
— *American Reference Books Annual, 2000*

"Recommended reference source."
— *Booklist, American Library Association, Dec '98*

■

# Environmental Health Sourcebook, 2nd Edition

*Basic Consumer Health Information about the Environment and Its Effect on Human Health, Including the Effects of Air Pollution, Water Pollution, Hazardous Chemicals, Food Hazards, Radiation Hazards, Biological Agents, Household Hazards, Such as Radon, Asbestos, Carbon Monoxide, and Mold, and Information about Associated Diseases and Disorders, Including Cancer, Allergies, Respiratory Problems, and Skin Disorders*

*Along with Information about Environmental Concerns for Specific Populations, a Glossary of Related Terms, and Resources for Further Help and Information*

Edited by Dawn D. Matthews. 673 pages. 2003. 0-7808-0632-8. $78.

ALSO AVAILABLE: *Environmentally Induced Disorders Sourcebook, 1st Edition.* Edited by Allan R. Cook. 620 pages. 1997. 0-7808-0083-4. $78.

■

# Environmentally Induced Disorders Sourcebook, 1st Edition

SEE *Environmental Health Sourcebook, 2nd Edition*

■

# Ethnic Diseases Sourcebook

*Basic Consumer Health Information for Ethnic and Racial Minority Groups in the United States, Including General Health Indicators and Behaviors, Ethnic Diseases, Genetic Testing, the Impact of Chronic Diseases, Women's Health, Mental Health Issues, and Preventive Health Care Services*

*Along with a Glossary and a Listing of Additional Resources*

Edited by Joyce Brennfleck Shannon. 664 pages. 2001. 0-7808-0336-1. $78.

■

# Eye Care Sourcebook, 2nd Edition

*Basic Consumer Health Information about Eye Care and Eye Disorders, Including Facts about the Diag-*

*nosis, Prevention, and Treatment of Common Refractive Problems Such as Myopia, Hyperopia, Astigmatism, and Presbyopia, and Eye Diseases, Including Glaucoma, Cataract, Age-Related Macular Degeneration, and Diabetic Retinopathy*

*Along with a Section on Vision Correction and Refractive Surgeries, Including LASIK and LASEK, a Glossary, and Directories of Resources for Additional Help and Information*

Edited by Amy L. Sutton. 543 pages. 2003. 0-7808-0635-2. $78.

*ALSO AVAILABLE: Ophthalmic Disorders Sourcebook, 1st Edition.* Edited by Linda M. Ross. 631 pages. 1996. 0-7808-0081-8. $78.

■

# Family Planning Sourcebook

*Basic Consumer Health Information about Planning for Pregnancy and Contraception, Including Traditional Methods, Barrier Methods, Hormonal Methods, Permanent Methods, Future Methods, Emergency Contraception, and Birth Control Choices for Women at Each Stage of Life*

*Along with Statistics, a Glossary, and Sources of Additional Information*

Edited by Amy Marcaccio Keyzer. 520 pages. 2001. 0-7808-0379-5. $78.

SEE ALSO *Pregnancy & Birth Sourcebook*

■

# Fitness & Exercise Sourcebook, 2nd Edition

*Basic Consumer Health Information about the Fundamentals of Fitness and Exercise, Including How to Begin and Maintain a Fitness Program, Fitness as a Lifestyle, the Link between Fitness and Diet, Advice for Specific Groups of People, Exercise as It Relates to Specific Medical Conditions, and Recent Research in Fitness and Exercise*

*Along with a Glossary of Important Terms and Resources for Additional Help and Information*

Edited by Kristen M. Gledhill. 646 pages. 2001. 0-7808-0334-5. $78.

# Food & Animal Borne Diseases Sourcebook

*Basic Information about Diseases That Can Be Spread to Humans through the Ingestion of Contaminated Food or Water or by Contact with Infected Animals and Insects, Such as Botulism, E. Coli, Hepatitis A, Trichinosis, Lyme Disease, and Rabies*

*Along with Information Regarding Prevention and Treatment Methods, and Including a Special Section for International Travelers Describing Diseases Such as Cholera, Malaria, Travelers' Diarrhea, and Yellow Fever, and Offering Recommendations for Avoiding Illness*

Edited by Karen Bellenir and Peter D. Dresser. 535 pages. 1995. 0-7808-0033-8. $78.

"Targeting general readers and providing them with a single, comprehensive source of information on selected topics, this book continues, with the excellent caliber of its predecessors, to catalog topical information on health matters of general interest. Readable and thorough, this valuable resource is highly recommended for all libraries."
— *Academic Library Book Review, Summer '96*

"A comprehensive collection of authoritative information." — *Emergency Medical Services, Oct '95*

# Food Safety Sourcebook

*Basic Consumer Health Information about the Safe Handling of Meat, Poultry, Seafood, Eggs, Fruit Juices, and Other Food Items, and Facts about Pesticides, Drinking Water, Food Safety Overseas, and the Onset, Duration, and Symptoms of Foodborne Illnesses,*

*Including Types of Pathogenic Bacteria, Parasitic Protozoa, Worms, Viruses, and Natural Toxins*

*Along with the Role of the Consumer, the Food Handler, and the Government in Food Safety; a Glossary, and Resources for Additional Help and Information*

Edited by Dawn D. Matthews. 339 pages. 1999. 0-7808-0326-4. $78.

"This book is recommended for public libraries and universities with home economic and food science programs." —*E-Streams, Nov '00*

"Recommended reference source."
—*Booklist, American Library Association, May '00*

"This book takes the complex issues of food safety and foodborne pathogens and presents them in an easily understood manner. [It does] an excellent job of covering a large and often confusing topic."
—*American Reference Books Annual, 2000*

# Forensic Medicine Sourcebook

*Basic Consumer Information for the Layperson about Forensic Medicine, Including Crime Scene Investigation, Evidence Collection and Analysis, Expert Testimony, Computer-Aided Criminal Identification, Digital Imaging in the Courtroom, DNA Profiling, Accident Reconstruction, Autopsies, Ballistics, Drugs and Explosives Detection, Latent Fingerprints, Product Tampering, and Questioned Document Examination*

*Along with Statistical Data, a Glossary of Forensics Terminology, and Listings of Sources for Further Help and Information*

Edited by Annemarie S. Muth. 574 pages. 1999. 0-7808-0232-2. $78.

"Given the expected widespread interest in its content and its easy to read style, this book is recommended for most public and all college and university libraries."
— *E-Streams, Feb '01*

"Recommended for public libraries."
—*Reference & User Services Quarterly, American Library Association, Spring 2000*

"Recommended reference source."
—*Booklist, American Library Association, Feb '00*

"A wealth of information, useful statistics, references are up-to-date and extremely complete. This wonderful collection of data will help students who are interested in a career in any type of forensic field. It is a great resource for attorneys who need information about types of expert witnesses needed in a particular case. It also offers useful information for fiction and nonfiction writers whose work involves a crime. A fascinating compilation. All levels." — *Choice, Association of College and Research Libraries, Jan 2000*

"There are several items that make this book attractive to consumers who are seeking certain forensic data. . . . This is a useful current source for those seeking general forensic medical answers."
—*American Reference Books Annual, 2000*

## Gastrointestinal Diseases & Disorders Sourcebook

*Basic Information about Gastroesophageal Reflux Disease (Heartburn), Ulcers, Diverticulosis, Irritable Bowel Syndrome, Crohn's Disease, Ulcerative Colitis, Diarrhea, Constipation, Lactose Intolerance, Hemorrhoids, Hepatitis, Cirrhosis, and Other Digestive Problems, Featuring Statistics, Descriptions of Symptoms, and Current Treatment Methods of Interest for Persons Living with Upper and Lower Gastrointestinal Maladies*

Edited by Linda M. Ross. 413 pages. 1996. 0-7808-0078-8. $78.

". . . very readable form. The successful editorial work that brought this material together into a useful and understandable reference makes accessible to all readers information that can help them more effectively understand and obtain help for digestive tract problems."
— *Choice, Association of College & Research Libraries, Feb '97*

**SEE ALSO** *Diet & Nutrition Sourcebook, Digestive Diseases & Disorders, Eating Disorders Sourcebook*

■

## Genetic Disorders Sourcebook, 2nd Edition

*Basic Consumer Health Information about Hereditary Diseases and Disorders, Including Cystic Fibrosis, Down Syndrome, Hemophilia, Huntington's Disease, Sickle Cell Anemia, and More; Facts about Genes, Gene Research and Therapy, Genetic Screening, Ethics of Gene Testing, Genetic Counseling, and Advice on Coping and Caring*

*Along with a Glossary of Genetic Terminology and a Resource List for Help, Support, and Further Information*

Edited by Kathy Massimini. 768 pages. 2001. 0-7808-0241-1. $78.

**ALSO AVAILABLE:** *Genetic Disorders Sourcebook, 1st Edition.* Edited by Karen Bellenir. 642 pages. 1996. 0-7808-0034-6. $78.

"Recommended for public libraries and medical and hospital libraries with consumer health collections."
— *E-Streams, May '01*

"Recommended reference source."
— *Booklist, American Library Association, Apr '01*

"Important pick for college-level health reference libraries." — *The Bookwatch, Mar '01*

"Provides essential medical information to both the general public and those diagnosed with a serious or fatal genetic disease or disorder." — *Choice, Association of College and Research Libraries, Jan '97*

## Head Trauma Sourcebook

*Basic Information for the Layperson about Open-Head and Closed-Head Injuries, Treatment Advances, Recovery, and Rehabilitation*

*Along with Reports on Current Research Initiatives*

Edited by Karen Bellenir. 414 pages. 1997. 0-7808-0208-X. $78.

■

## Headache Sourcebook

*Basic Consumer Health Information about Migraine, Tension, Cluster, Rebound and Other Types of Headaches, with Facts about the Cause and Prevention of Headaches, the Effects of Stress and the Environment, Headaches during Pregnancy and Menopause, and Childhood Headaches*

*Along with a Glossary and Other Resources for Additional Help and Information*

Edited by Dawn D. Matthews. 362 pages. 2002. 0-7808-0337-X. $78.

"Highly recommended for academic and medical reference collections." — *Library Bookwatch, Sep '02*

■

## Health Insurance Sourcebook

*Basic Information about Managed Care Organizations, Traditional Fee-for-Service Insurance, Insurance Portability and Pre-Existing Conditions Clauses, Medicare, Medicaid, Social Security, and Military Health Care*

*Along with Information about Insurance Fraud*

Edited by Wendy Wilcox. 530 pages. 1997. 0-7808-0222-5. $78.

"Particularly useful because it brings much of this information together in one volume. This book will be a handy reference source in the health sciences library, hospital library, college and university library, and medium to large public library."
— *Medical Reference Services Quarterly, Fall '98*

Awarded "Books of the Year Award"
— *American Journal of Nursing, 1997*

"The layout of the book is particularly helpful as it provides easy access to reference material. A most useful addition to the vast amount of information about health insurance. The use of data from U.S. government agencies is most commendable. Useful in a library or learning center for healthcare professional students."
— *Doody's Health Sciences Book Reviews, Nov '97*

■

## Health Reference Series Cumulative Index 1999

*A Comprehensive Index to the Individual Volumes of the Health Reference Series, Including a Subject Index, Name Index, Organization Index, and Publication Index*

*Along with a Master List of Acronyms and Abbreviations*

Edited by Edward J. Prucha, Anne Holmes, and Robert Rudnick. 990 pages. 2000. 0-7808-0382-5. $78.

"This volume will be most helpful in libraries that have a relatively complete collection of the Health Reference Series." —American Reference Books Annual, 2001

"Essential for collections that hold any of the numerous *Health Reference Series* titles." — Choice, Association of College and Research Libraries, Nov '00

∎

# Healthy Aging Sourcebook

*Basic Consumer Health Information about Maintaining Health through the Aging Process, Including Advice on Nutrition, Exercise, and Sleep, Help in Making Decisions about Midlife Issues and Retirement, and Guidance Concerning Practical and Informed Choices in Health Consumerism*

*Along with Data Concerning the Theories of Aging, Different Experiences in Aging by Minority Groups, and Facts about Aging Now and Aging in the Future; and Featuring a Glossary, a Guide to Consumer Help, Additional Suggested Reading, and Practical Resource Directory*

Edited by Jenifer Swanson. 536 pages. 1999. 0-7808-0390-6. $78.

"Recommended reference source." —Booklist, American Library Association, Feb '00

SEE ALSO *Physical & Mental Issues in Aging Sourcebook*

∎

# Healthy Children Sourcebook

*Basic Consumer Health Information about the Physical and Mental Development of Children between the Ages of 3 and 12, Including Routine Health Care, Preventative Health Services, Safety and First Aid, Healthy Sleep, Dental Care, Nutrition, and Fitness, and Featuring Parenting Tips on Such Topics as Bedwetting, Choosing Day Care, Monitoring TV and Other Media, and Establishing a Foundation for Substance Abuse Prevention*

*Along with a Glossary of Commonly Used Pediatric Terms and Resources for Additional Help and Information.*

Edited by Chad T. Kimball. 647 pages. 2003. 0-7808-0247-0. $78.

∎

# Healthy Heart Sourcebook for Women

*Basic Consumer Health Information about Cardiac Issues Specific to Women, Including Facts about Major Risk Factors and Prevention, Treatment and Control Strategies, and Important Dietary Issues*

*Along with a Special Section Regarding the Pros and Cons of Hormone Replacement Therapy and Its Impact on Heart Health, and Additional Help, Including Recipes, a Glossary, and a Directory of Resources*

Edited by Dawn D. Matthews. 336 pages. 2000. 0-7808-0329-9. $78.

"A good reference source and recommended for all public, academic, medical, and hospital libraries." — Medical Reference Services Quarterly, Summer '01

"Because of the lack of information specific to women on this topic, this book is recommended for public libraries and consumer libraries." —American Reference Books Annual, 2001

"Contains very important information about coronary artery disease that all women should know. The information is current and presented in an easy-to-read format. The book will make a good addition to any library." — American Medical Writers Association Journal, Summer '00

"Important, basic reference." — Reviewer's Bookwatch, Jul '00

SEE ALSO *Heart Diseases & Disorders Sourcebook, Women's Health Concerns Sourcebook*

∎

# Heart Diseases & Disorders Sourcebook, 2nd Edition

*Basic Consumer Health Information about Heart Attacks, Angina, Rhythm Disorders, Heart Failure, Valve Disease, Congenital Heart Disorders, and More, Including Descriptions of Surgical Procedures and Other Interventions, Medications, Cardiac Rehabilitation, Risk Identification, and Prevention Tips*

*Along with Statistical Data, Reports on Current Research Initiatives, a Glossary of Cardiovascular Terms, and Resource Directory*

Edited by Karen Bellenir. 612 pages. 2000. 0-7808-0238-1. $78.

ALSO AVAILABLE: *Cardiovascular Diseases & Disorders Sourcebook, 1st Edition.* Edited by Karen Bellenir and Peter D. Dresser. 683 pages. 1995. 0-7808-0032-X. $78.

"This work stands out as an imminently accessible resource for the general public. It is recommended for the reference and circulating shelves of school, public, and academic libraries." —American Reference Books Annual, 2001

"Recommended reference source." —Booklist, American Library Association, Dec '00

"Provides comprehensive coverage of matters related to the heart. This title is recommended for health sciences and public libraries with consumer health collections." —E-Streams, Oct '00

SEE ALSO *Healthy Heart Sourcebook for Women*

∎

# Household Safety Sourcebook

*Basic Consumer Health Information about Household Safety, Including Information about Poisons, Chemicals, Fire, and Water Hazards in the Home*

*Along with Advice about the Safe Use of Home Maintenance Equipment, Choosing Toys and Nursery Furni-*

ture, Holiday and Recreation Safety, a Glossary, and Resources for Further Help and Information

Edited by Dawn D. Matthews. 606 pages. 2002. 0-7808-0338-8. $78.

"This work will be useful in public libraries with large consumer health and wellness departments."
— American Reference Books Annual, 2003

"As a sourcebook on household safety this book meets its mark. It is encyclopedic in scope and covers a wide range of safety issues that are commonly seen in the home." — E-Streams, Jul '02

■

# Immune System Disorders Sourcebook

Basic Information about Lupus, Multiple Sclerosis, Guillain-Barré Syndrome, Chronic Granulomatous Disease, and More

Along with Statistical and Demographic Data and Reports on Current Research Initiatives

Edited by Allan R. Cook. 608 pages. 1997. 0-7808-0209-8. $78.

■

# Infant & Toddler Health Sourcebook

Basic Consumer Health Information about the Physical and Mental Development of Newborns, Infants, and Toddlers, Including Neonatal Concerns, Nutrition Recommendations, Immunization Schedules, Common Pediatric Disorders, Assessments and Milestones, Safety Tips, and Advice for Parents and Other Caregivers

Along with a Glossary of Terms and Resource Listings for Additional Help

Edited by Jenifer Swanson. 585 pages. 2000. 0-7808-0246-2. $78.

"As a reference for the general public, this would be useful in any library." — E-Streams, May '01

"Recommended reference source."
— Booklist, American Library Association, Feb '01

"This is a good source for general use."
— American Reference Books Annual, 2001

■

# Injury & Trauma Sourcebook

Basic Consumer Health Information about the Impact of Injury, the Diagnosis and Treatment of Common and Traumatic Injuries, Emergency Care, and Specific Injuries Related to Home, Community, Workplace, Transportation, and Recreation

Along with Guidelines for Injury Prevention, a Glossary, and a Directory of Additional Resources

Edited by Joyce Brennfleck Shannon. 696 pages. 2002. 0-7808-0421-X. $78.

"This publication is the most comprehensive work of its kind about injury and trauma."
— American Reference Books Annual, 2003

"This sourcebook provides concise, easily readable, basic health information about injuries. . . . This book is well organized and an easy to use reference resource suitable for hospital, health sciences and public libraries with consumer health collections."
— E-Streams, Nov '02

"Practitioners should be aware of guides such as this in order to facilitate their use by patients and their families." — Doody's Health Sciences Book Review Journal, Sep-Oct '02

"Recommended reference source."
— Booklist, American Library Association, Sep '02

"Highly recommended for academic and medical reference collections." — Library Bookwatch, Sep '02

■

# Kidney & Urinary Tract Diseases & Disorders Sourcebook

Basic Information about Kidney Stones, Urinary Incontinence, Bladder Disease, End Stage Renal Disease, Dialysis, and More

Along with Statistical and Demographic Data and Reports on Current Research Initiatives

Edited by Linda M. Ross. 602 pages. 1997. 0-7808-0079-6. $78.

■

# Learning Disabilities Sourcebook, 2nd Edition

Basic Consumer Health Information about Learning Disabilities, Including Dyslexia, Developmental Speech and Language Disabilities, Non-Verbal Learning Disorders, Developmental Arithmetic Disorder, Developmental Writing Disorder, and Other Conditions That Impede Learning Such as Attention Deficit/ Hyperactivity Disorder, Brain Injury, Hearing Impairment, Klinefelter Syndrome, Dyspraxia, and Tourette Syndrome

Along with Facts about Educational Issues and Assistive Technology, Coping Strategies, a Glossary of Related Terms, and Resources for Further Help and Information

Edited by Dawn D. Matthews. 621 pages. 2003. 0-7808-0626-3. $78.

ALSO AVAILABLE: Learning Disabilities Sourcebook, 1st Edition. Edited by Linda M. Shin. 579 pages. 1998. 0-7808-0210-1. $78.

"Teachers as well as consumers will find this an essential guide to understanding various syndromes and their latest treatments. [An] invaluable reference for public and school library collections alike."
— Library Bookwatch, Apr '03

Named "Outstanding Reference Book of 1999."
— New York Public Library, Feb 2000

"An excellent candidate for inclusion in a public library reference section. It's a great source of information. Teachers will also find the book useful. Definitely worth reading."
— Journal of Adolescent & Adult Literacy, Feb 2000

"Readable . . . provides a solid base of information regarding successful techniques used with individuals who have learning disabilities, as well as practical suggestions for educators and family members. Clear language, concise descriptions, and pertinent information for contacting multiple resources add to the strength of this book as a useful tool." — *Choice, Association of College and Research Libraries, Feb '99*

"Recommended reference source."
— *Booklist, American Library Association, Sep '98*

"A useful resource for libraries and for those who don't have the time to identify and locate the individual publications." — *Disability Resources Monthly, Sep '98*

▪

## Leukemia Sourcebook

*Basic Consumer Health Information about Adult and Childhood Leukemias, Including Acute Lymphocytic Leukemia (ALL), Chronic Lymphocytic Leukemia (CLL), Acute Myelogenous Leukemia (AML), Chronic Myelogenous Leukemia (CML), and Hairy Cell Leukemia, and Treatments Such as Chemotherapy, Radiation Therapy, Peripheral Blood Stem Cell and Marrow Transplantation, and Immunotherapy*

*Along with Tips for Life During and After Treatment, a Glossary, and Directories of Additional Resources*

Edited by Joyce Brennfleck Shannon. 587 pages. 2003. 0-7808-0627-1. $78.

▪

## Liver Disorders Sourcebook

*Basic Consumer Health Information about the Liver and How It Works; Liver Diseases, Including Cancer, Cirrhosis, Hepatitis, and Toxic and Drug Related Diseases; Tips for Maintaining a Healthy Liver; Laboratory Tests, Radiology Tests, and Facts about Liver Transplantation*

*Along with a Section on Support Groups, a Glossary, and Resource Listings*

Edited by Joyce Brennfleck Shannon. 591 pages. 2000. 0-7808-0383-3. $78.

"A valuable resource."
— *American Reference Books Annual, 2001*

"This title is recommended for health sciences and public libraries with consumer health collections."
— *E-Streams, Oct '00*

"Recommended reference source."
— *Booklist, American Library Association, Jun '00*

▪

## Lung Disorders Sourcebook

*Basic Consumer Health Information about Emphysema, Pneumonia, Tuberculosis, Asthma, Cystic Fibrosis, and Other Lung Disorders, Including Facts about Diagnostic Procedures, Treatment Strategies, Disease Prevention Efforts, and Such Risk Factors as Smoking, Air Pollution, and Exposure to Asbestos, Radon, and Other Agents*

*Along with a Glossary and Resources for Additional Help and Information*

Edited by Dawn D. Matthews. 678 pages. 2002. 0-7808-0339-6. $78.

"This title is a great addition for public and school libraries because it provides concise health information on the lungs."
— *American Reference Books Annual, 2003*

"Highly recommended for academic and medical reference collections." — *Library Bookwatch, Sep '02*

▪

## Medical Tests Sourcebook

*Basic Consumer Health Information about Medical Tests, Including Periodic Health Exams, General Screening Tests, Tests You Can Do at Home, Findings of the U.S. Preventive Services Task Force, X-ray and Radiology Tests, Electrical Tests, Tests of Blood and Other Body Fluids and Tissues, Scope Tests, Lung Tests, Genetic Tests, Pregnancy Tests, Newborn Screening Tests, Sexually Transmitted Disease Tests, and Computer Aided Diagnoses*

*Along with a Section on Paying for Medical Tests, a Glossary, and Resource Listings*

Edited by Joyce Brennfleck Shannon. 691 pages. 1999. 0-7808-0243-8. $78.

"Recommended for hospital and health sciences libraries with consumer health collections."
— *E-Streams, Mar '00*

"This is an overall excellent reference with a wealth of general knowledge that may aid those who are reluctant to get vital tests performed."
— *Today's Librarian, Jan 2000*

"A valuable reference guide."
— *American Reference Books Annual, 2000*

▪

## Men's Health Concerns Sourcebook, 2nd Edition

*Basic Consumer Health Information about the Medical and Mental Concerns of Men, Including Theories about the Shorter Male Lifespan, the Leading Causes of Death and Disability, Physical Concerns of Special Significance to Men, Reproductive and Sexual Concerns, Sexually Transmitted Diseases, Men's Mental and Emotional Health, and Lifestyle Choices That Affect Wellness, Such as Nutrition, Fitness, and Substance Use*

*Along with a Glossary of Related Terms and a Directory of Organizational Resources in Men's Health*

Edited by Robert Aquinas McNally. 644 pages. 2004. 0-7808-0671-9. $78.

***ALSO AVAILABLE:*** Men's Health Concerns Sourcebook, 1st Edition. Edited by Allan R. Cook. 738 pages. 1998. 0-7808-0212-8. $78.

"This comprehensive resource and the series are highly recommended."
— *American Reference Books Annual, 2000*

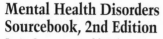

# Mental Health Disorders Sourcebook, 2nd Edition

*Basic Consumer Health Information about Anxiety Disorders, Depression and Other Mood Disorders, Eating Disorders, Personality Disorders, Schizophrenia, and More, Including Disease Descriptions, Treatment Options, and Reports on Current Research Initiatives*

*Along with Statistical Data, Tips for Maintaining Mental Health, a Glossary, and Directory of Sources for Additional Help and Information*

Edited by Karen Bellenir. 605 pages. 2000. 0-7808-0240-3. $78.

***ALSO AVAILABLE:*** *Mental Health Disorders Sourcebook, 1st Edition.* Edited by Karen Bellenir. 548 pages. 1995. 0-7808-0040-0. $78.

# Mental Retardation Sourcebook

*Basic Consumer Health Information about Mental Retardation and Its Causes, Including Down Syndrome, Fetal Alcohol Syndrome, Fragile X Syndrome, Genetic Conditions, Injury, and Environmental Sources*

*Along with Preventive Strategies, Parenting Issues, Educational Implications, Health Care Needs, Employment and Economic Matters, Legal Issues, a Glossary, and a Resource Listing for Additional Help and Information*

Edited by Joyce Brennfleck Shannon. 642 pages. 2000. 0-7808-0377-9. $78.

# Movement Disorders Sourcebook

*Basic Consumer Health Information about Neurological Movement Disorders, Including Essential Tremor,*

*Parkinson's Disease, Dystonia, Cerebral Palsy, Huntington's Disease, Myasthenia Gravis, Multiple Sclerosis, and Other Early-Onset and Adult-Onset Movement Disorders, Their Symptoms and Causes, Diagnostic Tests, and Treatments*

*Along with Mobility and Assistive Technology Information, a Glossary, and a Directory of Additional Resources*

Edited by Joyce Brennfleck Shannon. 655 pages. 2003. 0-7808-0628-X. $78.

# Obesity Sourcebook

*Basic Consumer Health Information about Diseases and Other Problems Associated with Obesity, and Including Facts about Risk Factors, Prevention Issues, and Management Approaches*

*Along with Statistical and Demographic Data, Information about Special Populations, Research Updates, a Glossary, and Source Listings for Further Help and Information*

Edited by Wilma Caldwell and Chad T. Kimball. 376 pages. 2001. 0-7808-0333-7. $78.

# Ophthalmic Disorders Sourcebook, 1st Edition

*SEE Eye Care Sourcebook, 2nd Edition*

# Oral Health Sourcebook

*SEE Dental Care & Oral Health Sourcebook, 2nd Edition*

# Osteoporosis Sourcebook

*Basic Consumer Health Information about Primary and Secondary Osteoporosis and Juvenile Osteoporosis and Related Conditions, Including Fibrous Dysplasia, Gaucher Disease, Hyperthyroidism, Hypophosphatasia, Myeloma, Osteopetrosis, Osteogenesis Imperfecta, and Paget's Disease*

*Along with Information about Risk Factors, Treatments, Traditional and Non-Traditional Pain Management, a Glossary of Related Terms, and a Directory of Resources*

Edited by Allan R. Cook. 584 pages. 2001. 0-7808-0239-X. $78.

"This would be a book to be kept in a staff or patient library. The targeted audience is the layperson, but the therapist who needs a quick bit of information on a particular topic will also find the book useful."
— *Physical Therapy, Jan '02*

"This resource is recommended as a great reference source for public, health, and academic libraries, and is another triumph for the editors of Omnigraphics."
— *American Reference Books Annual 2002*

"Recommended for all public libraries and general health collections, especially those supporting patient education or consumer health programs."
—*E-Streams, Nov '01*

"Will prove valuable to any library seeking to maintain a current, comprehensive reference collection of health resources. . . . From prevention to treatment and associated conditions, this provides an excellent survey."
—*The Bookwatch, Aug '01*

"Recommended reference source."
—*Booklist, American Library Association, July '01*

SEE ALSO *Women's Health Concerns Sourcebook*

■

# Pain Sourcebook, 2nd Edition

*Basic Consumer Health Information about Specific Forms of Acute and Chronic Pain, Including Muscle and Skeletal Pain, Nerve Pain, Cancer Pain, and Disorders Characterized by Pain, Such as Fibromyalgia, Shingles, Angina, Arthritis, and Headaches*

*Along with Information about Pain Medications and Management Techniques, Complementary and Alternative Pain Relief Options, Tips for People Living with Chronic Pain, a Glossary, and a Directory of Sources for Further Information*

Edited by Karen Bellenir. 670 pages. 2002. 0-7808-0612-3. $78.

ALSO AVAILABLE: *Pain Sourcebook, 1st Edition.* Edited by Allan R. Cook. 667 pages. 1997. 0-7808-0213-6. $78.

"A source of valuable information. . . . This book offers help to nonmedical people who need information about pain and pain management. It is also an excellent reference for those who participate in patient education."
— *Doody's Review Service, Sep '02*

"The text is readable, easily understood, and well indexed. This excellent volume belongs in all patient education libraries, consumer health sections of public libraries, and many personal collections."
— *American Reference Books Annual, 1999*

"A beneficial reference."  — *Booklist Health Sciences Supplement, American Library Association, Oct '98*

"The information is basic in terms of scholarship and is appropriate for general readers. Written in journalistic style . . . intended for non-professionals. Quite thorough in its coverage of different pain conditions and summarizes the latest clinical information regarding pain treatment."  — *Choice, Association of College and Research Libraries, Jun '98*

"Recommended reference source."
—*Booklist, American Library Association, Mar '98*

■

# Pediatric Cancer Sourcebook

*Basic Consumer Health Information about Leukemias, Brain Tumors, Sarcomas, Lymphomas, and Other Cancers in Infants, Children, and Adolescents, Including Descriptions of Cancers, Treatments, and Coping Strategies*

*Along with Suggestions for Parents, Caregivers, and Concerned Relatives, a Glossary of Cancer Terms, and Resource Listings*

Edited by Edward J. Prucha. 587 pages. 1999. 0-7808-0245-4. $78.

"An excellent source of information. Recommended for public, hospital, and health science libraries with consumer health collections."  — *E-Streams, Jun '00*

"Recommended reference source."
— *Booklist, American Library Association, Feb '00*

"A valuable addition to all libraries specializing in health services and many public libraries."
—*American Reference Books Annual, 2000*

■

# Physical & Mental Issues in Aging Sourcebook

*Basic Consumer Health Information on Physical and Mental Disorders Associated with the Aging Process, Including Concerns about Cardiovascular Disease, Pulmonary Disease, Oral Health, Digestive Disorders, Musculoskeletal and Skin Disorders, Metabolic Changes, Sexual and Reproductive Issues, and Changes in Vision, Hearing, and Other Senses*

*Along with Data about Longevity and Causes of Death, Information on Acute and Chronic Pain, Descriptions of Mental Concerns, a Glossary of Terms, and Resource Listings for Additional Help*

Edited by Jenifer Swanson. 660 pages. 1999. 0-7808-0233-0. $78.

"This is a treasure of health information for the layperson."  — *Choice Health Sciences Supplement, Association of College & Research Libraries, May 2000*

"Recommended for public libraries."
—*American Reference Books Annual, 2000*

"Recommended reference source."
— *Booklist, American Library Association, Oct '99*

SEE ALSO *Healthy Aging Sourcebook*

# Podiatry Sourcebook

*Basic Consumer Health Information about Foot Conditions, Diseases, and Injuries, Including Bunions, Corns, Calluses, Athlete's Foot, Plantar Warts, Hammertoes and Clawtoes, Clubfoot, Heel Pain, Gout, and More*

*Along with Facts about Foot Care, Disease Prevention, Foot Safety, Choosing a Foot Care Specialist, a Glossary of Terms, and Resource Listings for Additional Information*

Edited by M. Lisa Weatherford. 380 pages. 2001. 0-7808-0215-2. $78.

"Recommended reference source."
— *Booklist, American Library Association, Feb '02*

"There is a lot of information presented here on a topic that is usually only covered sparingly in most larger comprehensive medical encyclopedias."
— *American Reference Books Annual 2002*

■

# Pregnancy & Birth Sourcebook, 2nd Edition

*Basic Consumer Health Information about Conception and Pregnancy, Including Facts about Fertility, Infertility, Pregnancy Symptoms and Complications, Fetal Growth and Development, Labor, Delivery, and the Postpartum Period, as Well as Information about Maintaining Health and Wellness during Pregnancy and Caring for a Newborn*

*Along with Information about Public Health Assistance for Low-Income Pregnant Women, a Glossary, and Directories of Agencies and Organizations Providing Help and Support*

Edited by Amy L. Sutton. 600 pages. 2004. 0-7808-0672-7. $78.

*ALSO AVAILABLE: Pregnancy & Birth Sourcebook, 1st Edition. Edited by Heather E. Aldred. 737 pages. 1997. 0-7808-0216-0. $78.*

"A well-organized handbook. Recommended."
— *Choice, Association of College and Research Libraries, Apr '98*

"Recommended reference source."
— *Booklist, American Library Association, Mar '98*

"Recommended for public libraries."
— *American Reference Books Annual, 1998*

*SEE ALSO Congenital Disorders Sourcebook, Family Planning Sourcebook*

■

# Prostate Cancer Sourcebook

*Basic Consumer Health Information about Prostate Cancer, Including Information about the Associated Risk Factors, Detection, Diagnosis, and Treatment of Prostate Cancer*

*Along with Information on Non-Malignant Prostate Conditions, and Featuring a Section Listing Support and Treatment Centers and a Glossary of Related Terms*

Edited by Dawn D. Matthews. 358 pages. 2001. 0-7808-0324-8. $78.

"Recommended reference source."
— *Booklist, American Library Association, Jan '02*

"A valuable resource for health care consumers seeking information on the subject. . . .All text is written in a clear, easy-to-understand language that avoids technical jargon. Any library that collects consumer health resources would strengthen their collection with the addition of the *Prostate Cancer Sourcebook*."
— *American Reference Books Annual 2002*

■

# Public Health Sourcebook

*Basic Information about Government Health Agencies, Including National Health Statistics and Trends, Healthy People 2000 Program Goals and Objectives, the Centers for Disease Control and Prevention, the Food and Drug Administration, and the National Institutes of Health*

*Along with Full Contact Information for Each Agency*

Edited by Wendy Wilcox. 698 pages. 1998. 0-7808-0220-9. $78.

"Recommended reference source."
— *Booklist, American Library Association, Sep '98*

"This consumer guide provides welcome assistance in navigating the maze of federal health agencies and their data on public health concerns."
— *SciTech Book News, Sep '98*

■

# Reconstructive & Cosmetic Surgery Sourcebook

*Basic Consumer Health Information on Cosmetic and Reconstructive Plastic Surgery, Including Statistical Information about Different Surgical Procedures, Things to Consider Prior to Surgery, Plastic Surgery Techniques and Tools, Emotional and Psychological Considerations, and Procedure-Specific Information*

*Along with a Glossary of Terms and a Listing of Resources for Additional Help and Information*

Edited by M. Lisa Weatherford. 374 pages. 2001. 0-7808-0214-4. $78.

"An excellent reference that addresses cosmetic and medically necessary reconstructive surgeries. . . . The style of the prose is calm and reassuring, discussing the many positive outcomes now available due to advances in surgical techniques."
— *American Reference Books Annual 2002*

"Recommended for health science libraries that are open to the public, as well as hospital libraries that are open to the patients. This book is a good resource for the consumer interested in plastic surgery."
— *E-Streams, Dec '01*

"Recommended reference source."
— *Booklist, American Library Association, July '01*

# Rehabilitation Sourcebook

*Basic Consumer Health Information about Rehabilitation for People Recovering from Heart Surgery, Spinal Cord Injury, Stroke, Orthopedic Impairments, Amputation, Pulmonary Impairments, Traumatic Injury, and More, Including Physical Therapy, Occupational Therapy, Speech/ Language Therapy, Massage Therapy, Dance Therapy, Art Therapy, and Recreational Therapy*

*Along with Information on Assistive and Adaptive Devices, a Glossary, and Resources for Additional Help and Information*

Edited by Dawn D. Matthews. 531 pages. 1999. 0-7808-0236-5. $78.

"This is an excellent resource for public library reference and health collections."
— *American Reference Books Annual, 2001*

"Recommended reference source."
— *Booklist, American Library Association, May '00*

---

# Respiratory Diseases & Disorders Sourcebook

*Basic Information about Respiratory Diseases and Disorders, Including Asthma, Cystic Fibrosis, Pneumonia, the Common Cold, Influenza, and Others, Featuring Facts about the Respiratory System, Statistical and Demographic Data, Treatments, Self-Help Management Suggestions, and Current Research Initiatives*

Edited by Allan R. Cook and Peter D. Dresser. 771 pages. 1995. 0-7808-0037-0. $78.

"Designed for the layperson and for patients and their families coping with respiratory illness. . . . an extensive array of information on diagnosis, treatment, management, and prevention of respiratory illnesses for the general reader." — *Choice, Association of College and Research Libraries, Jun '96*

"A highly recommended text for all collections. It is a comforting reminder of the power of knowledge that good books carry between their covers."
— *Academic Library Book Review, Spring '96*

"A comprehensive collection of authoritative information presented in a nontechnical, humanitarian style for patients, families, and caregivers."
— *Association of Operating Room Nurses, Sep/Oct '95*

*SEE ALSO* Lung Disorders Sourcebook

---

# Sexually Transmitted Diseases Sourcebook, 2nd Edition

*Basic Consumer Health Information about Sexually Transmitted Diseases, Including Information on the Diagnosis and Treatment of Chlamydia, Gonorrhea, Hepatitis, Herpes, HIV, Mononucleosis, Syphilis, and Others*

*Along with Information on Prevention, Such as Condom Use, Vaccines, and STD Education; And Featuring a Section on Issues Related to Youth and Adolescents, a Glossary, and Resources for Additional Help and Information*

Edited by Dawn D. Matthews. 538 pages. 2001. 0-7808-0249-7. $78.

*ALSO AVAILABLE:* Sexually Transmitted Diseases Sourcebook, 1st Edition. Edited by Linda M. Ross. 550 pages. 1997. 0-7808-0217-9. $78.

"Recommended for consumer health collections in public libraries, and secondary school and community college libraries."
— *American Reference Books Annual 2002*

"Every school and public library should have a copy of this comprehensive and user-friendly reference book."
— *Choice, Association of College & Research Libraries, Sep '01*

"This is a highly recommended book. This is an especially important book for all school and public libraries." — *AIDS Book Review Journal, Jul-Aug '01*

"Recommended reference source."
— *Booklist, American Library Association, Apr '01*

"Recommended pick both for specialty health library collections and any general consumer health reference collection." — *The Bookwatch, Apr '01*

---

# Skin Disorders Sourcebook

*Basic Information about Common Skin and Scalp Conditions Caused by Aging, Allergies, Immune Reactions, Sun Exposure, Infectious Organisms, Parasites, Cosmetics, and Skin Traumas, Including Abrasions, Cuts, and Pressure Sores*

*Along with Information on Prevention and Treatment*

Edited by Allan R. Cook. 647 pages. 1997. 0-7808-0080-X. $78.

". . . comprehensive, easily read reference book."
— *Doody's Health Sciences Book Reviews, Oct '97*

*SEE ALSO* Burns Sourcebook

---

# Sleep Disorders Sourcebook

*Basic Consumer Health Information about Sleep and Its Disorders, Including Insomnia, Sleepwalking, Sleep Apnea, Restless Leg Syndrome, and Narcolepsy*

*Along with Data about Shiftwork and Its Effects, Information on the Societal Costs of Sleep Deprivation, Descriptions of Treatment Options, a Glossary of Terms, and Resource Listings for Additional Help*

Edited by Jenifer Swanson. 439 pages. 1998. 0-7808-0234-9. $78.

"This text will complement any home or medical library. It is user-friendly and ideal for the adult reader."
— *American Reference Books Annual, 2000*

"A useful resource that provides accurate, relevant, and accessible information on sleep to the general public. Health care providers who deal with sleep disorders patients may also find it helpful in being prepared to answer some of the questions patients ask."
— *Respiratory Care, Jul '99*

"Recommended reference source."
— *Booklist, American Library Association, Feb '99*

■

# Sports Injuries Sourcebook, 2nd Edition

*Basic Consumer Health Information about the Diagnosis, Treatment, and Rehabilitation of Common Sports-Related Injuries in Children and Adults*

*Along with Suggestions for Conditioning and Training, Information and Prevention Tips for Injuries Frequently Associated with Specific Sports and Special Populations, a Glossary, and a Directory of Additional Resources*

Edited by Joyce Brennfleck Shannon. 614 pages. 2002. 0-7808-0604-2. $78.

*ALSO AVAILABLE: Sports Injuries Sourcebook, 1st Edition.* Edited by Heather E. Aldred. 624 pages. 1999. 0-7808-0218-7. $78.

"This is an excellent reference for consumers and it is recommended for public, community college, and undergraduate libraries."
— *American Reference Books Annual, 2003*

"Recommended reference source."
— *Booklist, American Library Association, Feb '03*

■

# Stress-Related Disorders Sourcebook

*Basic Consumer Health Information about Stress and Stress-Related Disorders, Including Stress Origins and Signals, Environmental Stress at Work and Home, Mental and Emotional Stress Associated with Depression, Post-Traumatic Stress Disorder, Panic Disorder, Suicide, and the Physical Effects of Stress on the Cardiovascular, Immune, and Nervous Systems*

*Along with Stress Management Techniques, a Glossary, and a Listing of Additional Resources*

Edited by Joyce Brennfleck Shannon. 610 pages. 2002. 0-7808-0560-7. $78.

"Well written for a general readership, the *Stress-Related Disorders Sourcebook* is a useful addition to the health reference literature."
— *American Reference Books Annual, 2003*

"I am impressed by the amount of information. It offers a thorough overview of the causes and consequences of stress for the layperson. . . . A well-done and thorough reference guide for professionals and nonprofessionals alike."
— *Doody's Review Service, Dec '02*

# Stroke Sourcebook

*Basic Consumer Health Information about Stroke, Including Ischemic, Hemorrhagic, Transient Ischemic Attack (TIA), and Pediatric Stroke, Stroke Triggers and Risks, Diagnostic Tests, Treatments, and Rehabilitation Information*

*Along with Stroke Prevention Guidelines, Legal and Financial Information, a Glossary, and a Directory of Additional Resources*

Edited by Joyce Brennfleck Shannon. 606 pages. 2003. 0-7808-0630-1. $78.

■

# Substance Abuse Sourcebook

*Basic Health-Related Information about the Abuse of Legal and Illegal Substances Such as Alcohol, Tobacco, Prescription Drugs, Marijuana, Cocaine, and Heroin; and Including Facts about Substance Abuse Prevention Strategies, Intervention Methods, Treatment and Recovery Programs, and a Section Addressing the Special Problems Related to Substance Abuse during Pregnancy*

Edited by Karen Bellenir. 573 pages. 1996. 0-7808-0038-9. $78.

"A valuable addition to any health reference section. Highly recommended."
— *The Book Report, Mar/Apr '97*

". . . a comprehensive collection of substance abuse information that's both highly readable and compact. Families and caregivers of substance abusers will find the information enlightening and helpful, while teachers, social workers and journalists should benefit from the concise format. Recommended."
— *Drug Abuse Update, Winter '96/'97*

*SEE ALSO Alcoholism Sourcebook, Drug Abuse Sourcebook*

■

# Surgery Sourcebook

*Basic Consumer Health Information about Inpatient and Outpatient Surgeries, Including Cardiac, Vascular, Orthopedic, Ocular, Reconstructive, Cosmetic, Gynecologic, and Ear, Nose, and Throat Procedures and More*

*Along with Information about Operating Room Policies and Instruments, Laser Surgery Techniques, Hospital Errors, Statistical Data, a Glossary, and Listings of Sources for Further Help and Information*

Edited by Annemarie S. Muth and Karen Bellenir. 596 pages. 2002. 0-7808-0380-9. $78.

"Invaluable reference for public and school library collections alike."
— *Library Bookwatch, Apr '03*

■

# Transplantation Sourcebook

*Basic Consumer Health Information about Organ and Tissue Transplantation, Including Physical and Financial Preparations, Procedures and Issues Relating to Specific Solid Organ and Tissue Transplants, Rehabilitation, Pediatric Transplant Information, the Future* of Transplantation, and Organ and Tissue Donation Along with a Glossary and Listings of Additional Resources

Edited by Joyce Brennfleck Shannon. 628 pages. 2002. 0-7808-0322-1. $78.

"Along with these advances [in transplantation technology] have come a number of daunting questions for potential transplant patients, their families, and their health care providers. This reference text is the best single tool to address many of these questions. . . . It will be a much-needed addition to the reference collections in health care, academic, and large public libraries."
— American Reference Books Annual, 2003

"Recommended for libraries with an interest in offering consumer health information." — E-Streams, Jul '02

"This is a unique and valuable resource for patients facing transplantation and their families."
— Doody's Review Service, Jun '02

■

# Traveler's Health Sourcebook

Basic Consumer Health Information for Travelers, Including Physical and Medical Preparations, Transportation Health and Safety, Essential Information about Food and Water, Sun Exposure, Insect and Snake Bites, Camping and Wilderness Medicine, and Travel with Physical or Medical Disabilities

Along with International Travel Tips, Vaccination Recommendations, Geographical Health Issues, Disease Risks, a Glossary, and a Listing of Additional Resources

Edited by Joyce Brennfleck Shannon. 613 pages. 2000. 0-7808-0384-1. $78.

"Recommended reference source."
— Booklist, American Library Association, Feb '01

"This book is recommended for any public library, any travel collection, and especially any collection for the physically disabled."
—American Reference Books Annual, 2001

■

# Vegetarian Sourcebook

Basic Consumer Health Information about Vegetarian Diets, Lifestyle, and Philosophy, Including Definitions of Vegetarianism and Veganism, Tips about Adopting Vegetarianism, Creating a Vegetarian Pantry, and Meeting Nutritional Needs of Vegetarians, with Facts Regarding Vegetarianism's Effect on Pregnant and Lactating Women, Children, Athletes, and Senior Citizens

Along with a Glossary of Commonly Used Vegetarian Terms and Resources for Additional Help and Information

Edited by Chad T. Kimball. 360 pages. 2002. 0-7808-0439-2. $78.

"Organizes into one concise volume the answers to the most common questions concerning vegetarian diets and lifestyles. This title is recommended for public and secondary school libraries." — E-Streams, Apr '03

"Invaluable reference for public and school library collections alike." — Library Bookwatch, Apr '03

"The articles in this volume are easy to read and come from authoritative sources. The book does not necessarily support the vegetarian diet but instead provides the pros and cons of this important decision. The Vegetarian Sourcebook is recommended for public libraries and consumer health libraries."
— American Reference Books Annual, 2003

■

# Women's Health Concerns Sourcebook, 2nd Edition

Basic Consumer Health Information about the Medical and Mental Concerns of Women, Including Maintaining Health and Wellness, Gynecological Concerns, Breast Health, Sexuality and Reproductive Issues, Menopause, Cancer in Women, the Leading Causes of Death and Disability among Women, Physical Concerns of Special Significance to Women, and Women's Mental and Emotional Health

Along with a Glossary of Related Terms and Directories of Resources for Additional Help and Information

Edited by Amy L. Sutton. 748 pages. 2004. 0-7808-0673-5. $78.

ALSO AVAILABLE: Women's Health Concerns Sourcebook, 1st Edition. Edited by Heather E. Aldred. 567 pages. 1997. 0-7808-0219-5. $78.

"Handy compilation. There is an impressive range of diseases, devices, disorders, procedures, and other physical and emotional issues covered . . . well organized, illustrated, and indexed." — Choice, Association of College and Research Libraries, Jan '98

SEE ALSO Breast Cancer Sourcebook, Cancer Sourcebook for Women, Healthy Heart Sourcebook for Women, Osteoporosis Sourcebook

■

# Workplace Health & Safety Sourcebook

Basic Consumer Health Information about Workplace Health and Safety, Including the Effect of Workplace Hazards on the Lungs, Skin, Heart, Ears, Eyes, Brain, Reproductive Organs, Musculoskeletal System, and Other Organs and Body Parts

Along with Information about Occupational Cancer, Personal Protective Equipment, Toxic and Hazardous Chemicals, Child Labor, Stress, and Workplace Violence

Edited by Chad T. Kimball. 626 pages. 2000. 0-7808-0231-4. $78.

"As a reference for the general public, this would be useful in any library." — E-Streams, Jun '01

"Provides helpful information for primary care physicians and other caregivers interested in occupational medicine. . . . General readers; professionals."
— Choice, Association of College & Research Libraries, May '01

"Recommended reference source."
— Booklist, American Library Association, Feb '01

"Highly recommended." — The Bookwatch, Jan '01

# Worldwide Health Sourcebook

*Basic Information about Global Health Issues, Including Malnutrition, Reproductive Health, Disease Dispersion and Prevention, Emerging Diseases, Risky Health Behaviors, and the Leading Causes of Death*

*Along with Global Health Concerns for Children, Women, and the Elderly, Mental Health Issues, Research and Technology Advancements, and Economic, Environmental, and Political Health Implications, a Glossary, and a Resource Listing for Additional Help and Information*

Edited by Joyce Brennfleck Shannon. 614 pages. 2001. 0-7808-0330-2. $78.

**"Named an Outstanding Academic Title."**
> —*Choice, Association of College & Research Libraries, Jan '02*

**"Yet another handy but also unique compilation in the extensive Health Reference Series, this is a useful work because many of the international publications reprinted or excerpted are not readily available. Highly recommended."** —*Choice, Association of College & Research Libraries, Nov '01*

**"Recommended reference source."**
> —*Booklist, American Library Association, Oct '01*

# Teen Health Series

*Helping Young Adults Understand, Manage, and Avoid Serious Illness*

## Diet Information for Teens

*Health Tips about Diet and Nutrition*

*Including Facts about Nutrients, Dietary Guidelines, Breakfasts, School Lunches, Snacks, Party Food, Weight Control, Eating Disorders, and More*

Edited by Karen Bellenir. 399 pages. 2001. 0-7808-0441-4. $58.

"Full of helpful insights and facts throughout the book. . . . An excellent resource to be placed in public libraries or even in personal collections."
— *American Reference Books Annual 2002*

"Recommended for middle and high school libraries and media centers as well as academic libraries that educate future teachers of teenagers. It is also a suitable addition to health science libraries that serve patrons who are interested in teen health promotion and education."
— *E-Streams, Oct '01*

"This comprehensive book would be beneficial to collections that need information about nutrition, dietary guidelines, meal planning, and weight control. . . . This reference is so easy to use that its purchase is recommended."
— *The Book Report, Sep-Oct '01*

"This book is written in an easy to understand format describing issues that many teens face every day, and then provides thoughtful explanations so that teens can make informed decisions. This is an interesting book that provides important facts and information for today's teens."
— *Doody's Health Sciences Book Review Journal, Jul-Aug '01*

"A comprehensive compendium of diet and nutrition. The information is presented in a straightforward, plain-spoken manner. This title will be useful to those working on reports on a variety of topics, as well as to general readers concerned about their dietary health."
— *School Library Journal, Jun '01*

## Drug Information for Teens

*Health Tips about the Physical and Mental Effects of Substance Abuse*

*Including Facts about Alcohol, Anabolic Steroids, Club Drugs, Cocaine, Depressants, Hallucinogens, Herbal Products, Inhalants, Marijuana, Narcotics, Stimulants, Tobacco, and More*

Edited by Karen Bellenir. 452 pages. 2002. 0-7808-0444-9. $58.

"The chapters are quick to make a connection to their teenage reading audience. The prose is straightforward and the book lends itself to spot reading. It should be useful both for practical information and for research, and it is suitable for public and school libraries."
— *American Reference Books Annual, 2003*

"Recommended reference source."
— *Booklist, American Library Association, Feb '03*

"This is an excellent resource for teens and their parents. Education about drugs and substances is key to discouraging teen drug abuse and this book provides this much needed information in a way that is interesting and factual." — *Doody's Review Service, Dec '02*

## Mental Health Information for Teens

*Health Tips about Mental Health and Mental Illness*

*Including Facts about Anxiety, Depression, Suicide, Eating Disorders, Obsessive-Compulsive Disorders, Panic Attacks, Phobias, Schizophrenia, and More*

Edited by Karen Bellenir. 406 pages. 2001. 0-7808-0442-2. $58.

"In both language and approach, this user-friendly entry in the *Teen Health Series* is on target for teens needing information on mental health concerns." — *Booklist, American Library Association, Jan '02*

"Readers will find the material accessible and informative, with the shaded notes, facts, and embedded glossary insets adding appropriately to the already interesting and succinct presentation."
— *School Library Journal, Jan '02*

"This title is highly recommended for any library that serves adolescents and parents/caregivers of adolescents." — *E-Streams, Jan '02*

"Recommended for high school libraries and young adult collections in public libraries. Both health professionals and teenagers will find this book useful."
— *American Reference Books Annual 2002*

"This is a nice book written to enlighten the society, primarily teenagers, about common teen mental health issues. It is highly recommended to teachers and parents as well as adolescents."
— *Doody's Review Service, Dec '01*

## Sexual Health Information for Teens

*Health Tips about Sexual Development, Human Reproduction, and Sexually Transmitted Diseases*

*Including Facts about Puberty, Reproductive Health, Chlamydia, Human Papillomavirus, Pelvic Inflam-*

matory *Disease, Herpes, AIDS, Contraception, Pregnancy, and More*

Edited by Deborah A. Stanley. 391 pages. 2003. 0-7808-0445-7. $58.

# Skin Health Information For Teens

## Health Tips about Dermatological Concerns and Skin Cancer Risks

*Including Facts about Acne, Warts, Hives, and Other Conditions and Lifestyle Choices, Such as Tanning, Tattooing, and Piercing, That Affect the Skin, Nails, Scalp, and Hair*

Edited by Robert Aquinas McNally. 430 pages. 2003. 0-7808-0446-5. $58.

# Sports Injuries Information For Teens

## Health Tips about Sports Injuries and Injury Protection

*Including Facts about Specific Injuries, Emergency Treatment, Rehabilitation, Sports Safety, Competition Stress, Fitness, Sports Nutrition, Steroid Risks, and More*

Edited by Joyce Brennfleck Shannon. 425 pages. 2003. 0-7808-0447-3. $58.